Y0-DVL-330

TRAUMATIC BRAIN INJURY

TRAUMATIC BRAIN INJURY

MECHANISMS OF DAMAGE, ASSESSMENT, INTERVENTION, AND OUTCOME

Edited by Erin D. Bigler

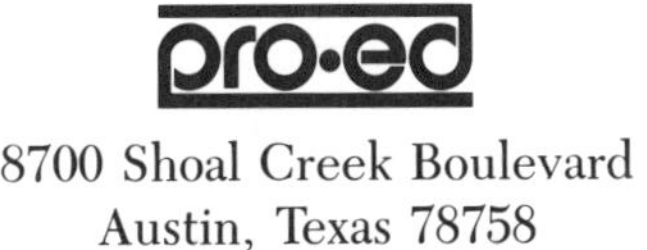
pro-ed
8700 Shoal Creek Boulevard
Austin, Texas 78758

Printed in the United States of America

Library of Congress Cataloging-in-Publication Data

Traumatic brain injury.

Text is an outgrowth of 14 articles published in the Journal of learning disabilities in 1987.
Includes bibliographies and index.
1. Brain damage. I. Bigler, Erin D., 1949–
II. Journal of learning disabilities. [DNLM: 1. Brain
Injuries—diagnosis. 2. Brain Injuries—therapy.
WL 354 T7778]
RC387.5.T73 1990 617'.481044 90-3855
ISBN 0-89079-201-1

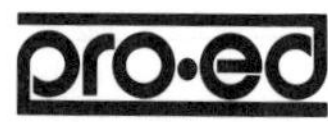

8700 Shoal Creek Boulevard
Austin, Texas 78758

10 9 8 7 6 5 4 3 2 1 89 90 91 92 93 94

Contents

PART III. INTERVENTION ISSUES

PART IV. OUTCOME ISSUES

PART V. CONCLUSIONS AND FUTURE DIRECTIONS

Preface

In 1987 the *Journal of Learning Disabilities* initiated a series dealing with traumatic brain injury (TBI) (see Bigler, 1987; Wiederholt, 1987). This series spanned five issues and included 14 articles. This text is an outgrowth of that series. The logical segregation of contents would be to divide topics into four main areas: mechanisms of injury, assessment issues, intervention and treatment issues, and outcome variables. By utilizing such a division, this text attempts to achieve a comprehensive review of all aspects of traumatic brain injury.

Since approximately 40% of all head injury patients are below the age of 18, many of these individuals will be receiving some form of remediation within the framework of the public school setting. Several of the chapters in this book deal with this particular issue. For example, Cathy Telzrow's chapter on the management of academic and educational problems in head injury focuses on the behavior of brain injured children as they return to the classroom and the special demands that this places upon the teacher, parent, and school. In a companion chapter, Ann Deaton writes about behavioral strategies in the treatment of brain injured children, who typically present with disruptive and maladaptive behavior. Similarly, Tona McGuire and Carrie Sylvester review traditional and innovative psychologic and psychiatric treatment methods for the brain injured individual. Muriel Lezak and Kevin O'Brien discuss further the emotional, social, and physical changes after brain injury.

However, before one can treat and manage behavioral problems of the brain injured individual, one must have a basic understanding of the neuropathology of acquired cerebral injury, which is the subject of Chapter 2. Likewise, the incidence and risk factors involved in cerebral injury need further review and attention than are given in the brief introduction. To meet this need, Felicia Goldstein and Harvey Levin review the incidence, clinical characteristics, and risk factors associated with pediatric head injury. Richard Naugle reviews epidemiological variables with adult brain injury. Similarly, once a brain injury has occurred, there is a need to assess the effects of that injury and provide some index concerning the deficits present. Several chapters address this topic area. Linda Ewing-Cobbs and Jack Fletcher review traditional neuropsychological methods of assessment of head injury in children. C. Munro Cullum, Julia Kuck, and Ronald Ruff address similar issues but in the adult TBI patient. George Hynd and John Obrzut review methods of neuropsychological inference from traditional psychoeducational tests in the assessment of the effects of cerebral injury of the child. And, in the assessment section, Thomas Marquardt, Julie Stoll, and Harvey Sussman discuss disorders of communication that result from brain injury.

A most important recent development in the comprehensive treatment of the brain injured individual has been in the area of cognitive rehabilitation. George Prigatano, who has been at the forefront of this development, reviews the various methods of direct remediation training as well as compensatory training methods in the amelioration of cognitive impairment. Also, he and Pamela Klonoff address psychotherapy issues in the treatment of TBI patients. Rodger Wood updates current thinking and treatment for disorders of attention in brain injured individuals and, in a related area, Elizabeth Glisky and Daniel Schacter demonstrate an effective treatment program for an amnesic patient.

To add a very personal insight into the acute and chronic effects of brain injury on a family, Darlene Martin, a nursing professor and mother of a head injured son, provides a family perspective. Last, because liability and litigation issues play a prominent role in many cases of acquired brain injury and these issues have an impact not only on the patient and family, but also upon those providing care and treatment, it is important that these issues be addressed as well. This is the focus of Reed Martin's chapter.

Obviously, the primary goal for those individuals with residual effects of brain injury is to improve their quality of life. It is to this goal that this book is dedicated. It is anticipated that a better understanding of the nature of brain injury, the neuropathologic processes that occur, and their effects on cognitive and behavioral outcome, as well as the diagnostic evaluation and treatment methods available, will result in an appreciation of this multifactorial problem of brain injury and provide for better long-term treatment and outcome.

I would like to thank Lee Wiederholt and Judy Voress for their help from the inception of this series to its completion.

REFERENCES

Bigler, E.D. (1987). Acquired cerebral trauma: An introduction to the special series. *Journal of Learning Disabilities, 20*, 449–512.

Wiederholt, J.L. (1987). A preface to the special series on acquired cerebral trauma. *Journal of Learning Disabilities, 20*, 449–512.

1

Introduction

ERIN D. BIGLER

The statistics are staggering. Estimates suggest that in the United States each year there are upwards of 1 million cases of head injury requiring hospitalization (Berrol & Rosenthal, 1986: Kurtzke, 1982). In terms of all head injuries, regardless of hospitalization or severity of injury, the number may be as high as 3 million per year (Cartlidge & Shaw, 1981; Dikman & Reitan, 1977; Jennett, 1983a). At least 10% of the individuals who survive a significant head injury are likely to have residual deficits that result in total and permanent incapacity (Kingston, 1985). The majority of the remaining head injury victims are likely to suffer at least some transient cognitive, motor, or sensory aberration, and somewhere between 40% to 80% of these patients will have residual physical, intellectual, or behavioral deficits (Fisher, 1985; Levin, Benton, & Grossman, 1982; National Head Injury Foundation, 1982). The most frequently injured group of individuals is males between the ages of 15 and 24. Such individuals constitute 50% of all head injury cases. Furthermore, for this group the incidence rate of head injury is 600 per 100,000 population as compared to an overall general population incidence rate of 200 per 100,000 population (Fisher, 1985; Jennett, 1983a; Levin et al., 1982; Rivara & Mueller, 1986). In terms of the economic burden, the cost involved in rehabilitating traumatic brain injured (TBI) patients has been estimated to be between $5 and $10 billion annually (Anderson & McLaurin, 1980), and the economic loss may reach upwards of $25 to $30 billion (Johnston, 1987). Because new patients are added to the head injured ranks each day, this is a problem that continues to expand.

The tragedy of these statistics is that the injury occurs at a time in most individuals' lives when the demands to be productive (e.g., school, work, establishing a career) and independent (e.g., emerging adolescence or adulthood, establishing a family, etc.) are the most pervasive. The resultant physical, cognitive, and/or behavioral deficits may be permanent (Klonoff, Costa, & Snow, 1986; Rimel & Jane, 1983), and patients may never return to their previous level of independence and productivity. Over the past two decades the initial medical and physical treatment of head injury has become fairly well understood and regimented (Jennett, 1986; Miller & Jones, 1985). However, it is the long-term effects of brain injury, and particularly the cognitive and behavioral deficits (i.e., the learning disabilities), that constitute the current challenge of treatment, rehabilitation, and research. Since "the brain is the sum total of all we are," as Nobel Prize laureate Sir John Eccles (1983, p. vii) states, injury to this structure, which constitutes our very being, is inherently going to have a multifaceted impact upon all aspects of behavior. Accordingly, it is necessary to have an understanding at many levels of the mechanisms of brain injury and its effects upon behavior.

It is only recently that patients with head injury have received comprehensive treatment programs that have dealt with the various cognitive and behavioral outcome deficits that accompany brain injury. Thus, for the brain injured patient, the clinical acumen available for long-term treatment is limited but improving. For example, Jennett (1983b) points out that,

> Although head injury is 10 times more frequent than spinal injuries, there is much less chance that the victim of head injury will be fortunate enough to find a coherent and expertly conceived rehabilitation program. The problems of paraplegia are fairly stereotyped and well understood, with solutions available for most of them. By comparison, the disabilities after head injury are complex and varied, and are seldom fully recognized; even when they are, their management is often difficult. The main reason for this is that the mental deficits dominate—and these interfere both with the patient's ability to cope and with the capacity for cooperation with those trying to help the patient. (p. vii)

Prior to the recent advances in emergency medicine, many patients with TBI died (Lillehei & Hoff, 1985). However, since the 1960s and the advent of fully staffed emergency programs, the development of regional trauma centers, and availability of neurosurgeons, along with the development of critical and acute care management of the brain injured patient, the individual with a brain injury now stands a better chance of survival (Miller & Jones, 1985). Survival, though, has required the development of programs to meet the long-term needs of these individuals.

For the longest time clinicians dealing with the brain injured patient have been under the assumption that once a brain injury victim passes through the spontaneous recovery phase, there is little that can be done to assist the patient with recovery, because brain damage is "permanent." We now realize that these brain injury victims can be helped beyond this spontaneous recovery phase, and that there is a considerable amount of treatment and rehabilitation programming that can be developed for the individual with residual physical, cognitive, and behavioral deficits as a consequence of brain injury. It is also evident that unique applications of the principles of learning theory to the brain damaged individual (Gouvier, Webster, & Blanton, 1986; Horton & Sautter, 1986; Rosenthal & Geckler, 1986) may assist in the recovery process. Thus, in the 1980s we realize that the situation for brain injured individuals is far from hopeless, and that there are a variety of methodologies that can be applied in the evaluation and treatment of such individuals.

The last decade and a half has been an unprecedented era of technological advances that has led to brain imaging methods that now permit in vivo examination of the acute and chronic effects of brain injury. Prior to this era one had to either infer the degree and amount of structural brain damage or wait until a postmortem examination could be performed. Because of the current technology, we now have a much more accurate means of assessing structural damage, and this has permitted, in turn, a better understanding of the mechanisms of brain injury and the correlation between area of brain damage and related changes in behavior.

The behavioral effects of TBI are multifaceted. Consequently, any text that purports to address this topic must encompass a broad spectrum of issues. To meet such a broad-based approach, the current text examines brain injury mechanisms and epidemiological variables, methods of assessment, intervention and rehabilitation techniques, and outcome variables. Since the potential behavioral changes that accompany TBI can be so varied, assessment procedures need to be comprehensive yet specific enough to detail particular problems. Assessment issues differ between children and adults, and these differences need clarification. Rehabilitation efforts need to incorporate assessment findings and integrate this information into the overall treatment program. This includes managing the psychological dimensions of personality change secondary to TBI as well as the emotional adjustment that the TBI individual must deal with. Finally, because TBI does produce permanent changes in many individuals, it is important to understand the various outcome variables that play a role in the long-term recovery from TBI. The chapters that follow address these various issues.

REFERENCES

Anderson, D., & McLaurin, R. (1980). Report on the national head and spinal cord survey. *Journal of Neurosurgery, 53*, (suppl.) 1–43.

Berrol, S., & Rosenthal, M. (1986). From the editors. *The Journal of Head Trauma Rehabilitation, 1*, viii.

Cartlidge, N.E.F., & Shaw, D.A. (1981). *Head injury.* London: W.B. Saunders.

Dikman, S., & Reitan, R.M. (1977). Emotional sequelae of head injury. *Annals of Neurology, 2*, 492–494.

Eccles, J.C. (1983). Foreword. In P. Black (Ed.), *Brain dysfunction in children* (pp. vii–viii). New York: Raven Press.

Education for All Handicapped Children Act. (1977). *Federal Register, 42*, 65082–65085.

Fisher, J.M. (1985). Cognitive and behavioral consequences of closed head injury. *Seminars in Neurology, 5*, 197–204.

Gouvier, D., Webster, J.S., & Blanton, P.D. (1986). Cognitive retraining with brain-damaged patients. In D. Wedding, A.M. Horton, & J. Webster (Eds.), *The neuropsychology handbook* (pp. 278–324). New York: Springer.

Horton, A.M., & Sautter, S.W. (1986). Behavioral neuropsychology: Behavioral treatment for the brain-injured. In D. Wedding, A.M. Horton, & J. Webster (Eds.), *The neuropsychology handbook* (pp. 259–277). New York: Spinger.

Jennett, B. (1983a). Scale and scope of the problem. In M. Rosenthal, E.R. Griffith, M.R. Bond, & J.D. Miller (Eds.), *Rehabilitation of the head injured adult* (pp. 3–8). Philadelphia: F.A. Davis.

Jennett, B. (1983b). Foreword. In M. Rosenthal, E.R. Griffith, M.R. Bond, & J.D. Miller (Eds.), *Rehabilitation of the head injured adult* (p. vii). Philadelphia: F.A. Davis.

Jennett, B. (1986). Head trauma. In A.K. Asbury, G.M. McKhann, & W.I. McDonald (Eds.), *Disease of the nervous system* (pp. 1282–1291). Philadelphia: W.B. Saunders.

Johnston, M.V. (1987, February). *The economics of brain injury.* Paper presented at the Third Annual Houston Conference on Neurotrauma, Houston, TX.

Kingston, W.J. (1985). Head injury. *Seminars in Neurology, 5*, 197–270.

Klonoff, P.S., Costa, L.D., & Snow, W.G. (1986). Predictors and indicators of quality of life in patients with closed-head injury. *Journal of Clinical and Experimental Neuropsychology, 8*, 469–485.

Kurtzke, J. (1982). The current neurologic burden of illness and injury in the United States. *Neurology, 32*, 1207–1214.

Levin, H.S., Benton, A.L., & Grossman, R.G. (1982). *Neurobehavioral consequences of closed head injury.* New York: Oxford University Press.

Lillehei, K.D., & Hoff, J.T. (1985). Advances in the management of closed head injury. *Annals of Emergency Medicine. 14*, 789–795.

Miller, J.D., & Jones, P.A. (1985). The work of a regional head injury service. *Lancet, 1*, 1141–1144.

National Head Injury Foundation. (1982). *The silent epidemic.* (Available from the National Head Injury Foundation, 18A Vernon St., Framingham, MA).

Rimel, R.W., & Jane, J.A. (1983). Characteristics of the head-injured patient. In M. Rosenthal, E.R. Griffith, M.R. Bond, & J.D. Miller (Eds.), *Rehabilitation of the head injured adult* (pp. 9–21). Philadelphia: F.A. Davis.

Rivara, F.P., & Mueller, B.A. The epidemiology and prevention of pediatric head injury. *Journal of Head Trauma Rehabilitation, 1*, 7–15.

Rosenthal, M., & Geckler, C. (1986). Family therapy issues in neuropsychology. In D. Wedding, A.M. Horton, & J. Webster (Eds.), *The neuropsychology handbook* (pp. 325–344). New York: Springer.

PART I

MECHANISMS OF INJURY: PATHOLOGIC CONSEQUENCES

2

Neuropathology of Traumatic Brain Injury

ERIN D. BIGLER

To best understand the cognitive and behavioral sequelae of cerebral injury, one must first have a foundation in the pathophysiology and neuropathology of cerebral trauma. The initial pathology in cerebral injury may set the basis for chronic residual cerebral dysfunction that may have profound effects on the recovery and outcome of the individual. Typically, the cognitive and behavioral effects that accompany brain injury relate directly to the actual brain sites damaged and/or the cerebral systems involved, although there is typically some degree of nonspecific impairment as well. By knowing these areas or extent of damage, some predictive value may be gained concerning behavioral and cognitive outcome from brain injury. First, what constitutes a significant brain injury is defined, and this is followed by an overview of the neuropathology of cerebral trauma. Our understanding of the mechanisms of cerebral injury has been greatly advanced by technological improvements that permit the in vivo visualization of the brain. These technological advances also are discussed.

DEFINITION OF HEAD INJURY

Most bodily organs and organ systems have an inherent tendency to withstand minor infection, metabolic derangement, and trauma, resulting in complete recovery without any permanent damage or defect. This is also true of the brain. One only has to look at the number of falls and minor blows to the head that a toddler experiences in the first few years of life, or witness the repeated impact that a football player experiences during a game, to realize that such minor blows to the head do not necessarily produce permanent alteration in physiological or cognitive functioning, and accordingly, that there is no evidence of "brain injury" in such cases. However, a more serious blow to the head may produce significant alteration of brain function with potential for permanent sequelae. From these analogies it can be seen that the definition of brain injury is not a simple one but actually incorporates multiple factors.

There have been several attempts, as reviewed recently by Levin, Benton, and Grossman (1982), to develop a system of classification defining all types of head injury, but such classification attempts have all possessed some difficulties and lack agreement concerning what constitutes brain injury, particularly in "mild" cases (Prigatano & Pepping, 1987). This is true, in part, because of the complexity of brain function as it relates to human behavior, along with the multifaceted fashion in which the brain may be injured. Typically most classifications attempt to establish the definition around some initial alteration in the level of consciousness. However, it is well known that cerebral injuries can occur without major changes or alterations in the level of consciousness. Other schemes have employed the presence of certain neurologic abnormalities (e.g., paralysis, aphasia) or the presence of diagnostic radiological signs (skull fracture or hematoma on computerized axial tomography scan) in patients who have had some type of head injury. Each of these factors introduces variables that preclude a single definition of head injury. What follows is an attempt to offer a definitional guideline of what constitutes a head injury.

As pointed out previously, an alteration in the level of consciousness has been the traditional benchmark of definitions of brain injury. While the great majority of all head injuries do result in some alteration of level of consciousness, alteration in level of consciousness may not occur with some brain injuries (Jennett, 1986; Levin et al., 1982). Also, in some cases a blow to the head of sufficient magnitude to produce a hematoma may only produce an alteration in the level of consciousness with the expansion of the hematoma (see Figure 2.14). Thus, alteration in the level of consciousness or a "concussion" (brief loss of consciousness followed by prompt recovery without any localizing neurological signs; Bakay & Glasauer, 1980) is not a necessary or sufficient event to define the presence of brain injury; nonetheless, level of consciousness does provide one very important data point in terms of establishing the magnitude and degree of initial brain injury and also provides some predictive information regarding outcome.

In an attempt to quantify level of consciousness, Teasdale and Jennett (1974) developed the Glasgow Coma Scale (GCS), the first empirically substantiated and clinically validated rating scale. The GCS evaluates three components of wakefulness independently of one another: (a) the stimulus required to induce eye opening, (b) the best motor response, and (c) the best verbal response. Based on the criteria of the GCS, coma is defined as the absence of eye opening, inability to obey commands, and failure to utter recognizable words. Such a definition is applied to patients with GCS scores of 8 or less. The "worst" score attainable on the GCS is a score of 3, which indicates no eye opening to any stimulus, including pain; flaccid paralysis without motor response, and no verbal utterances. A maximum score of 15 occurs on the GCS when the patient can spontaneously open his or her eyes, follow simple motor commands, and demonstrate normal orientation to time, place, and person.

The GCS ratings offer some index as to the level and degree of the severity of brain injury on admission to the hospital. For example, Clifton et al. (1980) found that 53% of 558 patients admitted to the hospital having suffered "a head injury" had a GCS rating of 13 to 14 (least severe), 17% had an intermediate score (9 to 12), and 30% had severe ratings (8 or less). Related studies (e.g., Bond, 1983) suggest that such rating scales do indicate the initial severity of brain injury and do predict survival (there is better survival rate with patients who have a GCS score of above 8). These rating scales do not necessarily predict level of outcome, although there is a relationship between lower GCS scores and poor outcomes. In general, it can be stated that patients with GCS scores of 8 or less for 6 hours or more tend to have a poorer outcome, typically with generalized disability (Jennett et al., 1979). For example, Heiden, Small, Caton, Weiss, and Kurtze (1983) studied 213 patients with severe head injury (GCS ratings of 8 and below). When evaluated at 1-year posttrauma, only 19% had "good recovery," defined as "able to pursue normal occupational and social activities with minor physical deficits" (p. 4), while 16% had moderate disability (independent but disabled), and 11% were severely disabled (awake but dependent and requiring assistance with daily living skills). Two percent remained in a persistent vegetative state and over half (52%) died within the year following injury. Thus, 71% of the patients in the study who lived were at least moderately impaired 1 year posttrauma based on an initial GCS score of 8 or below. Lobato et al. (1986) have suggested that the negative effects of a low GCS can be somewhat tempered when there is a normal computerized axial tomography (CT) scan, and such patients show a better outcome than similarly matched closed head injury (CHI) patients with abnormal CT findings.

When one thinks of brain injury, one typically thinks that there has to be some "blow" to the head or some other externally imposed physical trauma. This does not necessarily have to occur for there to be a significant brain injury. For example, in a motor vehicle accident, the rapid deceleration on impact may set up a variety of forces in the cranium that can produce a significant brain injury from acceleration-deceleration effects (Jennett, 1986). As Jennett pointed out, a significant brain injury can occur "without a fracture of the skull or a blemish on the scalp..." (p. 1282). Thus, the sustaining of some blow or traumatic event to the head should not be considered a necessary condition in the definition of brain injury.

Posttraumatic amnesia (PTA) has been used as another indicator of brain injury and provides another index as to the severity of brain injury (Brooks, 1983). Russell (1971) suggested a scheme over 50 years ago that provided an index as to the degree of amnesia that may accompany cerebral injury. This is outlined in Table 2.1. PTA is not to be confused with coma and recovery from coma. PTA assumes that the patient is alert and functioning and has recovered from the comatose state but has persistent, severe deficits in retaining new information and processing new memories (i.e., anterograde amnesia). There also may be a retrograde amnesia for a period of time preceding the accident. Several lines of research have consistently demonstrated that PTA lasting longer than 1 week (very severe PTA) is associated with poor outcome and persistent mental/cognitive dysfunction (Brooks, 1983). However, the specificity of PTA ratings and brain injury is limited because PTA of 5 minutes to 1 hour (mild) has been associated with significant brain injury as well (Brooks, 1983; Jennett, 1986).

TABLE 2.1
Levels of Severity of Posttraumatic Amnesia (PTA)

Duration of PTA	Severity Description
less than 5 minutes	very mild
5 minutes to 1 hour	mild
1 to 24 hours	moderate
1 to 7 days	severe
more than 7 days	very severe

Last, with the advent of imaging procedures such as computerized axial tomography (CT) and magnetic resonance imaging (MRI), in addition to the traditional electroencephalogram (EEG), the patient with head injury can be evaluated in terms of the anatomical (CT and/or MRI) or electrophysiological (EEG) basis of traumatic injury. There are several classification schemes using the EEG to define the degree of brain injury (Kiloh, McComas, & Osselton, 1979), and CT and MRI studies may demonstrate the presence of cerebral contusion, hemorrhage, edema, and other structural lesions that may occur (Raichle, 1986). Recently, the addition of computerized technology to EEG assessments has yielded even more diagnostically sensitive measures to the detection of abnormal physiological functioning. To date, the best researched procedure is the brain electrical activity mapping (BEAM) technique, pioneered by Duffy (Duffy & McAnulty, 1985). The BEAM technique is particularly sensitive in detecting abnormal physiological patterns in "mild" head injury cases as well as secondary sites of dysfunction in cases of lateralized brain injury.

Thus, the third dimension that needs to be added to the definition of brain injury is whether the patient shows any physical evidence of neurological injury on direct examination using CT, MRI, or EEG in addition to the original change in level of consciousness and presence or absence of PTA. Likewise, direct physical examination of the patient may show clinical syndromes such as aphasia, paralysis, or sensory deficit.

In summary, a single definitional statement cannot be made that encompasses the complexity of brain injury. Thus, the sufficient and necessary factors that need to be present for the presence of significant brain injury should be in the context of one or any combination of the following: (a) alteration in the level of consciousness sufficient to produce a Glasgow Coma Scale rating of 14 or lower; (b) posttraumatic amnesia of 5 minutes or greater; (c) physiologic evidence (e.g., EEG), radiologic evidence (e.g., CT, MRI), or objective physical findings (e.g., paralysis, aphasia, sensory deficit).

CAUSES OF HEAD INJURY

Head injury occurs in a diverse fashion. The majority of head injuries occur as a consequence of motor vehicle accidents (Figure 2.1), followed by motorcycle and bicycle accidents (Rivara & Mueller, 1986). Exact statistics are difficult to come by, but head injuries resulting from falls from heights, pedestrian injuries, and assaults also contribute a frequent source (Kaufman, Makela, Lee, Haid, & Gildenberg, 1986; Levin et al., 1982). It also should be noted that in pediatric head injury, child abuse—particularly that caused by violent shaking—is a significant source of cerebral injury (Alexander, Schor, & Smith, 1986; Cohen, Kaufman, Myers, & Towbin, 1986; Dykes, 1986).

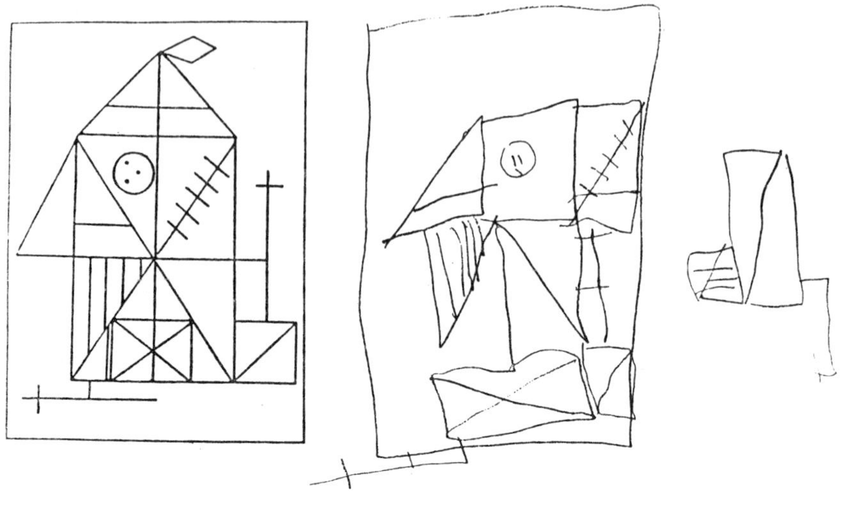

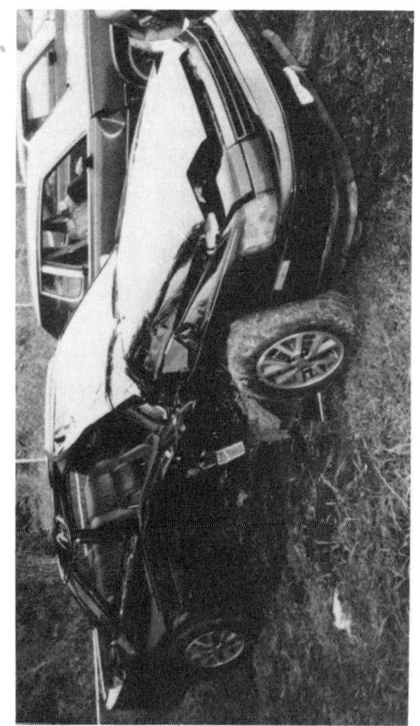

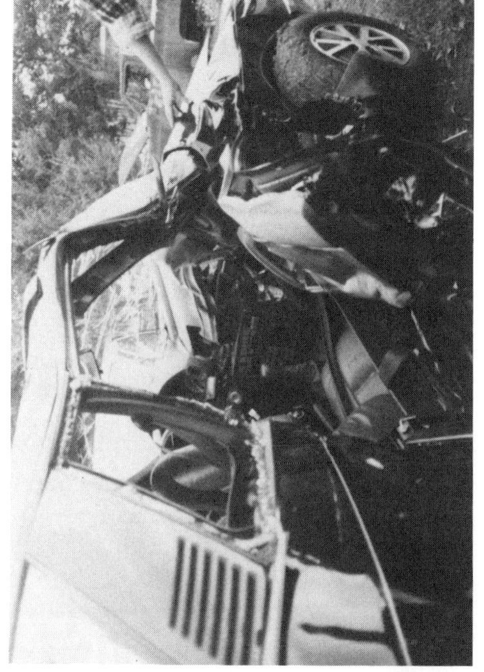

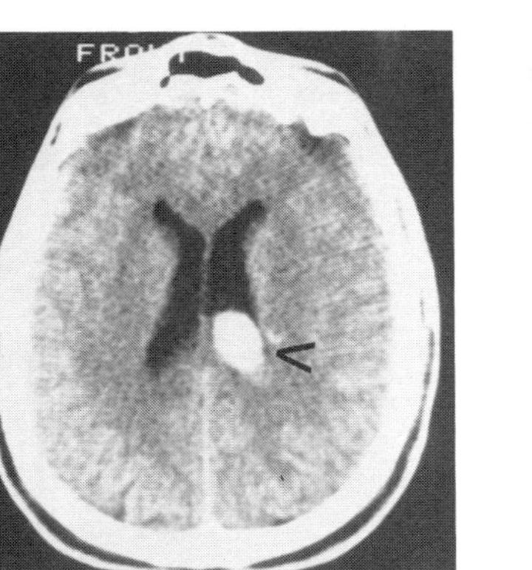
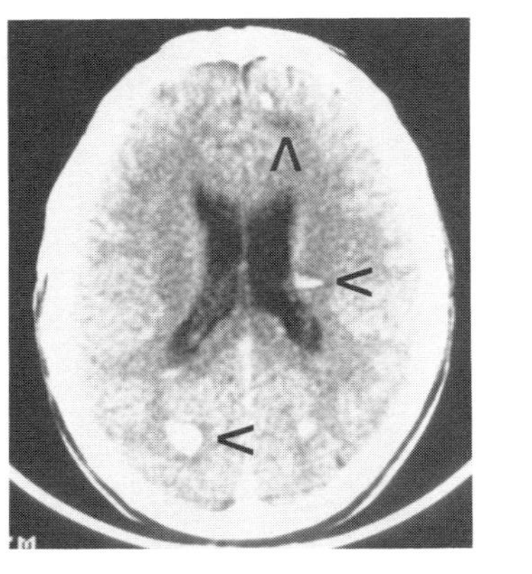
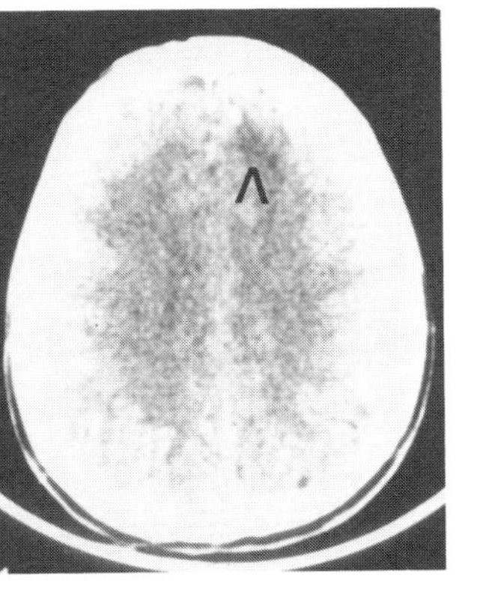

Figure 2.1. By viewing the actual damage to a motor vehicle, one can gain a greater appreciation for the dynamic impact forces that take place intracerebrally. Accordingly, this figure depicts the damaged car (facing page, left), the patient's performance on the Rey-Osterrieth Complex Figure Design (facing page, right), and the CT scans on admission to the hospital (above). The patient was a passenger in the car which was struck on the passenger's side when the driver pulled out in front of oncoming traffic across a three-lane highway. The police estimated speed of impact to be approximately 50 miles per hour. The patient was wearing a shoulder-strap safety belt. He was rendered unconscious on impact. CT scans on admission demonstrated multiple areas of hemorrhage throughout the frontal lobes with a large hemorrhagic contusion in the right frontal area. Neuropsychological studies completed 3 weeks postinjury reflected prominent deficits in perceptual-motor functioning along with impaired visual memory and an overall reduction in level of cognitive functioning. The patient's WAIS-R results indicated a VIQ score of 101, PIQ score of 69, and an FSIQ score of 84. (At the time of injury this patient had been a high school senior taking several honors classes, and his last California Achievement Test Total Battery score placed him at the 91st percentile; thus, premorbid intellectual/cognitive functions would have been expected to be in the bright normal to superior range—that is, 120+.) His Wechsler Memory Scale Memory Quotient (MQ) was 95, but particular deficits were noted on the visual memory subtest. The Rey-Osterrieth figure presented above demonstrates constructional praxic deficits along with impaired retention of visual information (the bottom Rey-Osterrieth figure was the patient's attempt to recall the original drawing after a 10-minute delay). The marked deficits in Performance abilities on the WAIS-R along with the greater visual than verbal memory deficits and constructional apraxic deficits suggest greater right hemispheric involvement. The lowered levels of overall intellectual and memory function suggest some degree of nonspecific impairment as well.

NEUROIMAGING IN THE DETERMINATION OF NEUROPATHOLOGY

Since the introduction of computerized axial tomography (CT scan) in 1973 (Hounsfield, 1973), an in vivo direct image of the brain can be obtained. With increased computer sophistication and improved imaging techniques, the CT scan image now approximates the actual appearance of the cerebral structures being imaged (see Figure 2.2). Magnetic resonance imaging (MRI), or, as it was previously called, nuclear magnetic resonance (NMR), utilizes a different principle (i.e., magnetic fields of atomic nuclei) from the X-ray beam assisted CT scanning technique (Hershey & Zimmerman, 1986; Jenkins, Teasdale, Hadley, Macpherson, & Rowan, 1986; Snow, Zimmerman, Gandy, & Deck, 1986; Zimmerman, Bilaniuk, Hackney, Goldberg, & Grossman, 1986), but likewise can generate an exquisite image of the brain (see Figure 2.2). The details of these procedures are beyond the scope of this article, but have been fully discussed in the referenced work by Raichle (1986). The advent of these procedures has revolutionized our ability to image the brain in the living individual and has resulted in a better understanding of the mechanisms of brain pathology (Han et al., 1984). It is now standard practice that anyone with a significant head injury will have some imaging technique performed to evaluate the neuropathological effects. The most common procedures are the CT or MRI. In the sections that follow, several CT or MRI results will be presented that depict the type of brain pathology that occurs as a result of brain injury. Figure 2.2 depicts the normal appearance of the brain. By using Figure 2.2 as the standard, the most common neuropathological changes associated with cerebral trauma can be readily identified in the subsequent illustrations.

NEUROPATHOLOGY

Skull-Brain Interface

The frontal lobes sit in the anterior fossa of the cranial cavity region of the skull with the antero-dorsal aspect of the bone swinging around each of the frontal lobes, encapsulating them (see Figure 2.3). Similarly, the temporal bone, laterally, and the greater wing of the sphenoid bone, anteriorly and medially, form the middle cranial fossa that bounds the temporal lobes (see Figure 2.3). Arising medially in the cranial fossa is the crista galli, which is a bony protuberance originating from the ethmoid bone (see Figure 2.3). This partially separates the anterior ventral aspect of both frontal lobes and also provides an anchor for the falx cerebri, a double fold of the dura mater that

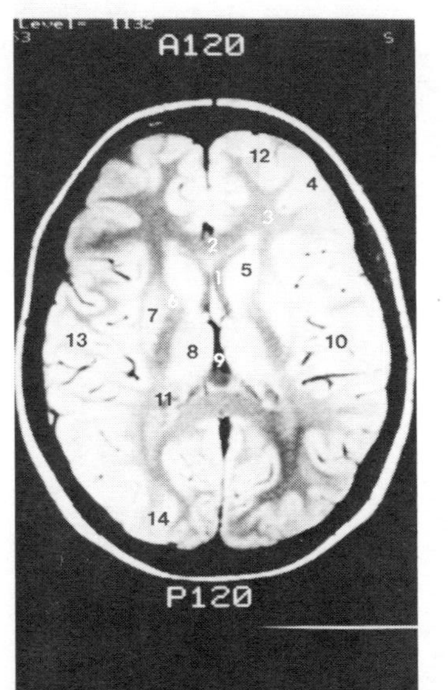

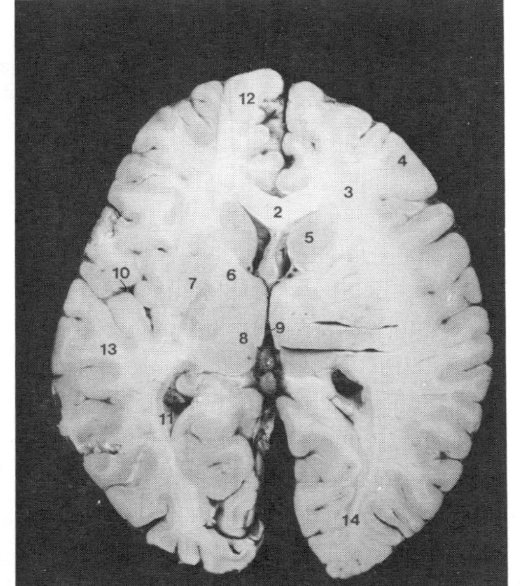

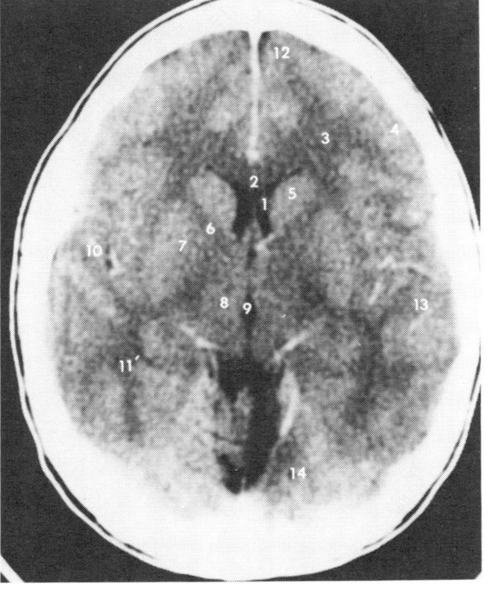

Figure 2.2. MRI scan (left), postmortem anatomic section at the level of the thalamus (middle), and CT scan (right). Note the great similarity between the MRI and CT scans and the actual anatomic sections. 1. anterior horn of lateral ventricle. 2. corpus callosum (genu). 3. white matter (pathways). 4. gray matter (cell bodies). 5. caudate nucleus. 6. internal capsule. 7. putamen-globus pallidus complex — it should be noted that the lacerations in the right lateral aspect of the thalamus and putamen-globus pallidus complex in this anatomic specimen were inadvertently imposed at the time of brain sectioning. 8. thalamus. 9. third ventricle. 10. Sylvian fissure. 11. posterior horn of the lateral ventricle. 12. frontal lobe. 13. temporal lobe. 14. occipital lobe.

Note the general symmetry present in the brain in the MRI and CT scans used in this demonstration. The darker the brain structure appears, the less dense it is and, conversely, the lighter the structure, the greater the density. As such, since the ventricles are cavities filled with cerebral spinal fluid, they would be the least dense, followed by white matter structures that are composed of myelinated fiber pathways, with the lightest areas being regions of tightly compacted cell bodies (gray matter). Deviations from this general pattern of symmetry or changes in the density may be a sign of pathology.

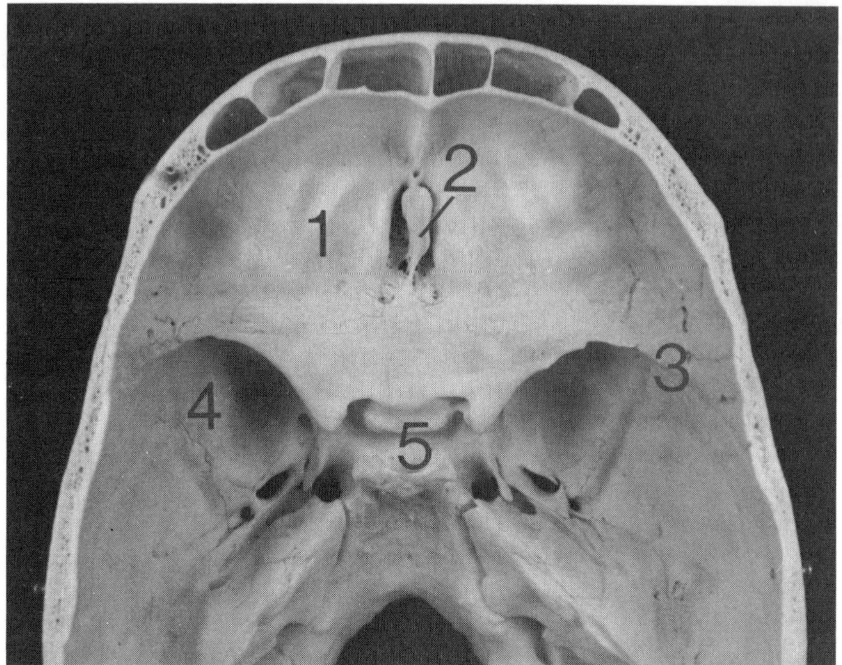

Figure 2.3. Horizontal view looking down into the anterior and middle fossa region of the skull. 1. orbital plate of the frontal bone forming the floor of the anterior cranial fossa. 2. orbital groove-crista galli. 3. sphenoid bone. 4. middle (temporal) cranial fossa. 5. hypophysial (pituitary) fossa. These areas represent the bone regions where there is greatest likelihood of brain contusions to arise from the damaging effects of the brain-skull interface.

separates the two cerebral hemispheres. The surface of the skull in the sphenoid wing and ethmoid bone region is quite irregular, being jagged and rough in some locations (see Figure 2.3). As a result, with cerebral trauma, it is quite common for contusions (bruising) to occur in the adjacent cerebral regions that are situated in relation to these skull regions; that is, where there is the greatest brain-bone interface (Figure 2.4) Accordingly, the frontal and temporal lobes are the regions most likely to be damaged because of the peculiarities of the skull-brain interface. This occurs regardless of the site or the direction of the initial impact. There is some relationship between the site of skull fracture and underlying hemorrhage (Dacey, Alves, Rimel, Winn, & Jane, 1986), and thus in some cases the area of skull fracture may indicate the most likely area of direct injury.

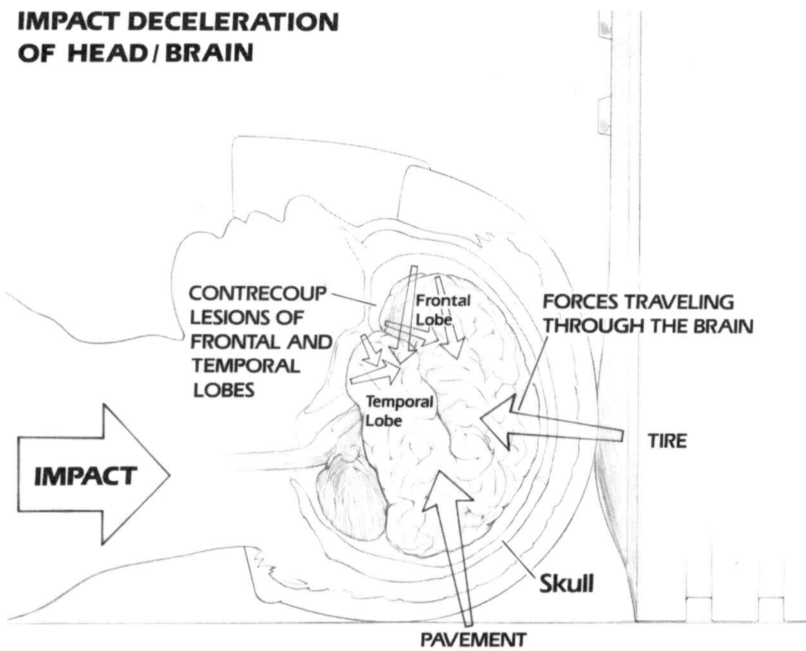

Figure 2.4. This illustration shows the effects of a frontal and temporal lobe injury in a 20-year-old motorcyclist who was struck by a car. As depicted, this individual was thrown from the cycle and simultaneously struck his head on the pavement while being struck by the tire of the automobile that hit him. As a consequence of this trauma, he suffered the expected frontal-temporal lobe damage common to such closed head injuries (note that he was wearing a helmet). At age 12 he had been evaluated in school, and his Wechsler Intelligence Scale for Children–Revised indicated the following intellectual quotients: Verbal IQ score = 123, Performance IQ score = 121, FSIQ score = 125. When tested 3 months post-injury, his Wechsler Adult Intelligence Scale–Revised results indicated a significant drop in overall intellectual functioning with the following scores obtained: VIQ score = 97, PIQ score = 102, FSIQ score = 99. This figure depicts the dynamic forces that impact on the brain, placing the frontal-temporal regions at greatest risk for injury. (Drawing by Medical Communication Services, Dallas, Texas.)

One of the most common neuropathological consequences of the damaging effects that can result from the skull-brain interface is the vulnerability of the hippocampus and other medial temporal lobe limbic structures. Because of its precarious position with respect to the skull, the hippocampus is frequently damaged with the accompanying neurobehavioral syndrome of a posttraumatic memory disorder (Levin et al., 1982). A variety of changes in emotional behavior may be associated with damage in these areas as well (Salazar, Grafman, Schlesselman, et al., 1986; Salazar, Grafman, Vance, et al., 1986).

Diffuse Axonal Injury (DAI)

There is clear neuropathological evidence to suggest that the predominant pattern of injury in cerebral trauma is of a diffuse, nonspecific nature (Adams, Graham, & Gennarelli, 1985; Jennett, 1986). When focal effects are present, they are typically superimposed on more generalized damage. The most common substrate for the diffuse effects of cerebral injury comes from the neuronal shear-strain effects (Adams et al., 1985; Auerbach, 1986). The shear-strain effects occur as a result of the twisting effects on brain tissue that result from the rapid acceleration (e.g., being thrown forward) and subsequent deceleration that accompany high velocity impact. The strain action occurs as a consequence of stretching of neuronal fibers that interconnect different brain regions. This stretching action may actually rupture or shear connections (Figure 2.5). The generalized damage that occurs as a result of torn axonal fibers, damage to supportive glial cell structure (the connective-supportive cells of the brain), and degeneration of neuronal fibers distal (i.e., away from) to the focal area of shearing or contusion is referred to as diffuse axonal injury (DAI). DAI effects may be widely distributed, but most frequently these lesions occur in deep white matter areas and in the brain stem (see Figure 2.6). The anatomic substrate for DAI is a series of microscopic lesions but their accumulative effect may allow detection by CT or MRI studies of the brain. For example, Figure 2.7 shows a postmortem lateral view of the brain of a young adult male (approximately 24 years of age) who sustained a severe closed head injury 2 years before. This gross specimen clearly demonstrates the visible effects of DAI. Note the thinning of the corpus callosum (see area labeled 1; it should be about twice the size seen), which signifies loss of neuronal and glial tissue in that structure. Similarly, the ventricular cavity is significantly enlarged (two to three times the normal size), again in response to the general loss of cerebral tissue. This case also demonstrates the appearance of a focal tissue (see area labeled 2) loss as a result of a contusion. The contusion was the result of focal shear-strain effects as described above.

The contusion depicted in Figure 2.7 was not a surface contusion. The most frequent areas for surface contusions to occur are in the frontal and temporal regions, as discussed in the previous section. Figure 2.8 demonstrates, in a postmortem specimen, the appearance of frontal and temporal lobe surface contusions in a patient who had sustained a severe closed head injury (unrelated to cause of death) three decades previous to death. In this ventral view one can see the chronic effects of such contusions. The damage is in the form of necrotic (degenerated) brain tissue. In this patient, the damage resulted in intellectual and emotional changes characteristic of a frontal lobe syndrome (emotional lability, impulsive behavior, and impaired higher cognitive abilities; see Bigler, 1984). Because of the vulnerability of

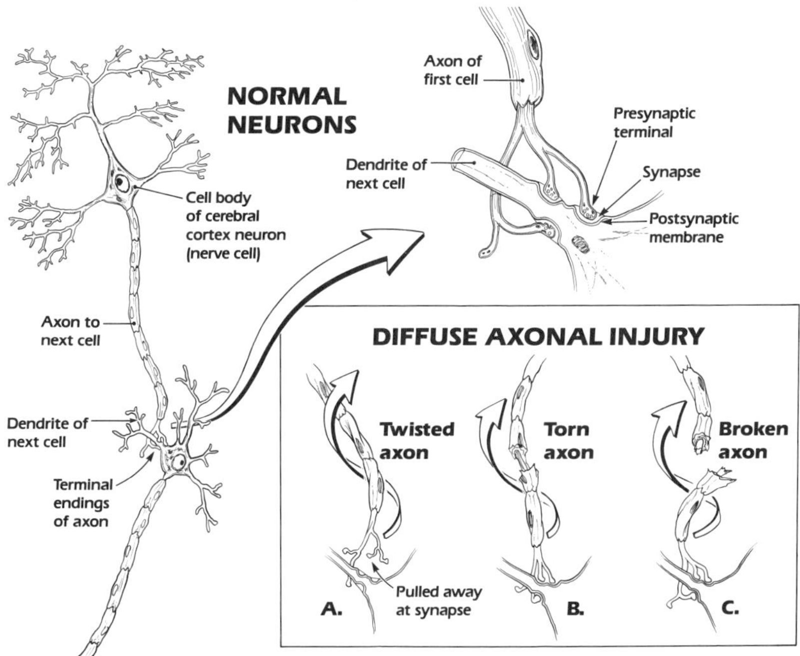

Figure 2.5. Schematic drawing depicting the various mechanisms of diffuse axonal injury (DAI). The drawing on the left is a characterization of a "typical" neuron which displays the major components of the neuron structure. The drawing in the upper right is a close-up demonstrating synaptic interaction. The box inset in the lower right depicts various hypothetical ways the axon can be affected by traumatic brain injury. As shown, axonal integrity may be compromised by shearing/strain effects generated by rapid acceleration/deceleration of brain tissue. The effects of such trauma may anatomically derange the axonal via specific damage of the axon shaft or surrounding myelin or by disrupting synaptic integrity. (Drawing by Medical Communication Services, Dallas, Texas.)

the frontal and temporal regions to injury and their role in controlling intellect and cognition, it is not uncommon that these are the most prominent sequelae following head injury.

Because of the technological advances in brain imaging since the 1970s, the structural integrity of the brain can be studied in situ via CT or MRI scanning. For example, Figure 2.9 demonstrates the appearance of a focal contusion and DAI in a 26-year-old college graduate who had sustained a severe cerebral injury (GCS of 5) some 4 years before. The CT scan shows areas of contusion (encircled) secondary to shear-strain effects in the white matter of the frontal lobes. The cortical sulci are also prominent for this age,

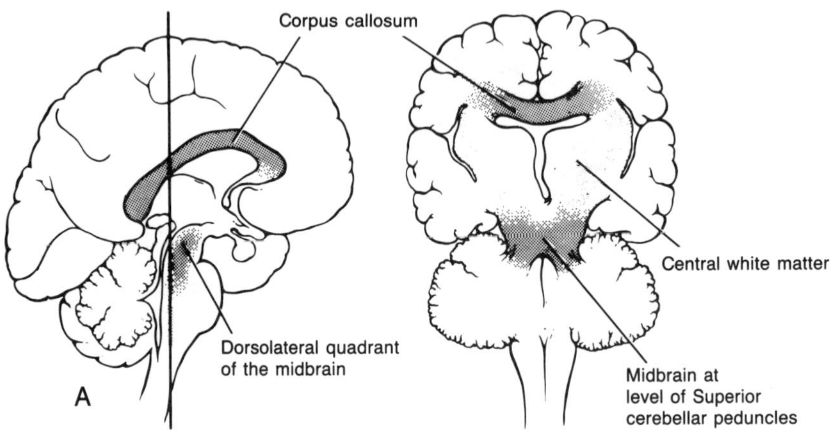

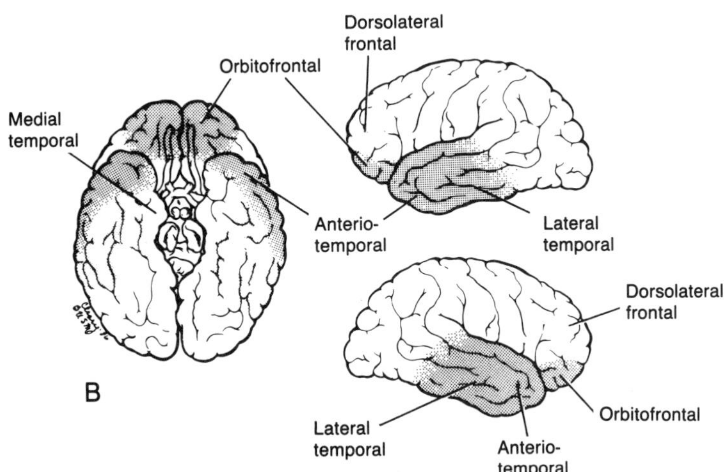

Figure 2.6. A. Brain regions particularly involved by diffuse axonal injury (DAI), including corpus callosum and parasagittal white matter, as well as dorsolateral quadrants of the midbrain. B. Areas predominantly affected by cortical contusions. Darker shading represents more frequently involved areas. Anteriotemporal and orbitofrontal regions are particularly involved. Note relative sparing of dorsolateral frontal lobe and medial temporal lobe. *Note.* From "Neuroanatomical Correlates of Attention and Memory Disorders in Traumatic Brain Injury: An Application of Neurobehavioral Subtypes" by S.H. Auerbach, 1986, *Journal of Head Trauma Rehabilitation, 1,* pp. 3–4. Copyright 1986 by Aspen Systems. Reprinted by permission.

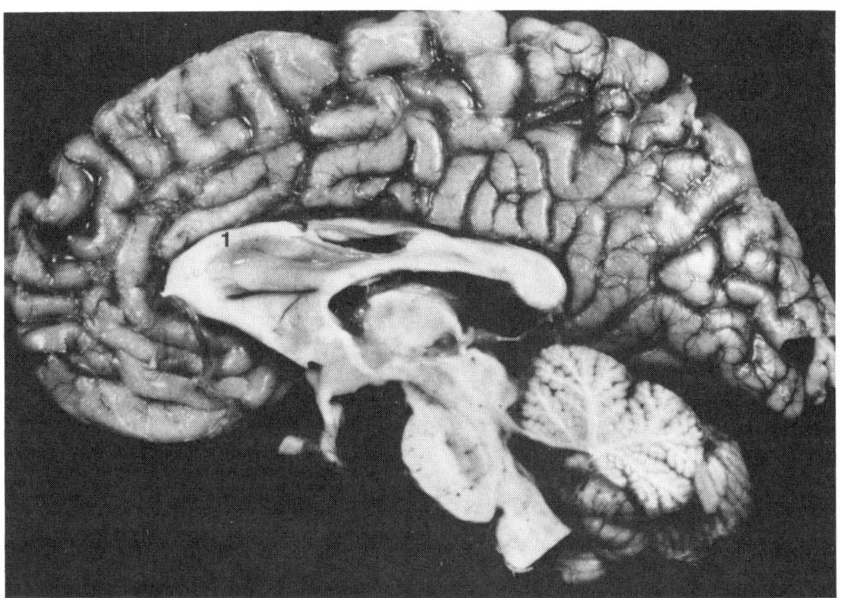

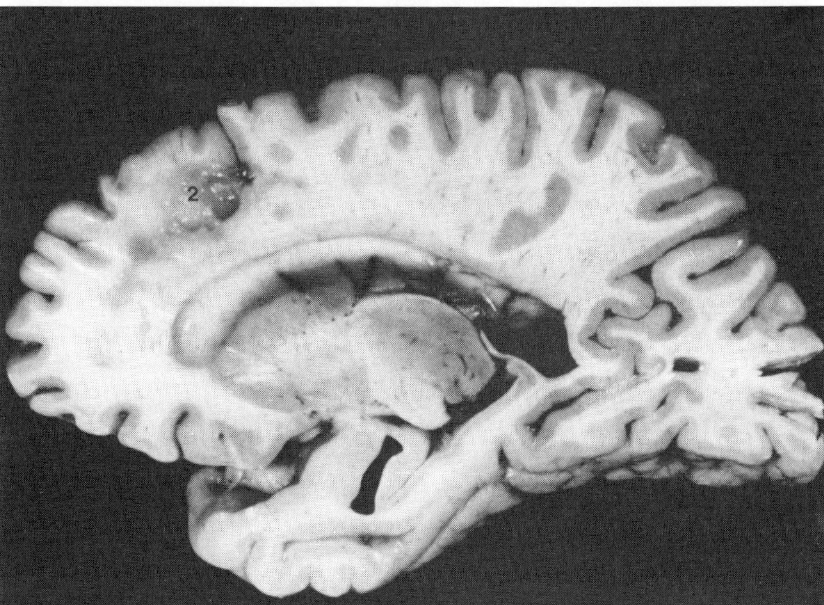

Figure 2.7. Postmortem sagittal views following an unrelated aspiration pneumonia in patient who suffered a severe closed head injury 2 years prior. Gross pathologic effects (top) can be seen in terms of the diminished size of the corpus callosum (1). The mid-sagittal view (bottom) demonstrates an area of focal contusion in the central white matter of the frontal lobe (2) and ventricular dilation.

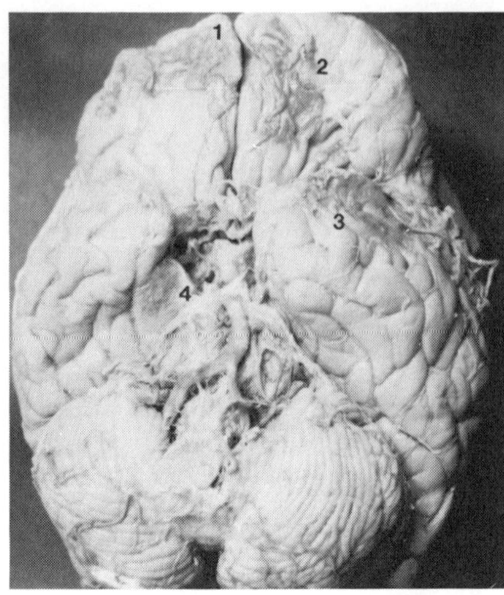

Figure 2.8. Postmortem ventral view of the brain demonstrating old contusions in the inferior frontal (1 & 2), anterior and lateral temporal lobe (3), and medial temporal lobe (4). These are the areas most likely to be damaged as a result of the effects by contusions at the brain-skull interface. The damage present is in the form of necrotic scar tissue. Because this damage is most frequently in the frontal and temporal lobe regions, injured individuals typically demonstrate behavioral changes in the form of impaired judgment, impulsivity, emotional lability, impaired memory processing, and impaired abstract reasoning.

suggestive of diffuse cortical atrophy. In such patients it is commonplace for there to be a significant reduction in intellect and memory. This patient had a Wechsler Adult Intelligence Scale–Revised (WAIS-R; Wechsler, 1981) Verbal IQ (VIQ) score of 82, Performance IQ (PIQ) score of 69, and Full Scale IQ (FSIQ) score of 75. His Wechsler Memory Scale Memory Quotient (WMS MQ; Wechsler, 1945), which has essentially the same statistical properties as the WAIS-R (i.e., $\overline{X} = 100$, $SD = 15$), was 69. These scores represent substantial declines in cognitive abilities considering that his college GPA in finance was 3.75. The deficits are permanent and no improvement is anticipated or expected.

As indicated in Figure 2.9, DAI may result in tissue loss to the point that diffuse cortical atrophy becomes a by-product, and this can be detected by CT or MRI studies. The atrophy occurs as a result of volume loss of the brain substance due to the cumulative effects of degenerated neuronal and glial tissue secondary to DAI. The atrophic patterns in such DAI patients are characteristically more prominent in the frontal and temporal regions, as depicted in the series of CT scans presented in Figure 2.10. In this patient,

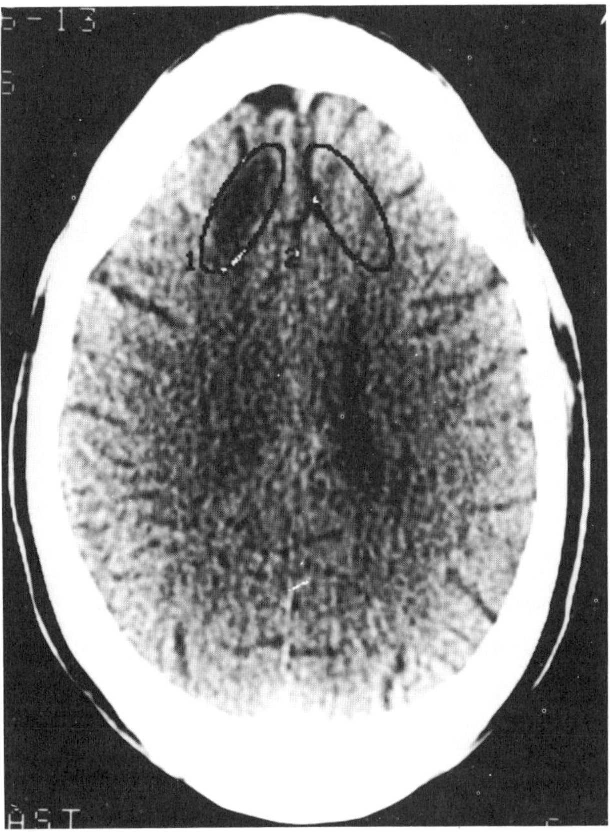

Figure 2.9. Horizontal CT scan depicting left frontal white matter contusion in a patient who suffered a severe closed head injury 4 years previously. The region encircled on the left clearly demonstrates diminished tissue density (dark area), which signifies cell loss in this region. There is also some density change in the right frontal region. Such lesions interrupt various critical pathways of the frontal lobes. Note there is some generalized atrophy as well. This patient suffered from significant intellectual and memory deterioration as a result of this injury (see text).

an 18-year-old high school graduate, the CT demonstrates prominent sulcal widening in the frontal and temporal regions and a particularly prominent Sylvian fissure. In the normal brain the sulci, the fissures or clefts of the brain, are very narrow with the outer boundary of each gyrus that forms the sulcus touching another boundary. Because of this compactness, the sulci typically cannot be visualized on a routine CT scan. When they are visualized, particularly in an individual of 50 years of age or younger, it may be a sign of cortical atrophy, as is the case in the patient presented in Figure 2.10. As previously indicated, such diffuse effects almost always result in some degradation of intellect and memory as well as a variety of related behavioral deficits. In this patient, who graduated in the top 10% of his high school class, his postinjury intellectual performance reflected a precipitous drop from what would have been expected had there not been a brain injury. His WAIS-R VIQ score was 84, PIQ score was 67, and FSIQ score was 75. His WMS MQ was 69. Behaviorally he demonstrated impaired attention, impulsive behavior, poor social monitoring, restlessness, and emotional lability, features commonly seen with this type of damage.

Another important effect of DAI is that pathways may be interrupted or disconnected; this is particularly true of interhemispheric pathways across the

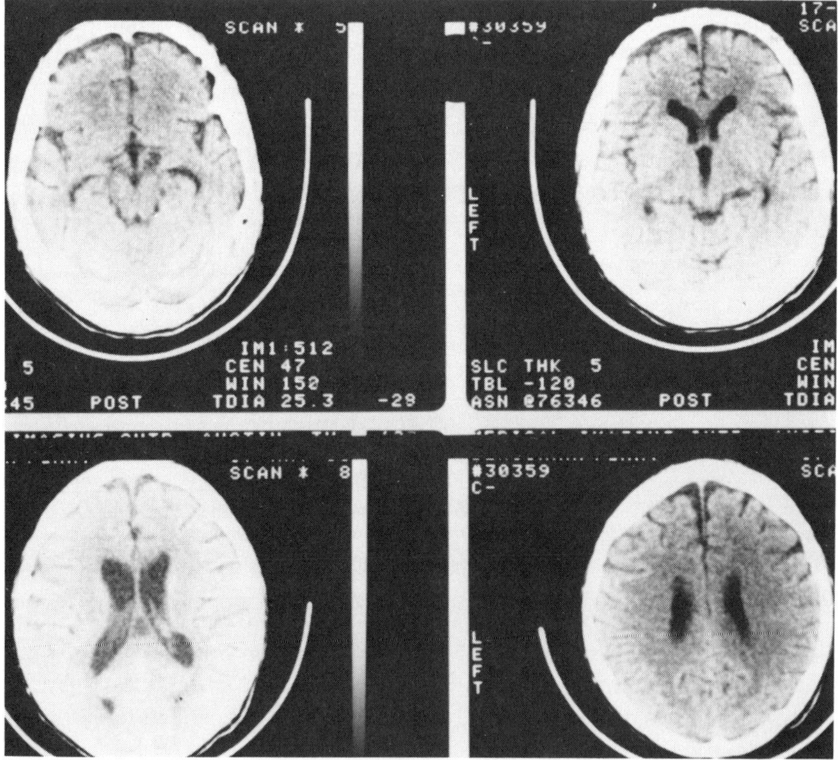

Figure 2.10. Classic CT configuration of generalized atrophy (with greater atrophy in the frontal regions) and ventricular dilation in an 18-year-old male patient who sustained a severe closed head injury 3 months previously (compare with the normal CT scan in Figure 2.2).

corpus callosum. In such cases, the two hemispheres may be functionally separated as a result of damage at the level of the corpus callosum (see Figure 2.11). It should also be noted that severe DAI may occur in the absence of skull fracture or cortical contusion (Jennet, 1986). In point of fact, Gennarelli, Adams, and Thibault (1982) have demonstrated in a nonhuman primate model that DAI can be produced by rapid acceleration of the head in the absence of any impact. They also demonstrated that DAI can be induced in cases of mild brain injury where the nonhuman primate had only transitory alterations in the level of consciousness.

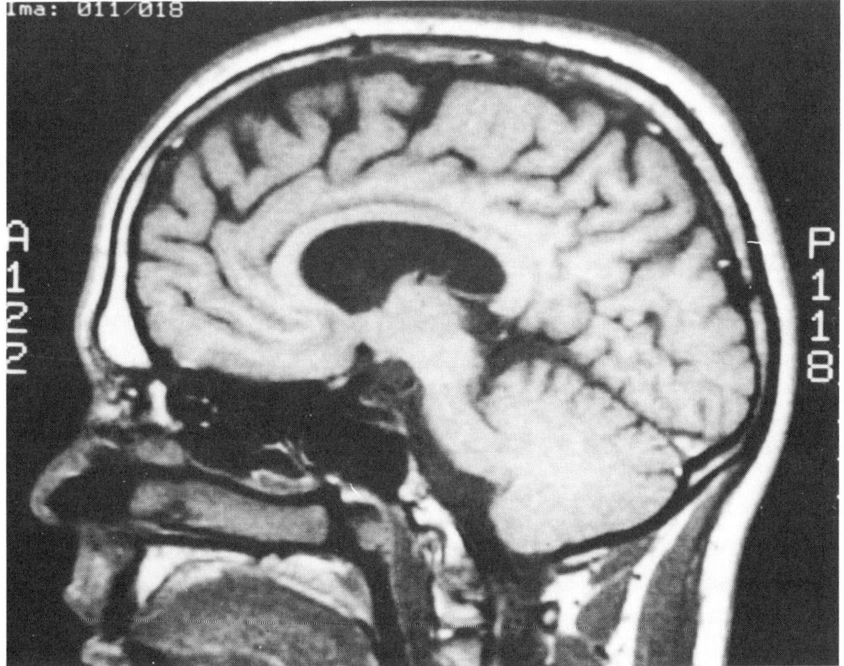

Figure 2.11. Sagittal MRI scan of a patient who 7 years previously sustained a serious closed head injury with initial coma lasting 1 week and with residual mild spastic left hemiparesis. Note the "thinning" of the corpus callosum and the corresponding enlargement of the ventricular space, situated beneath the corpus callosum. This patient sustained a significant contusion at the level of the corpus callosum with corresponding atrophy of this structure and compensatory enlargement of the ventricular system.

ISCHEMIA/HYPOXIA

DAI is a direct consequence of the shear-strain effect at the neuronal level, independent of any vascular or anoxic effects (Adams et al., 1985). However, alterations in blood flow dynamics are commonplace in cerebral injury, and such alterations may produce other significant damaging effects upon neuronal integrity. Accordingly, diffuse neuronal damage may occur as a result of widespread ischemic damage (tissue damage due to obstructed blood flow). There may be loss of adequate blood pressure to the brain (as a result of respiratory insufficiency or blood loss due to a laceration injury), and when cerebral blood perfusion drops below a critical level, ischemic hypoxia may occur. Cerebral perfusion can also be greatly affected by cerebral edema, or brain swelling, the most common metabolic consequence of brain injury (Jennett, 1986). Diminished cerebral perfusion, in turn, reduces cerebral blood flow dynamics, which may lead to brain tissue infarction (necrosis or cell degeneration due to loss of appropriate blood flow). These effects occur most frequently in the distal aspects of small vessels of the brain, and it leads to ischemic necrosis of underlying tissue.

Anoxia may also occur as the result of a variety of systemic (bodily) injuries directly involving the heart, cardiac output, or thoracic area, which affect breathing. In addition to the nonspecific effects of anoxia, there appears to be some predilection for anoxic damage to occur more selectively in the hippocampal region as well (Brierley, 1976; Graham, Adams, & Doyle, 1978; Squire, 1987). With hippocampal damage, prominent memory deficits may result, as the hippocampus is the critical structure for processing short-term memory. Because of the potential nonspecific effects of anoxia and ischemic brain damage in cerebral trauma, these effects typically will be additive to the more direct shear-strain effects of DAI.

CEREBRAL EDEMA

Cerebral edema (brain swelling) is commonplace in cerebral trauma cases; in fact, it is the most common secondary effect of brain injury. It may occur focally, such as that seen around a lateralized contusion, or it may occur in a generalized fashion (Yoshino, Yamaki, Higuchi, Horikawa, & Hirakawa, 1985). Sustained cerebral edema may lead to a variety of pathological consequences (Ito, Tomita, Yamazaki, Takada, & Inaba, 1986). These include compression of cerebral vessels that may lead to underlying infarction (as discussed above in the section on ischemia and hypoxia); structural compression of brain tissue itself, which leads to cell loss; herniation of brain tissue, which also leads to cell loss; and gradual strain effect on axonal fibers as the tissue expands and stretches, breaking axonal filaments. Uzzell, Obrist,

Dolinskas, and Langfitt (1986) found significant neuropsychological impairment, particularly in memory functioning, in all patients who sustained significantly elevated intracranial pressure. After approximately 3 months postinjury, follow-up CT scanning in such patients will typically demonstrate some degree of ventricular enlargement and/or cortical atrophy. These abnormal findings represent the diffuse degenerative changes that may result from cerebral edema.

The effects of cerebral edema are depicted in Figure 2.12. In this case serial CT scans demonstrate the structural changes that occur over time in response to severe closed head injury in a patient who likewise sustained a right frontal-temporal lobe contusion and diffuse cerebral edema. At the time of injury, this female child was 12 years of age. The CT on admission to the hospital (A) was generally within normal limits although a contusion is noted in the right frontal and temporal region (increased density as demonstrated by the splotchy, white areas) and there is a pocket of trapped air (arrow) as a result of the skull fracture. However, the CT scan 7 days later (B) demonstrates some resolution in the contusion and reabsorption of the blood that was present (this represents the normal healing/resolution process following a hemorrhage), but there is a significant midline shift to the left at this time, which represents the pathological effects of localized edema. Note the dilation of the left anterior horn and the collapse of the posterior horn of the ventricular system (compare this figure with the normal CT in Figure 2.2). This is due to edema effects across the right hemisphere, in large part a result of the right frontal and temporal contusion. The CT scan 11 days postinjury (C) demonstrates return to midline of the ventricular structures, but considerable dilation of those structures is beginning to develop. This dilation is the result of brain density changes secondary to DAI and the automatic increase in ventricular size due to outward expansion of the ventricular system (which is under pressure because it is being filled with cerebrospinal fluid) in response to diminished brain volume due to neuronal loss. The CT scan 2½ months postinjury (D) demonstrates ventricular dilation, particularly for the anterior right ventricular system. This is due to increased lateralized tissue loss secondary to the original right frontal-temporal lobe contusion and subsequent edematous effects, which have resulted in neuronal degeneration and loss of tissue. Also note the prominence of the interhemispheric fissure, which is indicative of some degree of frontal atrophy. These results demonstrate the importance of serial CT evaluation in the closed head injury patient and the progressive changes in the initial stages of recovery that may occur over time.

With such diffuse injuries, there are always concomitant cognitive changes of significant proportions. This child's last neuropsychological evaluation, some 2 years postinjury, continued to demonstrate significant residual deficits, particularly with respect to judgment, complex reasoning/problem solving, and memory. She obtained the following Wechsler Intelligence Scale

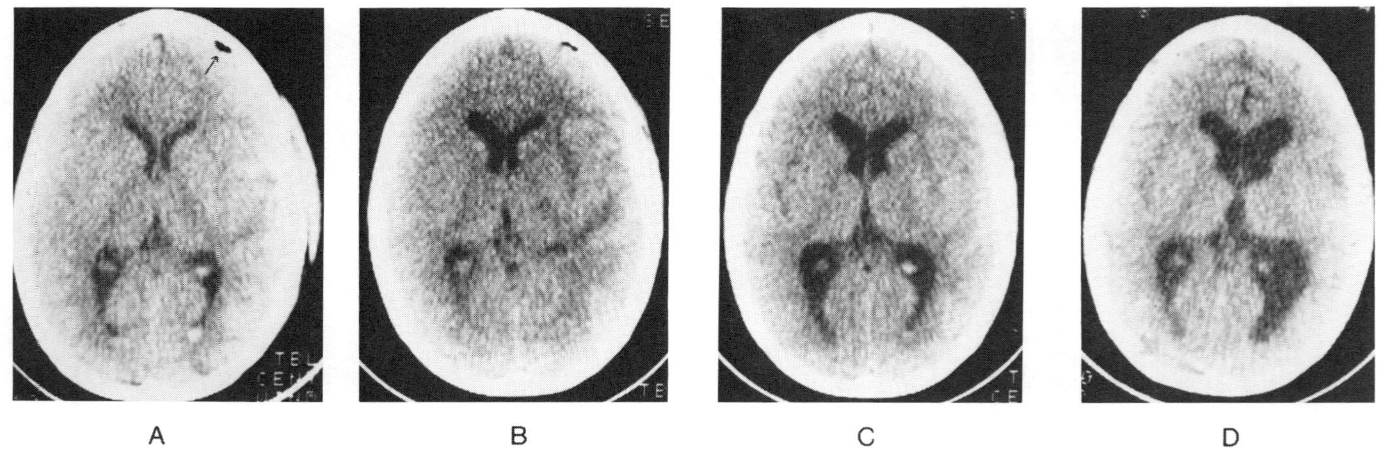

Figure 2.12. Sequential CT scans depicting the effects of a right frontal-temporal lobe contusion and subsequent edema. **(A)** CT on admission to the hospital. This CT was taken about 3 hours postinjury. It is generally within normal limits. The contusion (increased density manifested by the splotchy, white areas) can be visualized in the right frontal-temporal region. There is also a pocket of trapped air (arrow) as a result of the skull fracture. **(B)** CT scan taken 7 days postinjury that demonstrates some resolution of the contusion by the disappearance of blood (e.g., reabsorption), but a significant midline shift to the left is now quite apparent. Note the dilation or enlargement of the left anterior horn and the collapse of the right posterior horn. This is due to the massive swelling effects in the right hemisphere, which compresses cerebral spinal fluid out of the right ventricular system and shifts it to the left. **(C)** CT scan 11 days postinjury that indicates a shift back to midline of the ventricular structures, but now the entire ventricular system is enlarged. This ventricular enlargement is due to compensatory changes that are brought about by DAI. This occurs because a loss of brain tissue volume is beginning to develop. **(D)** CT scan 2½ months postinjury. At this point the chronic neuropathological effects have developed. Note generalized ventricular dilation with particular outward expansion of the right ventricular system. This is due to the greater lateralized effects of the right frontal-temporal lobe contusion and surrounding edema. Also note the prominence of the interhemispheric fissure, which is a sign of frontal atrophy.

for Children–Revised (WISC-R; Wechsler, 1974) results: VIQ=91, PIQ=86, FSIQ=87. The Wechsler Memory Scale (corrected for age) Memory Quotient was 89. Likewise, this child demonstrated marked deficits in terms of distractibility and impulsiveness. She consistently scored above the 90th percentile on standardized achievement tests prior to the brain injury, and, accordingly, the intellectual and memory results quoted above clearly reflect a substantial reduction in level of ability. Behaviorally, this child had no prior history of any emotional or behavioral problems and was described as a "model" child. Postinjury, numerous behavioral problems were present and she was very difficult to manage and keep on task. She was no longer goal oriented. Her attention span was very short, and she tended to be very garrulous and socially inappropriate. Some sexual acting out was evident.

HEMORRHAGE

Cerebral hemorrhage may occur as a consequence of cerebral trauma, as a result of skull fracture (typically resulting in an extradural hematoma—a blood clot between the skull and meninges), a tear in a meningeal artery (resulting in an epidural hematoma—a blood clot below and around the meninges), rupture of a brain surface vessel (creating a subdural or epidural hematoma), or a rupture of an internal vessel (producing an intracerebral hematoma—a blood clot within the brain). Such hemorrhagic masses typically produce mechanical distortion of the cerebral structures with resulting damaging compression effects, frequently similar to that seen with edema (see Figure 2.13). The effects of such compression may directly alter underlying structures by shifting or compression effects, and this in turn also may compress blood vessels (see Figure 2.14). The presence of a hematoma may produce focal effects (Shigemori et al., 1986) in and around the site of hemorrhage due to loss of appropriate blood flow as well as the effects of localized pressure and mechanical distortion. Also, the effect of the hematoma may produce some degree of generalized impairment. For example, Cullum and Bigler (1986) demonstrated that the mere presence of a hematoma, regardless of location, appeared to accentuate underlying cerebral damage and was associated with a greater residual cognitive deficit than that seen in patients who had sustained similar brain injury but who did not develop a hematoma (see Figures 2.15 and 2.16). It also should be noted that hematoma formation may occur some time after the injury. Thus it may not be an immediate consequence of the trauma (Bucci, Phillips, & McGillicuddy, 1986; Fukamachi et al., 1985; Soloniuk, Pitts, Lovely, & Bartkowski, 1986). The neuropathological effects of delayed hemorrhaging are essentially the same as for the immediate type.

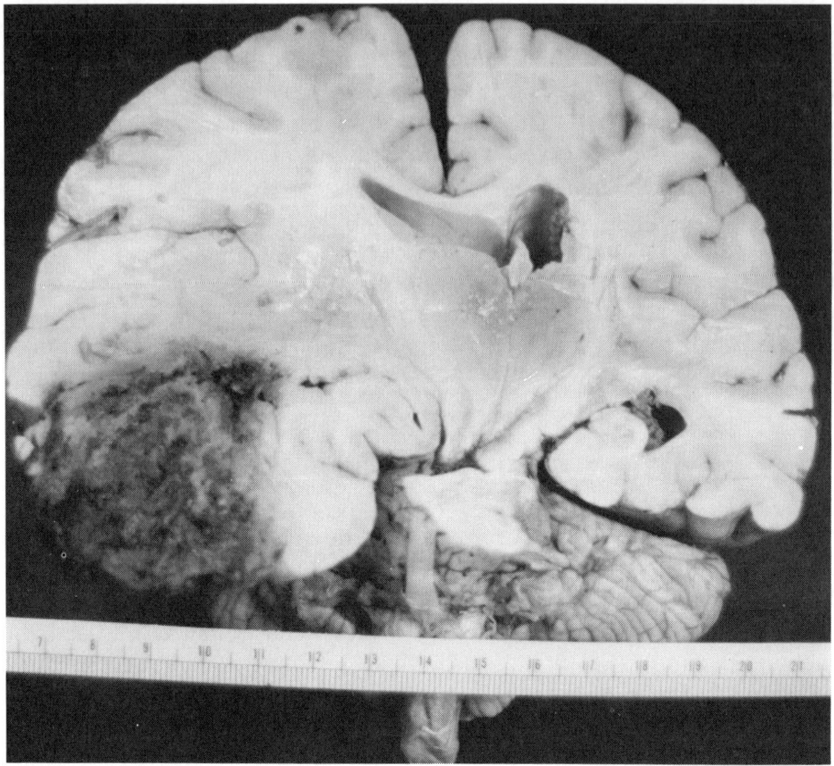

Figure 2.13. Postmortem coronal section depicting the effects of a hemorrhagic contusion. Note the almost complete obliteration of the right temporal lobe and the massive distortion that this induces throughout the brain. Note the collapse of the right lateral ventricle and the marked shift across midline at the level of the thalamus. Such marked distortions produce not only focal effects but also generalized damage as the result of increased pressure (edema) and compression effects.

FOCAL VERSUS NONFOCAL LESIONS

In cerebral lesions produced by focal hemorrhage or infarction associated with a cerebral vascular accident, the ensuing neurologic deficits may be related precisely to the area damaged. For example, a cerebral vascular accident (stroke) in the distribution of the middle cerebral artery over the inferior but lateral aspect of the left frontal lobe (Broca's area) would typically produce a "Broca's aphasia" in which the patient would have severe expressive language defects and contralateral (on opposite side) hemiplegia (paralysis), but would have intact verbal comprehension and typically intact visual-spatial abilities as well as intact left-sided motor functioning (Bigler, 1984). This syndrome is associated with a focal lesion in the inferior lateral aspect of the left frontal lobe without damage or effects in any other part of the cerebrum. Typically such "pure" focal syndromes do not occur in traumatic brain injury because the focal pathology is superimposed upon a background of nonspecific, generalized cerebral damage and dysfunction. There may be focal symptoms or syndromes that predominate, but they are typically only a subset of deficits superimposed upon some degree of generalized damage. It should also be pointed out that the site of greatest focal damage may actually occur, in a linear fashion, directly opposite the point of impact. This is the "coup/contre-coup" effect. As can be seen in Figure 2.17, there are two main areas of damage—one area in the left frontal lobe, the other in the right parietal-occipital region, which in linear trajectory is directly opposite the frontal injury. Such patients may develop "multi-focal" deficits. For example, this patient initially had expressive language deficits and right-side paralysis but left visual field and visual-spatial deficits. The former deficits were associated with the focal left frontal damage, the latter with the focal right occipital and parietal involvement.

Penetrating injuries such as those seen with gunshot wounds to the head (see Kaufman et al., 1986), as opposed to traumatic brain injury of the impact type, may produce focal effects without significant damage to areas outside the area of direct trauma (see Figures 2.18 and 2.19). Frequently, with large caliber gunshot wounds, the bullet will pass through the skull and brain, exiting opposite its point of entry. Thus, by knowing entrance and exit points, one can infer the area(s) of underlying damage. There are several complicating factors with penetrating injury. One is that bone fragments may penetrate the brain tissue, producing additional focal damage. The penetrating injury may also produce hemorrhaging.

CEREBRAL ATROPHY AND VENTRICULAR ENLARGEMENT

It is now well documented that as a consequence of cerebral injury there may be atrophy (shrinkage) of the cerebral cortex with corresponding enlargement of the ventricular system (Levin, Meyers, Grossman, & Sarwar, 1981; Lipper et al., 1985). In a study by Cullum and Bigler (1986) it was demonstrated that the average ventricular enlargement in patients with significant brain injury was nearly twice that of normal individuals; likewise, there were significant amounts of cortical atrophy. The atrophy tends to develop more in the frontal and temporal regions, although it may be widespread and diffuse as well (see Figure 2.10). It appears that the areas of greatest atrophy are related to the area or areas of contusion and/or prior hematoma. CT and MRI studies also

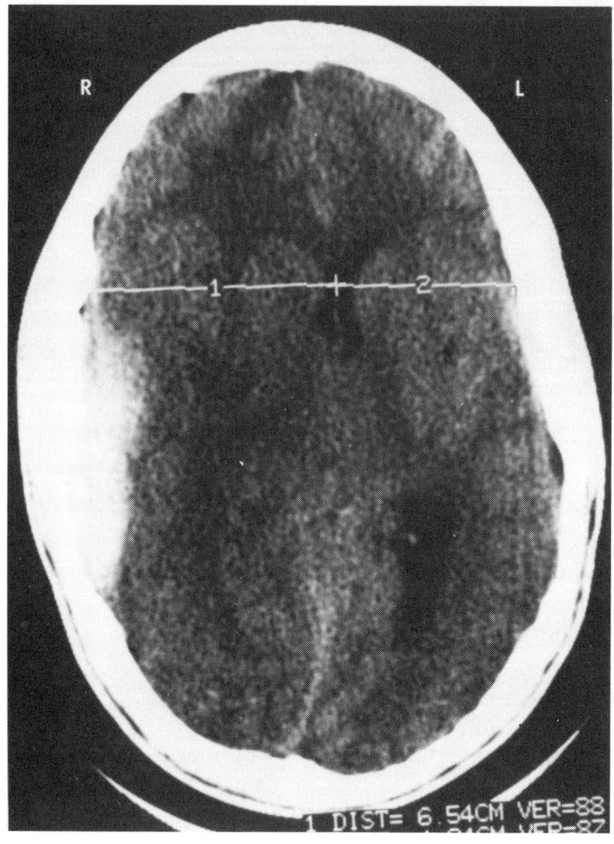

Figure 2.14. (this page and facing page) At age 16 this male patient sustained a severe head injury as a result of an assault. A large hematoma developed as a result of a tear in the right middle meningeal artery. The CT depicted on the left demonstrates the position of the hematoma (note that the CT and MRI are presented in the radiological position, which orients the patient's left on the viewer's right and vica versa) and the massive midline shift, as depicted by the unequal distances between the inner skull surface and the anterior horns of the lateral ventricles. Note that the tremendous shift has moved brain midline completely off center. The MRI depicted on the right is a ventral view that demonstrates tissue loss (increased "white" appearance) in the right temporal lobe. The MRI was taken 3 months postinjury and neurosurgical removal of the hematoma. This tissue loss was due to compression effects from the hematoma pressing the ventral temporal region against the middle cranial fossa. Prior to the injury, this adolescent male

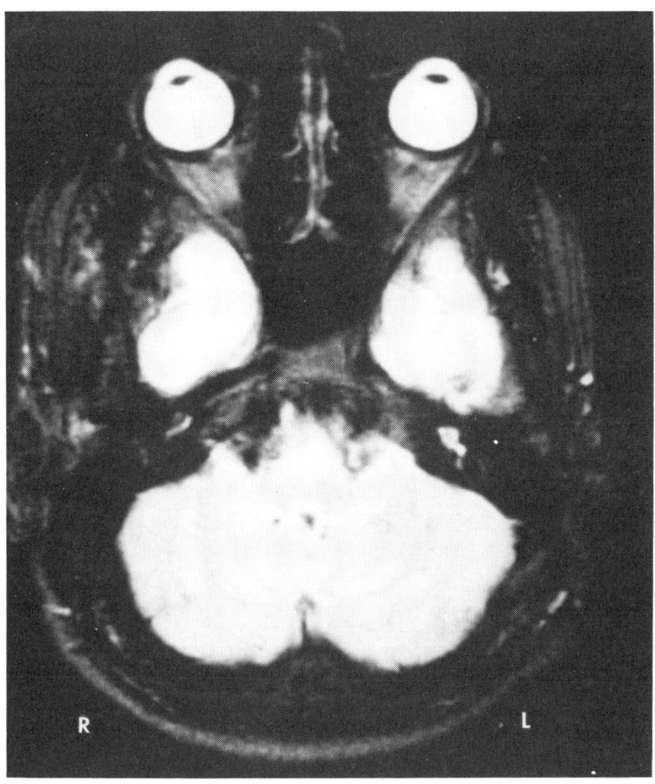

was a National Merit Scholar, who at age 12 years 1 month had a Stanford-Binet IQ score above 152. At 6 weeks postinjury, he obtained a Wechsler Adult Intelligence Scale–Revised (WAIS-R) Verbal IQ score of 127, Performance IQ score of 73, and a Full Scale IQ score of 103. His Wechsler Memory Scale (WMS) was only 69 with particular deficits in visual memory. The remainder of his neuropsychological studies were consistent with greater right hemispheric dysfunction. Two months following an intense rehabilitation program and as a result of spontaneous improvement, this patient demonstrated improved neuropsychological functioning (WAIS-R VIQ = 137, PIQ = 100, FSIQ = 126; WMS MQ = 121) but continued to demonstrate particular deficits in visual memory and visual-spatial processing, which, given his MRI findings of residual right temporal lobe damage, will probably remain (see Figure 2.16). This is an excellent demonstration of the damaging effects of a hematoma away from the actual site of hemorrhage.

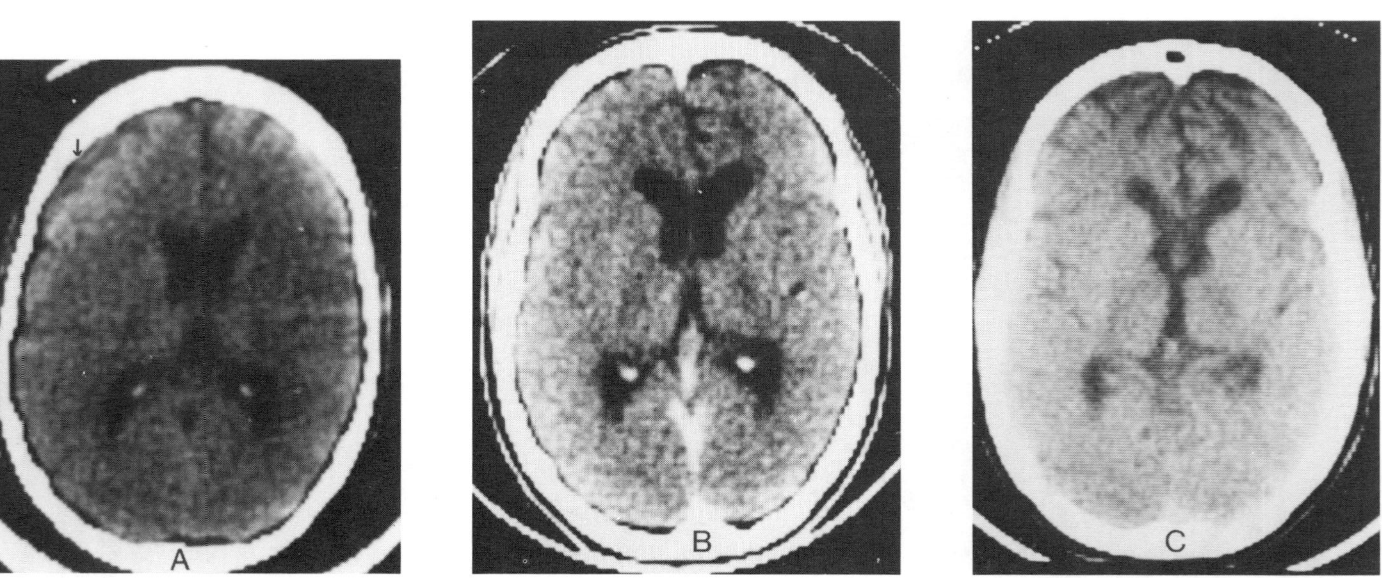

Figure 2.15. **(A)** CT depiction of a hematoma (arrow) in the left frontal region, which can be visualized as the thin dark line (1) over the lateral aspect of the frontal lobe. **(B)** Postsurgical "burrhole" aspiration removal of the hematoma 3 weeks postinjury with the CT scan now showing general restoration of orientation and positioning, and the absence of the hematoma. **(C)** CT scan 2 years posttrauma. Note the prominent frontal atrophy as demonstrated by the loss of brain density in the frontal regions (scatter dark areas) and the prominence of the interhemispheric fissure. The patient had a classic posttraumatic frontal lobe syndrome characterized by poor judgment, hyperemotionality and irritability, poor social skills, and impaired memory functioning as well as impaired abstract reasoning and complex problem solving.

have suggested that the change in ventricular size may be a more sensitive measure of structural deficits in brain injury than the presence of cortical atrophy. This is opposite of what is seen with the degenerative dementias (Bigler, Hubler, Cullum, & Turkheimer, 1985; Levin et al., 1985; Massman, Bigler, Cullum, & Naugle, 1986).

The cognitive effects of traumatically induced cerebral atrophy are related to various deficits in higher cortical function as well. Frequently these deficits affect complex reasoning/problem solving, memory, and social-emotional functioning. Psychometric studies have demonstrated significant reductions in intellect, language, and memory function (Cullum & Bigler, 1986; Levin et al., 1982).

"MILD" CEREBRAL TRAUMA

The effects of "mild" cerebral injury typically produce a "postconcussion" syndrome with a stereotypical constellation of symptoms that usually includes memory difficulties, problems with attention and concentration, lassitude, disturbance of sleep, irritability, depression, and headache (Gennarelli, 1986; Kwentus, Hart, Peck, & Kornstein, 1985; Prigatano & Pepping, 1987). These symptoms typically dissipate over time, reaching their peak in the weeks following the injury, but sometimes persist for 6 to 12 months. Some researchers have demonstrated residual cognitive deficits in such patients while others have not (Barth, Macciocchi, & Giordani, 1983; Gentilini et al., 1985). The differences in these studies probably relate to differences in what is defined as a "mild" injury. Gennarelli et al.'s (1982) primate studies provide theoretical evidence to suggest structural pathology at the microscopic level that could not be detected by CT or MRI studies in some of these patients with "mild" injury. An abundance of clinical literature also suggests that there may be permanent sequelae associated with "minor" cerebral injury (Gronwall & Wrightson, 1980; Kwentus et al., 1985). There also may be a relationship to systemic and spinal cord injuries in the evolution of cerebral damage/dysfunction in the patient who otherwise did not sustain a significant head injury (Wilmot, Cope, Hall, & Acker, 1985). In the most well-controlled study to date, Levin et al. (1987) demonstrated that a single uncomplicated minor head injury produced no permanent disability in the majority of patients studied. For this study "minor" head injury was defined to include the following:

> a history of cranial trauma resulting in a loss of consciousness of 20 minutes or less; an admission GCS score of 13 to 15 without subsequent deterioration (that is, the patient was disoriented and/or confused but had spontaneous eye opening and obeyed commands); no focal neurological deficit; no evidence of an intra-

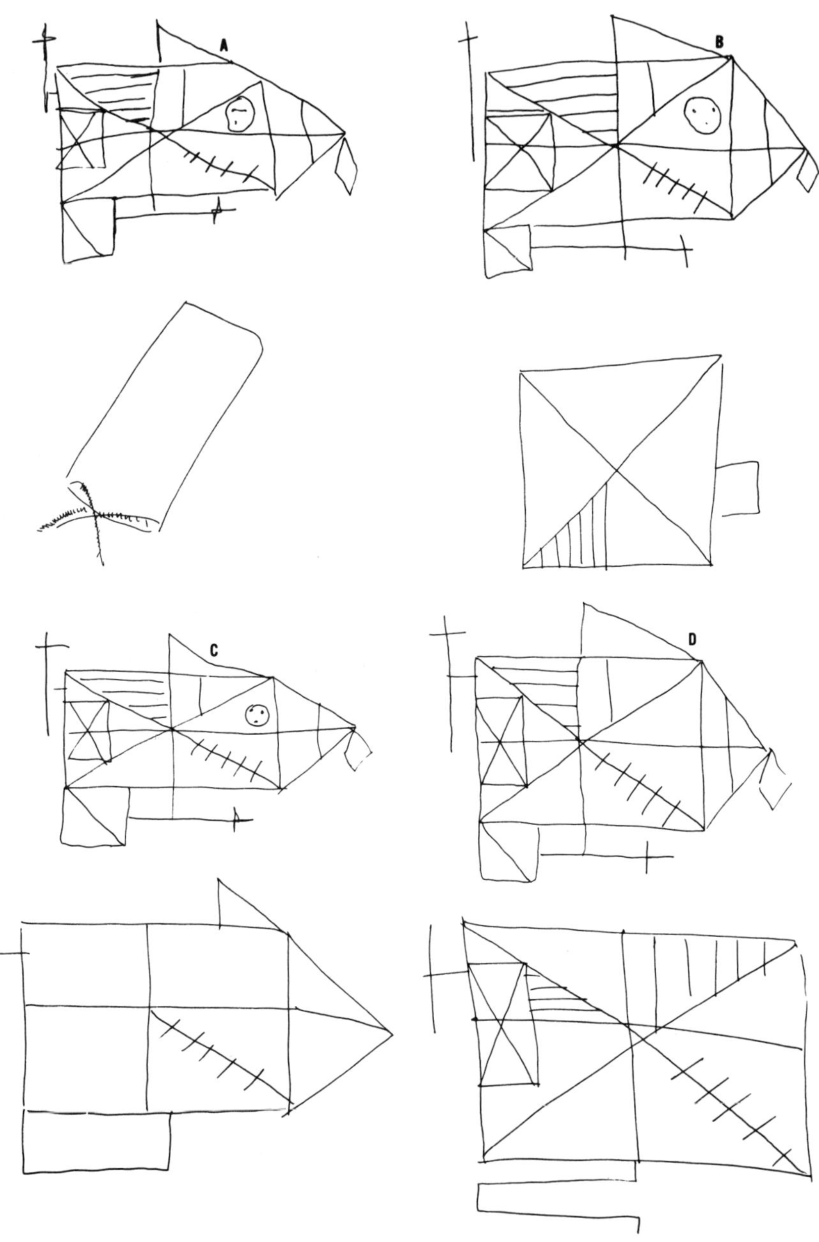
A
B
C
D

> cranial mass lesion such as a hematoma; no intracranial surgical procedures, such as repair of a depressed skull fracture; and absence of complications such as meningitis. (p. 235)

This research indicates that patients with minor head injury that meets the criteria listed above may not suffer permanent neurobehavioral sequelae. This group of patients all developed features of a postconcussion syndrome when tested at 1 week postinjury, but by 3 months postinjury the head injury patient group could not be statistically differentiated from a matched control group on a variety of neuropsychological measures.

CONCLUSIONS

This chapter has reviewed the basic neuropathology of acquired cerebral trauma. Traumatic brain injury may occur in a variety of ways with the most common being secondary to motor vehicle accidents. A significant brain injury is felt to have occurred in the presence of one or a combination of the following three events: (a) alteration in the level of consciousness sufficient to produce a Glasgow Coma Scale of 14 or lower; (b) posttraumatic amnesia of 5 minutes or greater; (c) the presence of physiologic findings (e.g., EEG), radiologic evidence (e.g., CT, MRI), or objective physical exam findings (e.g., paralysis, aphasia, sensory deficit). While any part of the brain may be damaged as a result of trauma, the frontal and temporal lobes are the areas most commonly affected. A major reason for this is related to the skull-brain interface in these regions. Diffuse axonal injury appears to be the substrate that produces the generalized effects of cerebral injury. Edema, ischemia, contusions, hypoxia, and hemorrhage may also be associated factors in pro-

---

Figure 2.16. (facing page) Significant visual memory defect in the patient discussed in Figure 2.14. Such pronounced visual memory deficits are most often associated with damage to the right hemisphere, particularly the right temporal lobe. The original stimulus design of the Rey-Osterrieth Complex Figure Design is presented in Figure 2.1 (top right). The top drawing in each case is the patient's direct copy of the figure. It is evident that even soon after the brain injury he was capable of adequately copying the figure, but in each case recall is significantly impaired. This is particularly significant in this patient, because his premorbid level of function was so high that prior to this traumatic brain injury he would have had little difficulty in drawing this figure from visual memory. **A.** 3 weeks posttrauma. **B.** 3 months posttrauma. **C.** 1 year posttrauma. **D.** 2 years posttrauma. Note the slight improvement over time, but even 2 years posttrauma visual memory impairment persists.

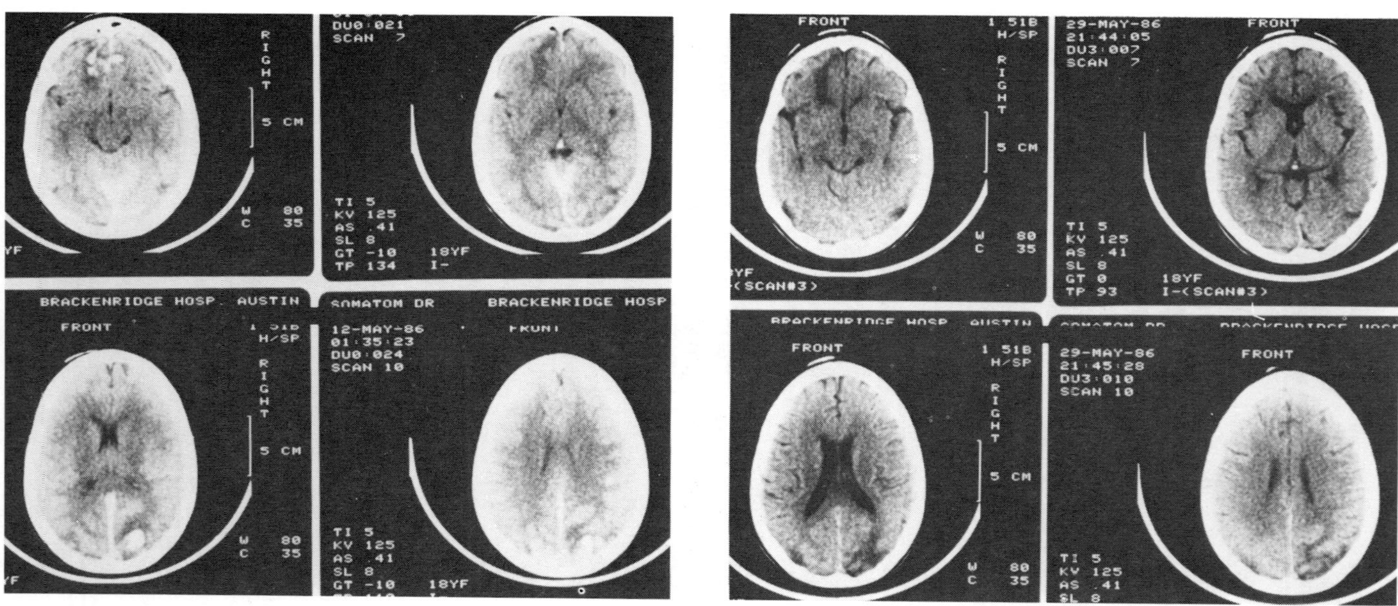

Figure 2.17. CT depiction of a coup/contre-coup lesion. The scans on the left demonstrate a focal contusion (the coup) in the left frontal region, with a second area of contusion (the contre-coup) in a direct linear trajectory in the right occipital area. This patient sustained a severe frontal injury in a motor vehicle accident, striking the left frontal region originally, and the contre-coup injury in the right occipital area is a result of the tearing/shearing effects that occur in a linear fashion away from the actual initial site of impact. The CT scans on the right depict the residual, lasting effects of such contusions. Note the decreased density in the left frontal and right occipital areas. These scans were taken 6 weeks postinjury. The lesion areas will constitute a chronic lesion site with permanent deficits. Note also the prominence of the Sylvian fissures and the frontal interhemispheric fissure, signs of some degree of generalized cerebral damage secondary to DAI in addition to the focal contusions.

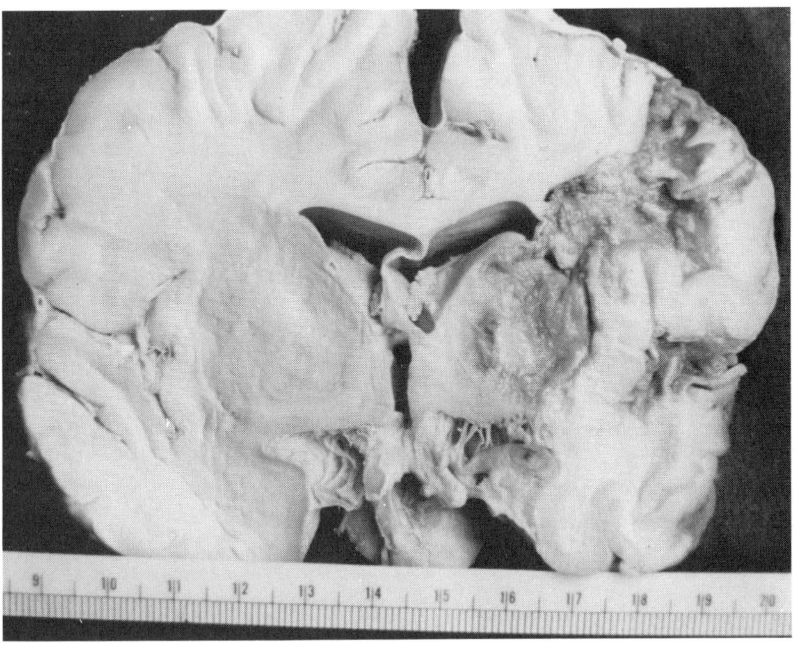

Figure 2.18. Postmortem coronal section depicting the pathway of a self-inflicted gunshot wound to the head. The individual shot himself through the roof of the mouth with the bullet exiting in the dorsal frontal region. Note the focal effects of such an injury.

ducing brain damage in cerebral trauma. The resultant structural effects of these brain damaging conditions can frequently be determined by CT and/or MRI studies of the brain. The most common CT or MRI finding in nonfocal brain injury is some degree of cortical atrophy and corresponding ventricular enlargement. Such neuropathological states typically result in reduced intellectual and cognitive abilities, particularly memory, along with the variety of behavioral changes, most commonly in the form of a frontal lobe syndrome (partially to fully expressed). It is hoped that a more complete understanding of the neuropathology of cerebral trauma will permit a better understanding of neurobehavioral consequences of cerebral injury.

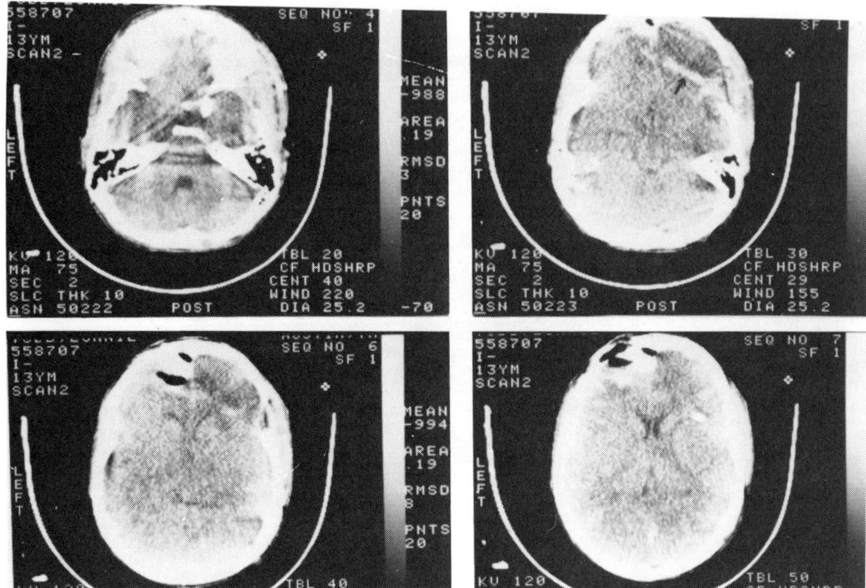

Figure 2.19. CT depiction of a self-inflicted gunshot wound. Note the pathway of the bullet (arrow). This was a 13-year-old male patient who attempted to take his life by shooting himself with a .22 caliber pistol by placing the muzzle of the gun in the right temple region and pulling the trigger. The patient never lost consciousness as the result of this injury, and the bullet made a clean exit out the left frontal region. The frontal lesion did produce a classic frontal lobe syndrome of impaired attention and increased impulsivity as well as impaired mental functioning and reduced level of intellectual ability. The patient's remote memory and fund of general information were generally intact, however. His intellectual test scores 3 months postinjury indicated the following on the Wechsler Intelligence Scale for Children–Revised: VIQ = 81, PIQ = 82, FSIQ = 79. The patient obtained an age-corrected score of 66 on the Wechsler Memory Scale.

REFERENCES

Adams, J.H., Graham, D.I., & Gennarelli, T.A. (1985). Contemporary neuropathological considerations regarding brain damage in head injury. In D.P. Becker & J.T. Povlishack (Eds.), *Central nervous system trauma status report—1985.* Washington, DC: National Institutes of Health—National Institute for Neurological and Communicative Disorders and Stroke.

Alexander, R.C., Schor, D.P., & Smith, W.L., Jr. (1986). Magnetic resonance imaging of intracranial injuries from child abuse. *Journal of Pediatrics, 109,* 975–979.

Auerbach, S.H. (1986). Neuroanatomical correlates of attention and memory disorders in traumatic brain injury: An application of neurobehavioral subtypes. *Journal of Head Trauma Rehabilitation, 1,* 1–12.

Bakay, L., & Glasauer, F.E. (1980). *Head*

injury. Boston: Little, Brown.

Barth, J., Macciocchi, S., & Giordani, B. (1983). Neuropsychological sequelae of minor head injury. *Neurosurgery, 13,* 529–537.

Bigler, E.D. (1984). *Diagnostic clinical neuropsychology.* Austin: University of Texas Press.

Bigler, E.D., Hubler, D.W., Cullum, C.M., & Turkheimer, E. (1985). *Journal of Nervous and Mental Disease, 173,* 347–352.

Bond, M.R. (1983). Effects on the family system. In M. Rosenthal, E.R. Griffith, M.R. Bond, & J.D. Miller (Eds.), *Rehabilitation of the head injured adult* (pp. 209–217). Philadelphia: F.A. Davis.

Brierley, J.B. (1976). Cerebral hypoxia. In W. Blackwood & J. Carsellis (Eds.), *Greenfield's neuropathology* (pp. 927–941). Edinburgh, London: Edward Arnold.

Brooks, D.N. (1983). Disorders of memory. In M. Rosenthal, E.R. Griffith, M.R. Bond, & J.D. Miller (Eds.), *Rehabilitation of the head injured adult* (pp. 185–196). Philadelphia: F.A. Davis.

Bucci, M.N., Phillips, T.W., & McGillicuddy, J.E. (1986). Delayed epidural hemorrhage in hypotensive multiple trauma patients. *Neurosurgery, 19,* 65–68.

Clifton, G.L., Grossman, R.G., Makela, M.E., Miner, M.E., Handel, S., & Sadhu, V. (1980). Neurological course and correlated computerized tomography findings after severe closed head injury. *Journal of Neurosurgery, 52,* 611–624.

Cohen, R.A., Kaufman, R.A., Myers, P.A., & Towbin, R.B. (1986). Cranial computed tomography in the abused child with head injury. *American Journal of Radiology, 146,* 97–102.

Cullum, C.M., & Bigler, E.D. (1986). Ventricle size, cortical atrophy and the relationship with neuropsychological status in closed head injury: A quantitative analysis. *Journal of Clinical and Experimental Neuropsychology, 8,* 437–452.

Dacey, R.G., Jr., Alves, W.M., Rimel, R.W., Winn, H.R., & Jane, J.A. (1986). Neurosurgical complications after apparently minor head injury. Assessment of risk in a series of 620 patients. *Journal of Neurosurgery, 2,* 203–210.

Duffy, F.H., & McAnulty, G.B. (1985). Brain electrical activity mapping (BEAM): The search for a physiological signature of dyslexia. In F.H. Duffy & N. Geschwind (Eds.), *Dyslexia: A neuroscientific approach to clinical evaluation* (pp. 105–122). Boston: Little, Brown.

Dykes, L.J. (1986). The whiplash shaken infant syndrome: What has been learned? *Child Abuse-Neglect, 10,* 211–221.

Fukamachi, A., Kohno, K., Nagaseki, Y., Misumi, S., Kunimine, H., & Wakao, T. (1985). The incidence of delayed traumatic intracerebral hematoma with extradural hemorrhages. *Journal of Trauma, 25,* 145–149.

Gennarelli, T.A. (1986). Mechanisms and pathophysiology of cerebral concussion. *Journal of Head Trauma Rehabilitation, 1,* 23–30.

Gennarelli, T.A., Adams, J.H., & Thibault, L.B. (1982). Diffuse axonal injury and traumatic coma in the primate. *Annals of Neurology, 12,* 564–574.

Gentilini, M., Michelli, P., Schoenhuber, R., Bortolotti, P., Tonelli, L., Falasca, A., & Merli, G.A. (1985). Neuropsychological evaluation of mild head injury. *Journal of Neurology, Neurosurgery, and Psychiatry, 48,* 137–140.

Graham, D.I., Adams, H., & Doyle, D. (1978). Ischemic brain damage in fatal nonmissile head injuries. *Journal of Neurological Science, 39*, 213–234.

Gronwall, D., & Wrightson, P. (1980). Duration of post-traumatic amnesia after mild head injury. *Journal of Clinical Neuropsychology, 2*, 51–60.

Han, J.S., Kaufman, B., Alfidi, R.J., Yeung, H.N., Benson, J.E., Haaga, J.R., El-Yousef, S.J., Clampitt, M.E., Bonstelle, C.T., & Huss, R. (1984). Head trauma evaluated by magnetic resonance and computed tomography: A comparison. *Radiology, 150*, 71–77.

Heiden, J., Small, R., Caton, W., Weiss, M., & Kurtze, T. (1983). Severe head injury. *Journal of the American Physical Therapy Association, 63*, 4–9.

Hershey, B.L., & Zimmerman, R.A. (1986). Magnetic resonance imaging of the child's brain. *Child's Nervous System, 2*, 115–120.

Hounsfield, G.N. (1973). Computerized transverse axial scanning (tomography). I. Description of system. *British Journal of Radiology, 46*, 1016–1022.

Ito, U., Tomita, H., Yamazaki, S., Takada, Y., & Inaba, Y. (1986). Brain swelling and brain edema in acute head injury. *Acta Neurochiro, 79*, 120–124.

Jenkins, A., Teasdale, G., Hadley, M.D. Macpherson, P., & Rowan, J.D. (1986). Brain lesions detected by magnetic resonance imaging in mild and severe head injuries. *Lancet, 2*, 445–446.

Jennett, B. (1986). Head trauma. In A.K. Asbury, G.M. McKhann, & W.I. McDonald (Eds.), *Disease of the nervous system* (pp. 1282–1291). Philadelphia: W.B. Saunders.

Jennett, B., Teasdale, G., Braakman, R., Minderhoud, J., Heiden, J., & Kurtze, T. (1979). Prognosis of patients with severe head injury. *Neurosurgery, 5*, 283–289.

Kaufman, H.H., Makela, M.E., Lee, K.F., Haid, R.W., Jr., & Gildenberg, P.L. (1986). Gunshot wounds to the head: A perspective. *Neurosurgery, 18*, 689–695.

Kiloh, L.G., McComas, A.J., & Osselton, J.W. (1979). *Clinical electroencephalography.* London: Butterworths.

Kwentus, J.A., Hart, R.P., Peck, E.T., & Kornstein, S. (1985). Psychiatric complications of closed head trauma. *Psychosomatics, 26*, 8–15.

Levin, H.S., Benton, A.L., & Grossman, R.G. (1982). *Neurobehavioral consequences of closed head injury.* New York: Oxford University Press.

Levin, H.S., Kalisky, Z., Handel, S.F., Goldman, A.M., Eisenberg, H.M., Morrison, D., & VonLaufen, A. (1985). Magnetic resonance imaging in relation to the sequelae and rehabilitation of diffuse closed head injury: Preliminary findings. *Seminars in Neurology, 5*, 221–232.

Levin, H.S., Mattis, S., Ruff, R.M., Eisenberg, H.M., Marshall, L.F., Tabaddor, K., High, W.M., & Frankowski, R.F. (1987). Neurobehavioral outcome following minor head injury: A three-center study. *Journal of Neurosurgery, 66*, 234–243.

Levin, H.S., Meyers, C.A., Grossman, R.G., & Sarwar, M. (1981). Ventricular enlargement after closed head injury. *Archives of Neurology, 38*, 623–629.

Lipper, M.H., Kishore, P.R., Enas, G.G., Domingues-da-Silva, A.A., Choi, S.C., & Becker, D.P. (1985). Computed tomography in the prediction of outcome in head injury. *American Journal of Radiology, 144*, 483–486.

Lobato, R.D., Sarabia, R., Rivas, J.J., Cordobes, F., Castro, S., Munoz, M.J., Cabrera, A., Barcena, A., & Lamas, E. (1986). Normal computerized tomography scans in severe head injury. Prognostic and clinical management implications. *Journal of Neurosurgery, 65,* 784–789.

Massman, P.J., Bigler, E.D., Cullum, C.M., & Naugle, R.I. (1986). The relationship between cortical atrophy and ventricular volume in Alzheimer's disease and closed head injury. *International Journal of Neuroscience, 30,* 87–99.

Prigatano, G.P., & Pepping, M. (1987). Neuropsychological status before and after mild head injury: A case report. *Barrow Neurological Institute Quarterly, 3,* 18–21.

Raichle, M.E. (1986). Neuroimaging. *Trends in Neurosciences, 9,* 525–529.

Rivara, F.P., & Mueller, B.A. (1986). The epidemiology and prevention of pediatric head injury. *Journal of Head Trauma Rehabilitation, 1,* 7–15.

Russell, W.R. (1971). *The traumatic amnesias.* New York: Oxford University Press.

Salazar, A.M., Grafman, J., Schlesselman, S., Vance, S.C., Mohr, J.P., Carpenter, M., Pevsner, P., Ludlow, C., & Weingartner, H. (1986). Penetrating war injuries of the basal forebrain: Neurology and cognition. *Neurology, 36,* 459–465.

Salazar, A.M., Grafman, J.H., Vance, S.C., Weingartner, H., Dillon, J.D., & Ludlow, C. (1986). Consciousness and amnesia after penetrating head injury: Neurology and anatomy. *Neurology, 36,* 178–187.

Shigemori, M., Kojyo, N., Yuse, T., Tokutomi, T., Nakashima, H., & Kuramoto, S. (1986). Massive traumatic haematoma of the corpus callosum. *Acta Neurochirurgica, 81,* 36–39.

Snow, R.B., Zimmerman, R.D., Gandy, S.E., & Deck, M.D. (1986). Comparison of magnetic resonance imaging and computed tomography in the evaluation of head injury. *Neurosurgery, 18,* 45–52.

Soloniuk, D., Pitts, L.H., Lovely, M., & Bartkowski, H. (1986). Traumatic intracerebral hematomas: Timing of appearance and indications for operative removal. *Journal of Trauma, 26,* 787–794.

Squire, L.R. (1987). *Memory and brain.* New York: Oxford University Press.

Teasdale, G., & Jennett, B. (1974). Assessment of coma and impaired consciousness: A practical scale. *Lancet, 2,* 81–84.

Uzzell, B.P., Obrist, W.D., Dolinskas, C.A., & Langfitt, T.W. (1986). Relationship of acute CBF and ICP findings to neuropsychological outcome in severe head injury. *Journal of Neurosurgery, 65,* 630–635.

Wechsler, D. (1945). *Wechsler memory scale.* New York: Psychological Corp.

Wechsler, D. (1974). *Wechsler intelligence scale for children–Revised.* New York: Psychological Corp.

Wechsler, D. (1981). *Wechsler adult intelligence scale–Revised.* New York: Psychological Corp.

Wilmot, C.B., Cope, D.N., Hall, K.M., & Acker, M. (1985). Occult head injury: Its incidence in spinal cord injury. *Archives of Physical Medicine and Rehabilitation, 66,* 227–231.

Yoshino, E., Yamaki, T., Higuchi, T., Horikawa, Y., & Hirakawa, K. (1985). Acute brain edema in fatal head injury: Analysis by dynamic CT scanning. *Journal of Neurosurgery, 63,* 830–839.

Zimmerman, R.A., Bilaniuk, L.T., Hackney, D.B., Goldberg, H.I., & Grossman, R.I. (1986). Head injury: Early results of comparing CT and high-field MR. *American Journal of Radiology, 147,* 1215–1222.

3

Epidemiology of Traumatic Brain Injury: Incidence, Clinical Characteristics, and Risk Factors

FELICIA C. GOLDSTEIN

HARVEY S. LEVIN

Investigation of the incidence and causes of pediatric closed head injury (CHI) has several important applications. First, characterization of environmental risk factors specific to children at various ages can have an impact in terms of strategies for prevention and public policy. For example, the knowledge that the death rate of children in motor vehicle accidents (MVA) is higher for those not wearing restraint devices (Scherz, 1981; Williams, 1981) has led to the enactment of child passenger laws that have played a major role in reducing the fatality of children aged 4 years and younger (Decker, Hutcheson, & Schaffner, 1984). Second, epidemiology helps to identify the clinical characteristics most likely to be encountered in subsets of the general population (Annegers, 1983), the medical and surgical sequelae produced from particular types of accidents such as falls (Smith, Burrington, & Woolf, 1975),

Preparation of this paper was supported by NIH grant NS 21889 (Javits Neuroscience Investigator Award, Neurobehavioral Outcome of Head Injury in Children) and a grant from the Dallas Rehabilitation Foundation. We thank Liz Zindler for assistance in manuscript preparation.

and the resultant neurosurgical interventions that may be necessary (i.e., which patients should be detained for observation) (Jennett & Teasdale, 1981). Finally, a knowledge of predisposing features sensitizes neuropsychologists to premorbid factors that should be considered when interpreting data of head injured children. To understand the role of brain trauma on emotional and intellectual outcome, it is necessary to appreciate the causes and potential psychological difficulties that may have preceded the injury (Rutter, 1981).

The purpose of this chapter is to review the epidemiological literature on pediatric closed head injury. Following a summary of incidence rates and etiologic/pathophysiologic correlates, we describe risk factors in children and their families. We will then consider issues that should be considered in future research. An argument will be made for the necessity of considering premorbid characteristics in relationship to neurobehavioral sequelae to assess the impact of CHI on the child's level of functioning.

INCIDENCE OF PEDIATRIC CHI

Estimates of CHI involving incidence (the number of new cases during a specified time period relative to the general population at risk) have been complicated by several methodological and conceptual problems. One difficulty concerns the lack of consistent definitions across studies of what constitutes a head injury (Kraus, 1987). As a result, patients who sustain facial lacerations, for example, without evidence of underlying brain pathology may be classified as head injured (Annegers, 1983; Frankowski, Annegers, & Whitman, 1985). In addition, there has been a tendency to list the etiology (e.g., "MVA") rather than the anatomic system (e.g., "ruptured spleen") as the cause of death (Annegers, 1983; Cooper, 1982). This classification system can produce an overestimation of mortality thought to be caused by head trauma per se and obscure the reasons for poor outcome. Finally, there is a major difficulty in locating cases of head trauma (e.g., children treated in emergency rooms who are not admitted to the hospital) such that estimates may reflect more the method used than the actual incidence. Figure 3.1 depicts the various potential outcomes from head injury and measures of data collection available to epidemiologists. Studies examining hospital admission records will tend to exclude cases that were not followed (e.g., mild or fatal injuries), whereas those utilizing telephone survey methods to identify patients not seeking medical attention will rely on the memory of respondents and miss clinical characteristics (Frankowski et al., 1985; Klauber, Barrett-Connor, Hofstetter, & Micik, 1986). Consequently, epidemiologic data can provide only a rough estimate of the actual occurrence of trauma within a given community.

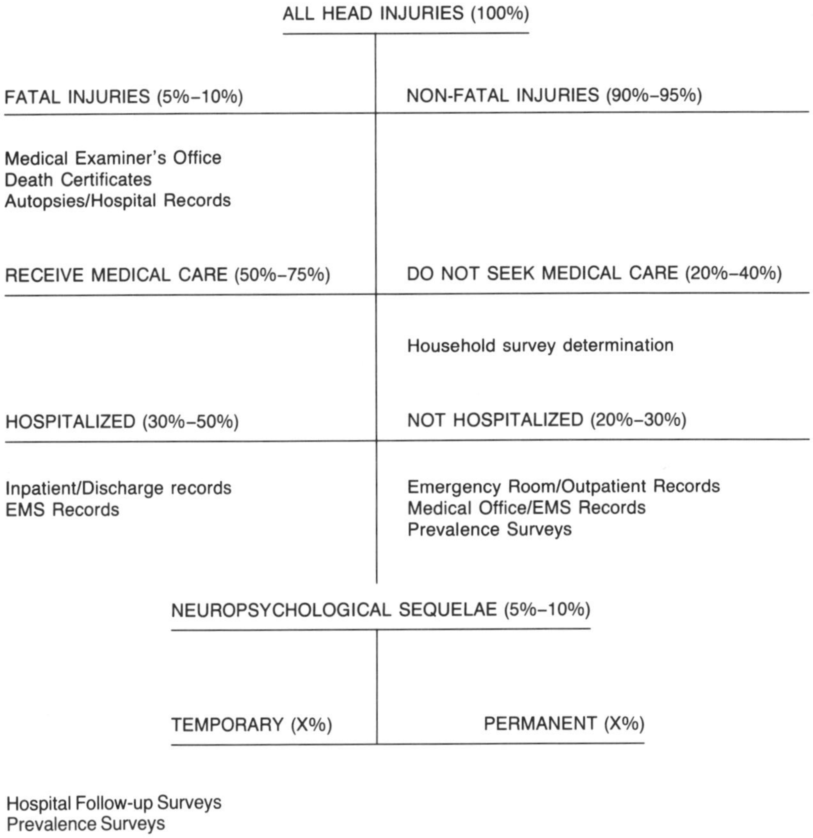

ALL HEAD INJURIES (100%)

FATAL INJURIES (5%–10%)

Medical Examiner's Office
Death Certificates
Autopsies/Hospital Records

NON-FATAL INJURIES (90%–95%)

RECEIVE MEDICAL CARE (50%–75%)

DO NOT SEEK MEDICAL CARE (20%–40%)

Household survey determination

HOSPITALIZED (30%–50%)

Inpatient/Discharge records
EMS Records

NOT HOSPITALIZED (20%–30%)

Emergency Room/Outpatient Records
Medical Office/EMS Records
Prevalence Surveys

NEUROPSYCHOLOGICAL SEQUELAE (5%–10%)

TEMPORARY (X%)

PERMANENT (X%)

Hospital Follow-up Surveys
Prevalence Surveys

Figure 3.1. Sources of case ascertainment, medical care, and approximate distribution of outcome of head injuries in a typical community. (Percentages for distribution of outcome are subjective estimates from the current literature. All percentages refer to the 100% base of all head injuries.) *Note.* From "Epidemiological and Descriptive Studies Part 1: The Descriptive Epidemiology of Head Trauma in the United States" by R.F. Frankowski, J.F. Annegers, & S. Whitman, 1985. In D.P. Becker & J.T. Povlishock (Eds), *Central Nervous System Trauma Status Report,* Bethesda, MD: National Institute of Neurological and Communicative Disorders and Stroke. Reprinted by permission.

Despite these methodological issues, there is little argument that head trauma constitutes a considerable source of mortality and morbidity in children and adolescents (Fletcher, Ewing-Cobbs, McLaughlin, & Levin, 1985; Frankowski, 1985; Levin, Benton, & Grossman, 1982). Although figures vary, it has been noted that more than 1 million children in the United States sustain closed head injuries each year and that one-sixth of these cases are admitted to hospitals (Eiben et al., 1984). Regardless of the methods used in various studies to assess mortality and morbidity, there is consistency in the demonstration that head injuries are most frequent in younger age groups (i.e., birth to 24 years) (Krause, 1987). Figures 3.2 and 3.3 show the estimated incidence of head trauma from two independent studies (Annegers, Grabow, Kurland, & Laws, 1980; Kraus et al., 1984). Annegers and colleagues (1980) conducted the first epidemiological effort that utilized clinical definitions (e.g., concussion with loss of consciousness) rather than diagnostic criteria (e.g., laceration of the scalp) to examine incidence rates in Olmsted County, Minnesota. While the researchers most likely excluded many mild injuries because they did not incorporate cases of confusion followed by normal consciousness without amnesia, the overall incidence per 100,000 was 270 in males and 116 in females. As shown in Figure 3.2, the researchers observed a general trend for the incidence of head trauma to rise sharply in the age range of 15 to 24 (most noticeable for males) followed by a second rise at the

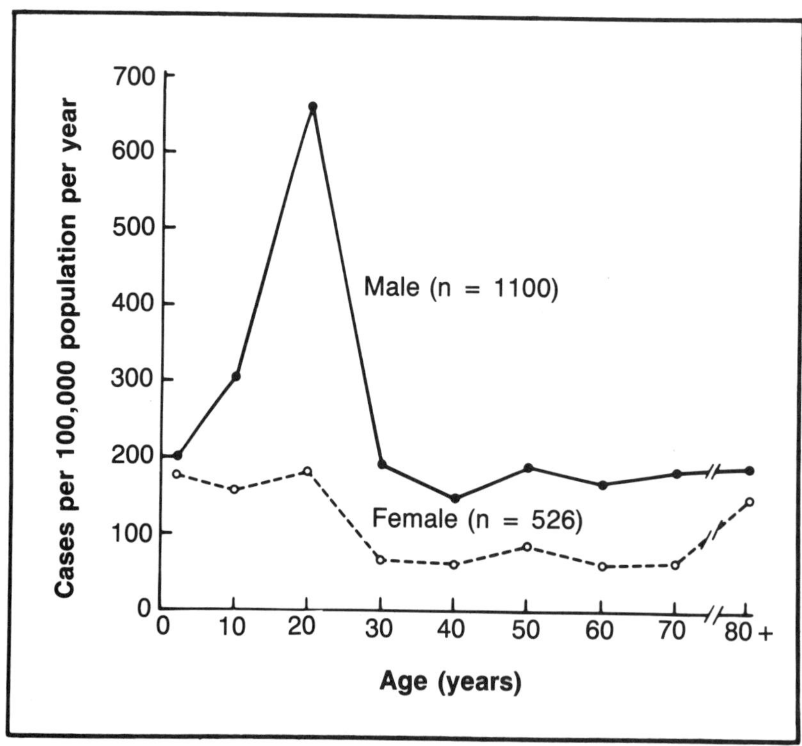

Figure 3.2. Incidence rates of head trauma in Olmsted County, Minnesota, 1964–1974. *Note.* From "The Incidence, Causes, and Secular Trends of Head Trauma in Olmsted County, Minnesota, 1935–1974" by J.F. Annegers, J.D. Grabow, L.T. Kurland, & E.R. Laws, 1980, *Neurology, 30,* pp. 912–919. Reprinted by permission.

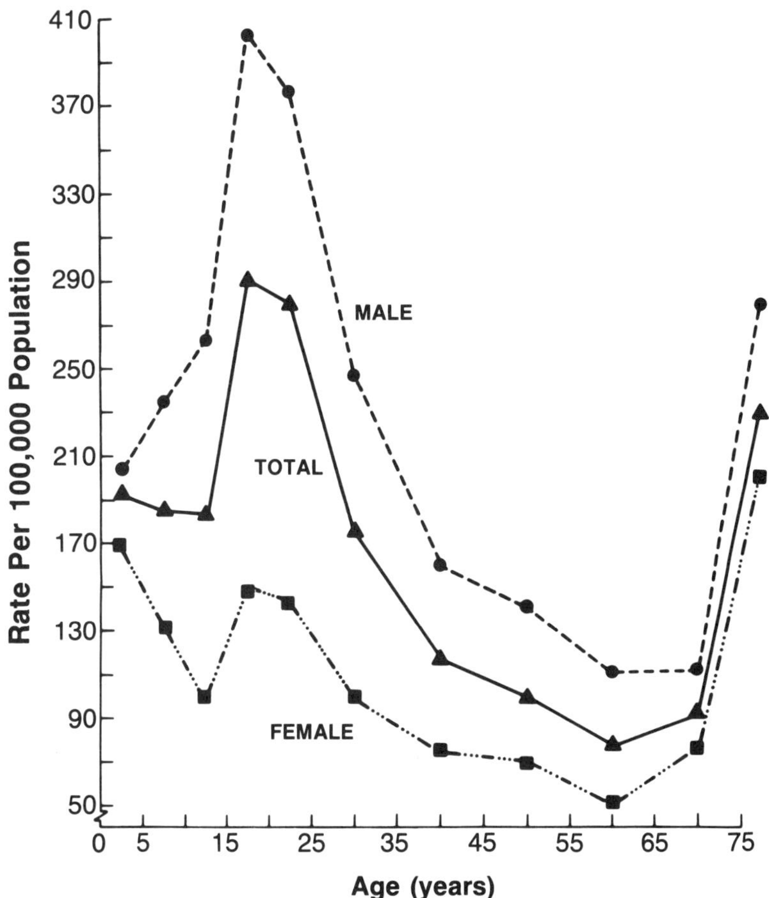

Figure 3.3. Age- and sex-specific incidence rates of brain injury per 100,000 population, San Diego County, California, 1981. *Note.* From "The Incidence of Acute Brain Injury and Serious Impairment in a Defined Population" by J.F. Kraus, M.A. Black, N. Hessol, P. Ley, W. Rokaw, C. Sullivan, S. Bowers, S. Knowlton, & L. Marshall, 1984, *American Journal of Epidemiology, 119,* pp. 186–201. Reprinted by permission.

age of 70 and beyond. This pattern was also observed by Kraus et al. (1984; see Figure 3.3), who studied records of patients who died or were admitted to the hospital in San Diego County, California, during 1981. As depicted, the incidence rates were highest between the ages of 15 and 24 and again after age 70. An estimate from combined studies (per 100,000) has cited figures of 150 for ages 0 to 4, an increase to 550 for ages 15 to 19, a drop to 160 at age 50, and then in increase by age 65 to 200 (Frankowski et al., 1985).

Annegers (1983) recently used the same clinical criteria as in the Olmsted County study to focus on pediatric head injury (0 to 14 years). The average annual incidence rates for males and females under 15 years of age was estimated to be 220/100,000. This figure is comparable to the 230/100,000 reported by Kalsbeek, McLaurin, Harris, and Miller (1980), which was based on hospital admission data, and the 185/100,000 cited by Kraus, Fife, Cox, Ramstein, and Conroy (1986), which was based on age-specific incidence rates for San Diego County in 1981. Annegers noted that if Olmsted County estimates were applied to the population of the United States, the annual number of cases would be approximately 110,000.

Annegers (1983) also estimated a head injury mortality rate of 10/100,000 children, which far exceeds the second major cause of death in pediatric patients, leukemia. In general, studies have demonstrated a lower mortality in children and adolescents as compared to adults. Figure 3.4 shows an increase in mortality from severe head injury with increasing age (Jennett & Teasdale, 1981). It is possible that associated medical conditions in the elderly, as well as the fact that children are more likely to be admitted to the hospital, could serve to lower mortality (Cooper, 1982).

Two general trends emerge in the pediatric epidemiological literature. First, as is apparent from Figures 3.2 and 3.3, males are more likely than females to sustain a head injury, with an average reported ratio of 2:1 (Klauber, Barrett-Connor, Marshall, & Bowers, 1981; Kraus, 1980; Kraus et al., 1984). Additionally, there is an age-specific difference in the peak incidence of head trauma between male and female children. Males show an increased incidence from ages 5 to 25, while females demonstrate a decline throughout the first 15 years. As Frankowski et al. (1985) noted, these patterns suggest that young males and females differ in both the degrees of risk as well as in the kinds of risk for head injury. Males also tend to have more severe head trauma (Annegers, 1983; Klauber et al., 1981), with a mortality ratio for male over female children estimated to be as high as 4:1 (Moyes, 1980).

THE RELATIONSHIPS AMONG ETIOLOGY, AGE, AND POTENTIAL PATHOPHYSIOLOGICAL MECHANISMS

Most studies assessing pediatric outcome have failed to take into account the various mechanisms of injury operating at different ages and their potential relationship to pathophysiology. The literature clearly suggests that the etiology of head injuries shifts as a function of age. Table 3.1 lists the percentages of children in Houston and Galveston, Texas, sustaining head trauma of different causes. In line with general research findings, falls constitute a major

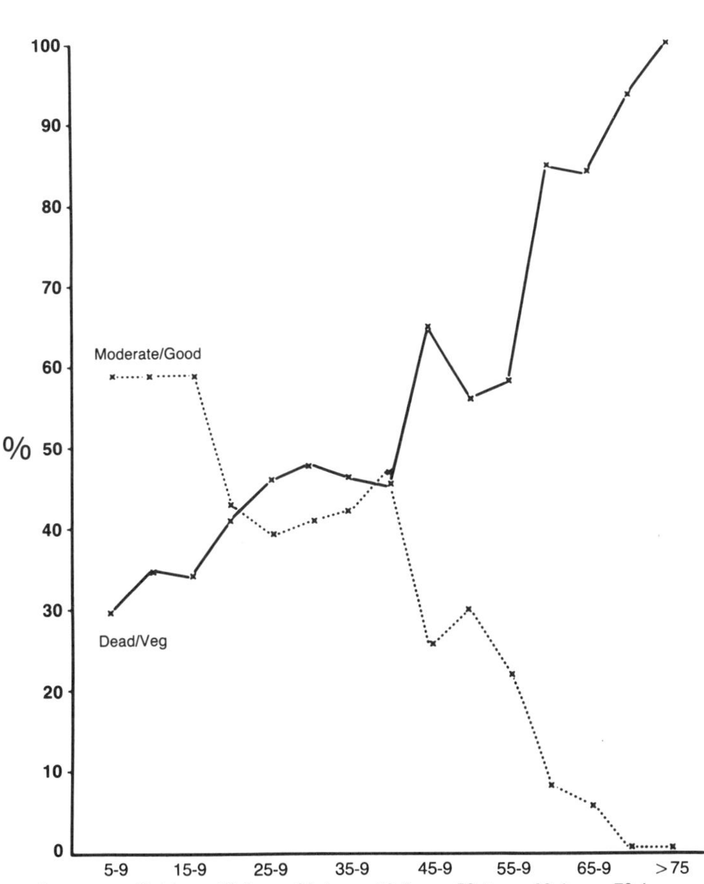

Figure 3.4. Outcome of severe head injury plotted against age at the time of injury. Based on cases from the International Coma Data Bank. The percentage of patients who died or remained persistently vegetative after a severe head injury increased as a function of age at injury. *Note.* From *Management of Head Injuries* by B. Jennett & G. Teasdale, 1981, Philadelphia: F.A. Davis. Reprinted by permission.

source of CHI in children under 5 years (Annegers, 1983; Kraus et al., 1984), with a peak incidence rate typically reported at age 2 (Smith et al., 1975). Rivara (1984) noted that cases of non-motor vehicle accidents were highest in infants and speculated that they may be at an increased risk for head versus trunk/extremity injuries due to relatively large head size and a high center

TABLE 3.1
Mechanisms of Injury for 1,123 Central Nervous System (CSN) Injuries Admitted to Comprehensive CNS Trauma Centers in Houston or Galveston, 1980–1982 (in percentages)

	Age (year)				
Mechanism	**Under 1 (*N* = 68)**	**1–4 (*N* = 221)**	**5–9 (*N* = 183)**	**10–14 (*N* = 134)**	**15–19 (*N* = 517)**
MVA*	26.0	17.2	25.7	37.3	51.8
Motorcycle	—	0.5	1.6	0.7	8.7
Pedestrian	1.5	20.4	39.3	15.7	6.0
Bicycle	—	0.9	9.3	9.0	1.9
Fall	61.8	50.7	18.6	20.1	9.7
Gunshot Wound	1.5	2.3	—	4.5	7.9
Assault	5.9	2.7	0.5	3.0	8.5
Other	3.3	5.3	5.0	9.7	5.5
Total	100.0	100.0	100.0	100.0	100.0

*MVA = Motor vehicle accident.

Note: From "Head Injury Mortality in Urban Populations and Its Relation to the Injured Child" by R.F. Frankowski. 1985. In B.F. Brooks (Ed.), *The Injured Child,* Austin: University of Texas Press. Reprinted by permission.

of gravity. With age, the role of recreational and sports-related injuries rises, and both pedestrian–motor vehicles and bicycle accidents predominate in the 5- to 14-year-old range (Klauber et al., 1981). Finally, motor vehicle injuries are more prevalent in the 15-year-old and older age group. Males are at greater risk than females for all types of etiologies (Annegers et al., 1980).

The finding of differences in mechanisms according to age undoubtedly plays a role in both the pathophysiology and severity of CHI. For example, skull fractures are extremely common in infants in contrast to older children and adults, with an average incidence across studies estimated to be approximately 40% (Choux, 1986). Choux has postulated that the flexibility of bones in the infant's skull and open sutures lead to a predisposition toward fractures.

Patients who sustain head trauma as a result of falls (with or without skull fracture) run the risk of developing delayed intracranial hematomas (DiRocco & Velardi, 1986). On the other hand, motor vehicle accidents are more likely to be the cause of concussion and are frequently encountered in school-age children and adolescents (Rivara, 1984). Intracranial mass lesions (i.e., hematomas, contusions) are common in older children and adolescents. An implication of these trends is that the nature of such injuries can produce different complications even when neurologic scores on indices such as the Glasgow Coma Scale (GCS) (Teasdale & Jennett, 1974) are equated (Levin et al., 1982). Kalsbeek and colleagues (1980) have noted that coma after a head injury produced by a fall is likely to result in brain compression due to intracerebral hematoma. On the other hand, coma caused by a motor vehicle accident is more often due to severe primary brain damage from acceleration/deceleration forces.

While it was previously noted that the mortality rate of young children following head trauma is lower than that of adults, the reasons for this finding are unclear (see Levin et al., 1982, for a review). It has been postulated that the above mentioned flexibility of children's skull bones leads to greater absorption of traumatic effects and lessens impact to the brain (Craft, 1972; Gurdjian & Webster, 1958). In addition, young adults are more likely to sustain severe brain damage as a result of high speed motor accidents, whereas pedestrian-car accidents at low speeds are prevalent in children. This may predispose adults toward more severe brain damage due to acceleration and rotation forces. Teasdale, Skene, Parker, and Jennett (1979) reported that the proportion of patients with severe CHI who developed intracranial hematomas rose with age. However, this finding did not explain the higher mortality in their older patients.

There is some evidence that the neurologic picture in children differs from that found in adults in terms of both initial severity and the possibility for delayed complications (Goethe & Levin, 1986; Levin, Ewing-Cobbs, & Benton, 1984). Gurdjian and Webster (1958) originally proposed that head injuries in the child would be more likely to cause shearing effects potentiating brain stem injury due to relatively shallow brain convolutions, thereby producing greater deformation upon impact. Bruce, Schut, Bruno, Wood, and Sutton (1978) found that 30% of their pediatric series sustaining severe head injuries had impaired oculovestibular function and bilaterally fixed pupils (measures of brain stem dysfunction). Moreover, fewer children sustained mass lesions (e.g., intracerebral hematomas) in contrast to typical findings in adults with comparable severity scores on the Glasgow Coma Scale (Jennett et al., 1977). The investigators found that one-third of their sample sustained diffuse cerebral swelling characterized by obliteration of the ventricles and cisterns followed by enlargement of ventricles to normal or larger size. The overall mortality rate was low (6%) despite extremely poor initial neurologic indices. Bruce and colleagues (1981) found increased cerebral blood flow in six children which was followed by a decrease in flow accompanying resolution of swelling. They concluded that CHI in children primarily caused diffuse cerebral swelling due to increased cerebral blood volume as the result of cerebrovascular congestion.

Recent work, however, suggests that intracranial hematomas and contusions are more common in children than previously thought. Berger, Pitts, Lovely, Edwards, and Bartkowski (1985) noted a high proportion of hematomas and mass lesions as well as a higher mortality rate (33%) in their pediatric sample of severe closed head injuries. Differences in these studies may reflect specific sampling biases (e.g., the lack of a centralized trauma care unit in the Berger et al. study).

Snoek, Minderhoud, and Wilmink (1984) reported delayed complications in 42 mild head injured children. Thirteen children developed posttraumatic seizures, with the majority of cases occurring within 1 hour after injury. The remaining children were seizure free but showed short-lived acute onset of symptoms such as loss of consciousness, focal neurologic signs, or extreme restlessness. Three of the children in their series died from complications due to uncontrollable unilateral or diffuse brain swelling. Other investigators (Oka, Kako, Matsushima, & Ando, 1977; Takahashi & Nakazawa, 1980) have also reported delayed impairment of consciousness and neurologic deficits associated with convulsions after mild head injury. The explanation for delayed complications in children will require detailed studies examining electroencephalographic (EEG) and computerized tomography (CT) scans, as well as application of magnetic resonance imaging (MRI) technology to detect lesions that may have been missed in earlier studies.

RISK FACTORS

Researchers have attempted to identify the antecedent risk factors associated with pediatric CHI. While the conclusions that can be reached are equivocal, those studies that do report positive findings indicate the importance of considering premorbid characteristics of both the child (e.g., personality/cognitive functioning) and family (e.g., socioeconomic status [SES], marital stability). As we will argue in the final section, interpretation of behavioral and cognitive outcome must be evaluated in conjunction with the child's developmental history and environmental circumstances.

Investigations of the personality characteristics of head injured children suggest that they may not represent a random sample of the general population (Rutter, Chadwick, Shaffer, & Brown, 1980). Craft, Shaw, and Cartlidge (1972) found a higher incidence of teacher-reported pre-existing behavioral problems (e.g., hyperactivity, antisocial actions) in head injured children versus classmates serving as controls. Whereas Klonoff (1971) did not observe evidence for greater premorbid behavioral disturbance in children sustaining CHI over controls, later research (Klonoff & Paris, 1974) reported a sex-related finding of positive premorbid factors (e.g., developmental problems, learning difficulties) in younger boys versus girls. The researchers suggested an increased vulnerability to head injury in boys that may be related not only to differences in stereotyped patterns (e.g., roughhouse play) but also to premorbid status.

More recent studies by Rutter and colleagues (Brown, Chadwick, Shaffer, Rutter, & Traub, 1981; Rutter, 1981) have demonstrated the necessity of screening for pre-existing psychosocial difficulties. The researchers examined patients with mild posttraumatic amnesia ([PTA] of at least 1 hour but less than 7 days) or severe (PTA of 7 days or more) CHI and included an orthopedic control group matched for age, sex, and social characteristics. Information was gathered concerning the child's behavior and adjustment prior to the injury (baseline screening) and then at various intervals after injury (4 months; 1 year; 2 years; 3 years). The mildly injured group showed a higher rate of behavioral disturbance at baseline in contrast to the other groups, suggesting that they were more disturbed prior to their injuries. Moreover, the mildly injured group, unlike those with severe injuries, failed to show a change in their behavior (e.g., an increase in behavioral disturbance over serial assessments). It has been hypothesized that features including impulsivity and overactivity may lead to risk-taking behaviors which, in turn, cause head injury. In addition, postinjury sequelae may reflect premorbid characteristics rather than being the direct result of brain trauma (Rutter, 1981).

Using similar methodology, Rutter and his research group also found that children who sustained mild injuries exhibited evidence of poorer premorbid academic achievement. Chadwick, Rutter, Brown, Shaffer, and Traub (1981) reported that their mild head injury group had a high rate of "reading backwardness" (lower scores on the Neale Analysis of Reading Ability) in contrast to controls and that they did not improve their scores over time. Mahoney et al. (1983) studied educational outcome in children with severe head injuries (coma duration of greater than 24 hours). While 18 out of 34 children returned to school with mild behavioral or cognitive sequelae, 11 (61%) had evidence of premorbid difficulties including language and learning problems, thus suggesting that they were functioning at their premorbid levels. These studies are based on small, selected samples of patients and are not meant to provide generalizations to the pediatric head injury population. Nonetheless, they do indicate the necessity of prescreening criteria in order to evaluate the effects of CHI on psychosocial and cognitive outcome.

It has been suggested that head injured children live in more congested areas, are from low SES backgrounds, and that their parents tend to be unemployed or to have emotional difficulties (Klonoff, 1971). However, this finding has not been consistently reported in the literature (Jamison & Kaye, 1974; Klauber et al., 1986). For example, Klauber and colleagues (1986) conducted a telephone survey of nonfatal childhood injuries (poisoning, burns, and head injuries) in San Diego County, California. Education and income of parents were unrelated to the incidence of head injury. Epidemiologic studies need to more closely examine the relationship of environmental features to incidence rates.

Finally, there has been conflicting evidence in the literature concerning whether children who sustain head injuries are at greater risk for a second injury. Early studies by Partington (1960) and Jamison and Kaye (1974) did not find a greater frequency of previous trauma in their head injured sample. More recent epidemiologic work based on population statistics, though, suggests the opposite trend. Annegers et al. (1980) found that the relative risk for a second head injury was age related. Observed over expected incidence rates doubled after a head injury sustained in children under 14 years of age, tripled through ages 15–24, and was five times the expected rate after age 25. Annegers (1983) reported that boys with head trauma have a 2:1 risk of subsequent injury. It may be that individuals develop behavioral patterns that predispose them to additional injuries (Annegers et al., 1980). Moreover, neuropsychological sequelae including slowed reaction time may also be contributory (Goethe & Levin, 1986).

SUGGESTIONS FOR FUTURE RESEARCH

A review of the epidemiology of pediatric closed head injury suggests several directions for future research. It has been noted that head injuries sustained by children of various ages can be distinguished both in the etiology (e.g., falls versus motor vehicle accidents) as well as in the pathophysiology (e.g., fractures versus intracranial lesions). Studies have typically grouped children according to a severity index such as the GCS score without considering the heterogeneity of the sample. As we discussed earlier, differences in the etiology of injuries can lead to diverse complications even when a global index score is equated (Levin et al., 1982). Moreover, the argument that younger children fare better than older children has not been compelling due to a failure to analyze mechanisms of injury and outcome. Future studies need to consider the relationships among etiology, pathophysiology, and sequelae in order to examine the effects of age on recovery and to isolate distinct patterns associated with a favorable outcome.

There is a strong trend in the epidemiological literature for males to be more susceptible to head injuries than females across all age groups. The reasons for this pattern are not well understood. It may be that greater activity levels, stereotyped differences in play, and premorbid characteristics (e.g., learning difficulties) contribute to this pattern. Research might carefully examine sex-related features that contribute to higher incidence rates in order to determine whether certain risk factors exist, and if so, whether these are avoidable.

Furthermore, there is a suggestion that head injured children may differ from the general pediatric population in terms of personality/cognitive characteristics. Rutter (1981) has discussed the importance of demonstrating a "dose-response" relationship in neuropsychological research. In order to conclude that head injury is the cause of observed impairments, one must establish a relationship between severity of injury and the presence/degree of deficit. In addition, a change in recovery should be seen over time. Failure to find a pattern may indicate that the deficit existed preinjury. Longitudinal research is important for assessing outcome. Moreover, Rutter et al. (1980) have argued that orthopedic matched controls are useful for taking into account the predisposing risk factors that may produce an accident as well as for helping in the assessment of psychosocial stresses following an injury.

Evaluation of intellectual and psychosocial functioning needs to be undertaken within the context of the child's premorbid level. With respect to intellectual and academic outcome, we have suggested previously (Goldstein & Levin, 1985) that statements that a child is performing within normal limits do not reflect the degree of loss if premorbid functioning was in the superior range. On the other hand, the finding of a borderline IQ in a child who was also borderline before injury may indicate that the injury is not as likely to interfere with ability to perform in school. Academic records, particularly achievement test scores, may be useful for assessing premorbid functioning. Using such an approach, Levin and Eisenberg (1979) found that although intellectual ability was within normal limits for many of the children in their head injured sample, comparison of Performance IQ with premorbid achievement records showed that only partial recovery was actually obtained. As shown in Figure 3.5, 12 patients had premorbid percentiles above 50, whereas Performance IQ percentiles were generally lower. Parental questionnaires and interviews as well as teacher checklists are also important for evaluating premorbid functioning in relation to outcome.

Finally, while epidemiological research indicates that mortality is lower in children versus adults, the issue of age and quality of outcome has not been discussed in this review. Cognitive and personality changes often persist despite resolution of focal neurologic deficits. Studies examining long-term neuropsychological sequelae will help to elucidate our understanding of pediatric closed head injury.

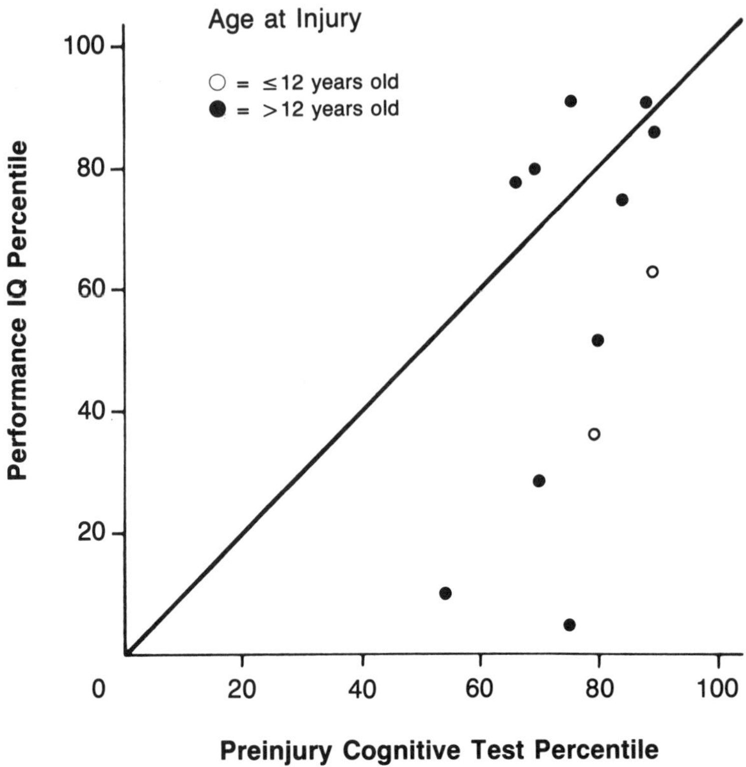

Figure 3.5. Percentile corresponding to Performance Scale IQ at the time of follow-up plotted against percentile of premorbid cognitive test given in school. *Note.* From "Neuropsychological Impairment after Closed Head Injury in Children and Adolescents" by H.S. Levin & M. Eisenberg, 1979, *Journal of Pediatric Psychology, 4,* pp. 389–402. Reprinted by permission.

REFERENCES

Annegers, J.F. (1983). The epidemiology of head trauma in children. In K. Shapiro (Ed.), *Pediatric head trauma* (pp. 1–10). Mount Kisco, NY: Futura.

Annegers, J.F., Grabow, J.D., Kurland, L.T., & Laws, E.R. (1980). The incidence, causes, and secular trends of head trauma in Olmsted County, Minnesota, 1935–1974. *Neurology, 30,* 912–919.

Berger, M.S., Pitts, L.H., Lovely, M., Edwards, M.S., & Bartkowski, H.M. (1985). Outcome from severe head injury in children and adolescents. *Journal of Neurosurgery, 62,* 194–199.

Brown, G., Chadwick, O., Shaffer, D., Rutter, M., & Traub, M. (1981). A prospective study of children with head injuries: III. Psychiatric sequelae. *Psychological Medicine, 11,* 63–78.

Bruce, D.A., Alavi, A., Bilaniuk, L., Dolinskas, C., Orbrist, W., & Uzzell, B. (1981). Diffuse cerebral swelling following head injuries in children: The syndrome of "malignant brain edema." *Journal of Neurosurgery, 54,* 170–178.

Bruce, D.A., Schut, L., Bruno, L.A., Wood, J.H., & Sutton, L.N. (1978). Outcome following severe head injury in children. *Journal of Neurosurgery, 48,* 679–688.

Chadwick, O., Rutter, M., Brown, G., Shaffer, D., & Traub, M. (1981). A prospective study of children with head injuries: II. Cognitive sequelae. *Psychological Medicine, 11,* 49–61.

Choux, M. (1986). Incidence, diagnosis, and management of skull fractures. In A.J. Raimondi, M. Choux, & C. DiRocco (Eds.), *Head injuries in the newborn and infant* (pp. 163–182). New York: Springer-Verlag.

Cooper, P.R. (1982). Epidemiology of head injury. In P.R. Cooper (Ed.), *Head injury* (pp. 1–14). Baltimore: Williams & Wilkins.

Craft, A.W. (1972). Head injury in children. In P.J. Vinken & G.W. Bruyn (Eds.), *Handbook of clinical neurology* (Vol. 23, pp. 445–458) New York: Elsevier.

Craft, A.W., Shaw, D.A., & Cartlidge, N.E. (1972). Head injuries in children. *British Medical Journal, 4,* 200–203.

Decker, M.D., Hutcheson, R.H., & Schaffner, W. (1984). The use and efficacy of child restraint devices. *The Journal of the American Medical Association, 252,* 2571–2575.

DiRocco, C., & Velardi, F. (1986). Epiemiology and etiology of craniocerebral trauma in the first two years of life. In A.J. Raimondi, M. Choux, & C. DiRocco (Eds.), *Head injuries in the newborn and infant* (pp. 125–139). New York: Springer-Verlag.

Eiben, C.F., Anderson, T.P., Lockman, L., Matthews, D.J., Dryja, R., Martin, J., Burrill, C., Gottesman, N., O'Brian, P., & Witte, L. (1984). Functional outcome of closed head injury in children and young adults. *Archives of Physical Medicine Rehabilitation, 65,* 168–170.

Fletcher, J.M., Ewing-Cobbs, L., McLaughlin, E.J., & Levin, H.S. (1985). Cognitive and psychosocial sequelae of head injury in children: Implications for assessment and management. In B.F. Brooks (Ed.), *The injured child* (pp. 30–39). Austin: University of Texas Press.

Frankowski, R.F. (1985). Head injury mortality in urban populations and its relation to the injured child. In B.F. Brooks (Ed.), *The injured child* (pp. 20–29). Austin: University of Texas Press.

Frankowski, R.F., Annegers, J.F., & Whitman, S. (1985). Epidemiological and descriptive studies Part I: The descriptive epidemiology of head trauma in the United States. In D.P. Becker & J.T. Povlishock (Eds.), *Central nervous system trauma status report—1985* (pp. 33–43). Bethesda, MD: National Institute of Neurological and Communicative Disorders and Stroke, National Institutes of Health.

Goethe, K.E., & Levin, H.S. (1986). Neuropsychological consequences of head injury in children. In R.E. Tarter & G. Goldstein (Eds.), *Advances in clinical neuropsychology* (Vol. 3, pp. 213–242). New York: Plenum Press.

Goldstein, F.C., & Levin, H.S. (1985). Intellectual and academic outcome following closed head injury in children and adolescents: Research strategies and empirical findings. *Developmental Neuropsychology, 1,* 195–214.

Gurdjian, E.S., & Webster, J.E. (1958). *Head injuries: Mechanisms, diagnosis, and management.* Boston: Little,

Brown.

Jamison, D.L., & Kaye, H.H. (1974). Accidental head injury in children. *Archives of Disease in Childhood, 49,* 376–381.

Jennett, B., & Teasdale, G. (1981) *Management of head injuries.* Philadelphia: F.A. Davis.

Jennett, B., Teasdale, G., Galbraith, S., Pickard, J., Grant, H., Braakman, R., Avezaat, C., Maas, A., Minderhoud, J., Vecht, C.J., Heiden, J., Small, R., Caton, W., & Kurtze, T. (1977). Severe head injuries in three countries. *Journal of Neurology, Neurosurgery, and Psychiatry, 40,* 291–298.

Kalsbeek, W.D., McLaurin, R.L., Harris, B.S., & Miller, J.D. (1980). The national head and spinal cord injury survey: Major findings. *Journal of Neurosurgery, 53* (Suppl.), 19–31.

Klauber, M.R., Barrett-Connor, E., Hofstetter, C.R., & Micik, S.H. (1986). A population-based study of nonfatal childhood injuries. *Preventive Medicine, 15,* 139–149.

Klauber, M.R., Barrettt-Connor, E., Marshall, L.F., & Bowers, S.A. (1981). The epidemiology of head injury: A prospective study of an entire community—San Diego County, California, 1978. *American Journal of Epidemiology, 113,* 500–509.

Klonoff, H. (1971). Head injuries in children: Predisposing factors, accident conditions, accident proneness and sequelae. *American Journal of Public Health, 61,* 2405–2417.

Klonoff, H., & Paris, R. (1974). Immediate, short-term, and residual effects of acute head injuries in children: Neuropsychological and neurological correlates. In R.M. Reitan & L.A. Davison (Eds.), *Clinical neuropsychology: Current status and applications* (pp. 179–210). New York: John Wiley.

Kraus, J.F. (1980). A comparison of recent studies on the extent of the head and spinal cord injury problem in the United States. *Journal of Neurosurgery, 53* (Suppl.), 35–43.

Kraus, J.F. (1987). Epidemiology of head injury. In P.R. Cooper (Ed.), *Head injury* (2nd ed., pp. 1–19). Baltimore: Williams & Wilkins.

Kraus, J.F., Black, M.A., Hessol, N., Ley, P., Rokaw, W., Sullivan, C., Bowers, S., Knowlton, S., & Marshall, L. (1984). The incidence of acute brain injury and serious impairment in a defined population. *American Journal of Epidemiology, 119,* 186–201.

Kraus, J.F., Fife, D., Cox, P., Ramstein, K., & Conroy, C. (1986). Incidence, severity, and external causes of pediatric brain injury. *American Journal of Diseases of Children, 140,* 687–693.

Levin, H.S., Benton, A.L., & Grossman, R.G. (1982). *Neurobehavioral consequences of closed head injury.* New York: Oxford University Press.

Levin, H.S., & Eisenberg, H.M. (1979). Neuropsychological impairment after closed head injury in children and adolescents. *Journal of Pediatric Psychology, 4,* 389–402.

Levin, H.S., Ewing-Cobbs, L., & Benton, A.L. (1984). Age and recovery from brain damage: A review of clinical studies. In S.W. Scheff (Ed.), *Aging and recovery of function in the central nervous system* (pp. 169–205). New York: Plenum Press.

Mahoney, W.J., D'Souza, B.J., Haller, A., Rogers, M.C., Epstein, M.H., & Freeman, J.M. (1983). Long-term outcome of children with severe head trauma and prolonged coma. *Pediatrics, 71,* 756–762.

Moyes, C.D. (1980). Epidemiology of serious head injuries in childhood. *Child Care Health Development, 6,* 1–6.

Oka, H., Kako, M., Matsushima, M., &

Ando, K. (1977). Traumatic spreading depression syndrome: Review of a particular type of head injury in 37 patients. *Brain, 100*, 287–298.

Partington, M.W. (1960). The importance of accident-proneness in the aetiology of head injuries in childhood. *Archives of Disease in Childhood, 35*, 215–223.

Rivara, F.P. (1984). Childhood injuries. III: Epidemiology of non-motor vehicle head trauma. *Developmental Medicine & Child Neurology, 26*, 81–87.

Rutter, M. (1981). Psychological sequelae of brain damage in children. *The American Journal of Psychiatry, 138*, 1535–1544.

Rutter, M., Chadwick, O., Shaffer, D., & Brown, G. (1980). A prospective study of children with head injuries: I. Design and methods. *Psychological Medicine, 10*, 633–645.

Scherz, R.G. (1981). Fatal motor vehicle accidents of child passengers from birth through 4 years of age in Washington State. *Pediatrics, 68*, 572–575.

Smith, M.D., Burrington, J.D., & Woolf, A.D. (1975). Injuries in children sustained in free falls: An analysis of 66 cases. *The Journal of Trauma, 15*, 987–991.

Snoek, J.W., Minderhoud, J.M., & Wilmink, J.T. (1984). Delayed deterioration following mild head injury in children. *Brain, 107*, 15–36.

Takahashi, H., & Nakazawa, S. (1980). Specific type of head injury in children: Report of 5 cases. *Child's Brain, 7*, 124–131.

Teasdale, G., & Jennett, B. (1974). Assessment of coma and impaired consciousness: A practical scale. *Lancet, 2*, 81–84.

Teasdale, G., Skene, A., Parker, L., & Jennett, B. (1979). Age and outcome of severe head injury. *Acta Neurochirurgica, 28* (Suppl.), 140–143.

Williams, A.F. (1981). Children killed in falls from motor vehicles. *Pediatrics, 68*, 576–578.

4

Epidemiology of Traumatic Brain Injury in Adults

RICHARD I. NAUGLE

It has been estimated that approximately 200 of every 100,000 people in the United States incur traumatic brain injuries each year (Kalsbeek, McLaurin, Harris, & Miller, 1980). Such a statement regarding the incidence of head injury might be interpreted to imply that those injuries occur randomly and that all members of the population are at equal risk. In fact, that is not the case. Research regarding the various factors associated with the frequency with which those injuries occur (i.e., the *epidemiology* of head injuries) has repeatedly demonstrated that some individuals are more susceptible to head trauma than are others. For example, victims are more frequently male and between the ages of 15 and 25. Some activities and situations are more conducive to head injuries than others. Motor vehicle accidents account for the majority of such injuries, and alcohol consumption plays a prominent role in their occurrence.

There are other, more subtle epidemiologic factors that are not as readily apparent. Psychiatric history, criminal record, learning disabilities, and previous head injuries have all been related to the incidence of accidents resulting in significant trauma. Race, socioeconomic status, and divorce have been implicated as well. Even seasonal trends and fluctuations over the course of the year, week, and day have been uncovered. The nature of the relationship between each of these variables and the incidence of head injury is discussed in this chapter.

First, some problems with epidemiologic research deserve mention. The study of the incidence, or frequency, with which new head injuries occur and the prevalence, or number, of head injured individuals at any given point in time is complicated by variations in the definition of what actually constitutes a head injury and the means by which affected patients are identified (Annegers, Grabow, Kurland, & Laws, 1980; Axelrod, 1986). Taken literally, *head injury* would refer to "acute physical damage to the face, scalp, skull, dura or brain caused by external, mechanical (kinetic) energy" (Frankowski, 1986, p. 152). Many of those injuries, however, are of little or no consequence to the victim; typically, bruises, cuts, and sometimes even simple fractures pose no real danger, and individuals with those injuries may recover with no significant aftereffects. Actual damage to the brain as a consequence of such injuries, however, causes profound and long-standing motor and sensory deficits and cognitive limitations that in turn result in significant impairments of day-to-day functioning. So profound are the consequences of many of those injuries and the extent to which they disrupt patients' lives that Jane and Rimel (1982) concluded that "these patients rarely, if ever, return to their original place in society" (p. 82).

Even minor head trauma such as a concussion has been shown to result in significant compromise (Gronwall & Wrightson, 1975; Rutherford, 1977; Symonds, 1962). By one estimate, as many as a third of the patients suffering "mild" head injuries are unable to return to the jobs they held prior to their accidents (Kraus et al., 1984). Because the behavioral and medical sequelae of head trauma are often monumental, the cost to society is staggering (Frankowski, 1986; Klauber, Barrett-Connor, Marshall, & Bowers, 1981; Kraus, 1978; Rimel, Giordani, & Barth, 1981).

In 1974 direct and indirect care costs for the brain injured population approximated $2.4 billion (Kalsbeek et al., 1980). By 1980 the figure had risen to approximately $3.9 billion annually (Anderson & McLaurin, 1980). Of that amount, medical costs accounted for about 35%, while disability payments and lost income accounted for about 65%. Ambulance costs, legal fees, and claim settlements are also often substantial (Parkinson, Stephenson, & Phillips, 1985). The issue of lost income and other indirect expenses is most salient for those patients in the 25–44 year age group, as those patients are affected in the midst of their prime wage-earning years (Anderson, Miller, & Kalsbeek, 1983). In light of the considerable behavioral, medical, and financial sequelae, traumatic head injury with presumed brain involvement has become the focus of increasing attention, and epidemiologists have directed their attention to those injuries resulting in emergency room treatment, hospitalization, and/or death (Jennett & MacMillan, 1981).

DETERMINATION OF TRAUMATIC BRAIN INJURY CASES

This section provides a definition of traumatic brain injury, a discussion of case ascertainment, and data on the incidence and prevalence of such cases.

Definition

In order to differentiate between head injuries that entail damage to and/or functional impairment of the brain and those that do not, some researchers have chosen to infer that traumatic *brain* injury results from any head trauma that involves any combination of clinical criteria such as loss of consciousness, retrograde amnesia, skull fracture, or the development of a hematoma, neurologic deficit, or seizure disorder (Annegers et al., 1980; Edna, 1983; Jagger, Levine, Jane, & Rimel, 1984; Klauber et al., 1981; Kraus et al., 1984; Wang, Schoenberg, Li, Yang, Cheng, & Bolis, 1986). Others have relied solely on causality codes of the International Classification of Diseases (ICD) system (Jennett & MacMillan, 1981; Simpson et al., 1981). As might be expected, the use of different definitions results in different incidence and prevalence estimates. Data collected by the National Center for Health Statistics in 1974 suggest that an estimated 8,111,000 (or 3,900/100,000) head injuries occur annually in the United States. This figure includes superficial contusions and lacerations to the scalp and face but excludes deaths resulting from head trauma (Kraus, 1978). Most other studies exclude trivial injuries and suggest an incidence rate of approximately 200/100,000 (see Table 4.1). Clearly, estimates of the incidence of brain injury must be interpreted with great caution and with full awareness of how, in each study, *injury* is defined.

Case Ascertainment

Understanding the means by which head trauma cases are located and data are collected is also important. One study involved a door-to-door survey, thereby including cases not originally seen by medical personnel but obviously excluding those who died as a result of their injuries or some other cause occurring between the date of the accident and the time at which the data were collected. Some research relies solely on hospital admission records (Barber & Webster, 1974; Edna, 1983; Jagger et al., 1984), but hospitalization rates for head injury vary across facilities and are dependent to some extent

TABLE 4.1
Overview of Epidemiologic Studies

Publication	Period Under Year(s)	Sample N	Male: Female Ratio	Annual Incidence	Sample Location	Definition*	Case Ascertainment Procedure
Annegers et al. (1980)[1]	1965–1974	3,587	2.30:1	270/100,000(M) 116/100,000(F)	Olmstead County	Clinical Criteria[a]	1,2,3
Barber et al. (1974)[2]	1966–1972	150	3.84:1		St. Louis, MO	Clinical Criteria	1
Cooper et al. (1983)[3]	1980–1981	1,209	2.80:1	249/100,000	Bronx, NY	Clinical Criteria	1,2,3
Desai et al. (1983)[4]	1979–1980	702	3.84:1		Cook County, IL	Clinical Criteria	1
Edna (1987)[5]	1979–1980	1,124	2.31:1	200/100,000	Norway	Clinical Criteria	1
Fife et al. (1986)[6]	1979–1980	2,870	1.84:1	152/100,000	Rhode Island	ICD Codes	1
Freedman et al. (1986)[7]	1980–1982	162	2.77:1		Oxford, GB	Clinical Criteria	1
Jagger et al. (1984)[8]	1978	735	2.40:1	208/100,000	N Central Virginia	Clinical Criteria	1
Jennett et al. (1981)[9]	1974	3,615	2.53:1	270/100,000 313/100,000	England & Wales Scotland	ICD Codes	1,3

[1] *Definition:* concussion with loss of consciousness, posttraumatic amnesia, or neurologic deficit or skull fracture. *Case ascertainment:* hospital admission records, emergency room visits, outpatient examinations, home visits, death certificates, and autopsy reports; excluded injuries to nonresidents.

[2] *Definition:* diagnosis of head injury. *Case ascertainment:* hospital admission records.

[3] *Definition:* loss of consciousness greater than 10 minutes, skull fracture or posttraumatic seizures, or neurologic deficit secondary to the head injury; includes immediate deaths. *Case ascertainment:* hospital records of neurosurgery, neurology, and pediatric wards, autopsy records, and emergency room records.

[4] *Definition:* blow to the head, altered consciousness, scalp laceration. *Case ascertainment:* hospital admission records.

[5] *Definition:* loss of consciousness, fracture, or intracranial hematoma. *Case ascertainment:* admission records of three hospitals; excluded birth trauma, deaths on arrival, and others not brought to the hospitals.

[6] *Definition:* ICD codes likely to include head injuries. *Case ascertainment:* hospital admission records.

[7] *Definition:* fracture, head injury with intracranial collection, secondary hydrocephalus and retained intracranial foreign bodies, cerebral spinal fluid leaks, or chronic subdural hematomas. *Case ascertainment:* neurosurgical unit admission records.

[8] *Definition:* loss of consciousness, posttraumatic amnesia, or skull fracture (99%), or presence of nausea, vomiting, diplopia, vertigo, headaches. *Case ascertainment:* hospitalization for at least overnight stay.

[9] *Definition:* ICD codes. *Case ascertainment:* hospital admission records, deaths by road accident, and head injury.

TABLE 4.1 (cont.)

Publication	Period Under Year(s)	Sample N	Male: Female Ratio	Annual Incidence	Sample Location	Definition*	Case Ascertainment Procedure
Kalsbeek et al. (1980)[10]	1970–1974	3,516	2.10:1	272/100,000(M) 132/100,000(F)	United States	ICD Codes	1
Klauber et al. (1981)[11]	1978	5,055	2.60:1	295/100,000	San Diego County	Clinical Criteria[b]	1,3
Klonoff et al. (1969)[12]	1967	352	1.62:1		Vancouver, BC	Clinical Criteria	1,2
Kraus et al. (1984)[13]	1981	3,358	2.20:1	180/100,000	San Diego County	Clinical Criteria	1,2,3,4
Parkinson et al. (1985)[14]	1978–1981	3,000	2.19:1		Winnepeg, Ontario	Clinical Criteria	1
Servadei et al. (1985)[15]	1981–1982	327	2.14:1	894/100,000	San Marino Republic	Clinical Criteria	1,2
Wang et al. (1986)[16]	1982	63,195	1.66:1	56/100,000	Urban People's Republic of China	Clinical Criteria	5

[10]*Definition:* ICD codes. *Case ascertainment:* estimates from hospital admission records.

[11]*Definition:* skull fracture, loss of consciousness, amnesia, neurologic deficit, or seizures; excluded gunshot wounds; includes injuries to tourists and other nonresidents and immediate deaths. *Case ascertainment:* hospital admission records and death resulting from head injury.

[12]*Definition:* head injury, fracture, concussion, contusion in patients aged 16 or older. *Case ascertainment:* emergency room and hospital admission records.

[13]*Definition:* physical damage to or functional impairment of the contents of the cranium due to acute mechanical energy sources; excludes skull fractures without evidence of brain injury, gunshot wounds, injuries to residents outside of the county; includes immediate deaths. *Case ascertainment:* hospital admission and emergency room records, coroner's cases, death certificates, nursing home and extended care facility records.

[14]*Definition:* "head injured patients" not including deaths on admission and deaths on transport. *Case ascertainment:* hospital admission records.

[15]*Definition:* skull fracture, loss of consciousness; includes trivial scalp wounds. *Case ascertainment:* hospital admission and emergency room records.

[16]*Definition:* loss of consciousness, posttraumatic amnesia, or clinical evidence of focal brain dysfunction. *Case ascertainment:* door-to-door survey.

* Clinical Criteria refers to any combination of clinical characteristics such as skull fracture, loss of consciousness, posttraumatic amnesia, posttraumatic seizures, subdural hematoma, etc., or the diagnosis of "head injury."

[a]Excludes injuries to nonresidents
[b]Includes injuries to tourists and other nonresidents

Case Ascertainment Procedures:
1 = review of hospital admission records; 2 = review of emergency room records; 3 = review of death certificates and/or autopsy reports; 4 = review of nursing home and extended care facilities; 5 = door-to-door survey.

on the availability of local health care services (or lack thereof), the distance and access to the hospitals, the training and expertise of the staff at each hospital and their admission policies as well as the means by which those admissions are recorded (Barber & Webster, 1974; Edna, 1987; Jennett & MacMillan, 1981). Also, by definition, studies using only hospital admission records neglect to include data on those less severe injuries that were treated in emergency rooms or those cases that were dead on arrival to the hospital. To correct for these sources of error, some studies have included emergency room records and, consequently, report substantially higher incidence rates than those that do not (e.g., Servadei et al., 1985). Others have included the review of death certificates for a particular period of time (Cooper, Tabaddor, Hauser, Schulman, Feiner, & Factor, 1983; Kraus et al., 1984; Ring et al., 1986). Still others have included both hospital and outpatient emergency room visits as well as death certificates and autopsy protocols (Annegers et al., 1980; Cooper et al., 1983), but these are the exception.

Clearly, each of these methodologies results in data that are very different from the others. The meaningful interpretation of incidence and prevalence estimates requires full awareness of the means by which the data were collected.

Incidence

Trauma as the result of accidents is the leading cause of death for those aged 1–44 in the United States and Canada, and head injuries constitute approximately 65% of these trauma cases (Klauber et al., 1981; Klonoff & Thompson, 1969). As stated earlier, most annual estimates suggest that approximately 200 out of every 100,000 people in the U.S. population suffer head injuries with consequent brain trauma (Frankowski, 1986), resulting in an estimated 410,000 new cases annually (Kraus et al., 1984). This is evident in separate studies of samples in central Virginia (Jagger et al., 1984), Rhode Island (Fife, Faich, Hollinshead, & Boynton, 1986), Olmstead County in Minnesota (Annegers et al., 1980), and San Diego County in Southern California (Klauber et al., 1981; Kraus et al., 1984). An overview of those estimates and others and the means by which they were reached is presented in Table 4.1. This corresponds rather closely to similarly derived estimates of the incidence of head injury in other industrialized countries such as Great Britain (Freedman, Saunders, & Briggs, 1986), Australia (Ring et al., 1986), Norway (Edna, 1987), and Canada (Klonoff & Thompson, 1969; Parkinson et al., 1985). Schoenberg (1978) points out that this figure *exceeds* the annual number of new cases of Reyes Syndrome, bacterial meningitis, encephalitis, paralytic polio, Guillain-Barre Syndrome, epilepsy, stroke, Parkinson's Disease, amyotrophic lateral sclerosis, multiple sclerosis, myasthenia gravis, and neurologic cancer combined! In contrast, the incidence rate reported for urban China is considerably lower, at 56/100,000 (Wang et al., 1986).

Case fatality ratios have suggested that approximately 7% to 16% of head injuries result in death (Klauber et al., 1981; Kraus et al., 1984). In those studies that include patients who die prior to treatment, the incidence rate is naturally higher than in those relying only on hospital admission records. When comatose patients are studied separately, the percentage of fatalities climbs to as high as 52% (Jennett, Teasdale, Braakman, Minderhoud, & Knill-Jones, 1976). In the San Diego County sample, the percentage of patients who expired as a consequence of their injuries was highest among those less than 5 years of age (17%) and older than 70 (17.5%) but low by comparison in children aged 10–14 (1.2%; Klauber et al., 1981). Of their 381 patients suffering fatal accidents, Klauber et al. (1981) found that 42% were dead at the scene of the accident, 19% died en route to the hospital, and 39% of the deaths occurred following hospitalization. Ninety-five percent of the subjects in their total sample survived long enough that they could be admitted for treatment, and, of those patients admitted, more than 97% survived. In other words, the case fatality ratio dropped from 5% during the prehospitalization period to 3% among those hospitalized. This suggests that, if a patient is able to survive long enough to be hospitalized, his or her chances for continued survival nearly double.

Prevalence

The proportion of individuals within the population who are head injured at any given time is more difficult to establish than the rate at which new cases occur, as records containing that information are not readily available. One study estimates the prevalence of head injuries in the United States at 800/100,000 (Kurtzke, 1982). In comparison, Wang et al. (1986) estimate that, among the urban areas of the People's Republic of China, the prevalence of head injury is approximately 709/100,000 when their sample is age-corrected to correspond to the 1960 U.S. population.

Clearly, head injury is a significant medical problem and warrants intensive study to determine any patterns of occurrence that might, in turn, suggest means by which those injuries could be prevented or at least reduced. The remainder of this chapter is devoted to elucidating the patterns, trends, and correlates of the incidence of head injury.

CAUSES OF TRAUMATIC BRAIN INJURY

Although several types of accidents result in head injuries, the percentage of patients affected by each of those causes is surprisingly stable across samples. Table 4.2 presents the percentages of patients injured as a consequence of

TABLE 4.2
Percentages of Head Injury Accidents Attributable to Various Causes

Study	Sample N	MVA	Sports/ Recreation	Home Accidents	Falls	Assault	Work	Other/ Unknown
Anderson et al. (1983)	3,516	49.0	NR	28.0	NR	NR	NR	23.0
Annegers et al. (1980)	3,587	46.0	9.0	NR	29.0	7.0[1]	NR	9.0
Cooper et al. (1983)	1,209	27.0	NR	NR	32.0	34.0	NR	7.0
Desai et al. (1983)	702	18.7	2.2	NR	26.8	44.2[1]	NR	8.1
Edna (1987)	1,124	44.8	14.2	12.8	NR	7.7	1.6	16.2
Fife et al. (1986)	2,870	39.0	NR	NR	35.0	9.0	NR	17.0
Kalsbeek et al. (1980)	1,210	49.0	NR	NR	28.0	NR	NR	23.0
Klauber et al. (1981)	5,055	53.0	NR	NR	30.6	10.8	NR	5.9
Klonoff et al. (1969)								
ER:	351	43.9	5.1	NR	19.9	12.5	10.0	8.6
Hospital:	279	52.7	2.9	NR	23.3	3.6	10.8	6.8
Kraus et al. (1984)	3,358	48.0	9.7	NR	20.6	17.7	NR	3.9
Parkinson et al. (1985)	3,113	31.7	4.1	NR	29.1	29.6	4.0	3.8
Ring et al. (1986)	991	53.4	3.6	NR	28.3	NR	2.8	11.9

TABLE 4.2 (cont.)

Study	Sample N	MVA	Sports/ Recreation	Home Accidents	Falls	Assault	Work	Other/ Unknown
Selecki et al. (1967)	1,112	38.0	11.0	17.0	NR	NR	NR	34.0
Servadei et al. (1985)	207	61.5	2.3	24.0	NR	2.0	8.2[2]	2.0
Steadman et al. (1970)[3]	484	64.0	3.0	10.0	54.1[4]	7.0	9.0	—
Wang et al. (1986)	495	31.7	15.4	NR	21.8	1.4	23.8	29.0
Whitman et al. (Evanston; 1984)								
Black:	62	32.0	11.0	NR	21.0	26.0	NR	10.0
White:	103	39.0	14.0	NR	31.0	10.0	NR	6.0
Whitman et al. (Chicago; 1984)								
Black:	617	31.0	3.0	NR	20.0	40.0	NR	6.0

[1]includes gunshot wounds

[2]includes injuries occurring at school

[3]categories overlap, so percentages do not total 100

[4]includes falls down stairs (25, 5.2%), from heights (46, 10%), from the ground (72, 14.9%), from bicycles/motorcycles (106, 22%), and from other motor vehicles (13, 2.7%)

motor vehicle accidents, falls, sports and recreation mishaps, home accidents, assaults, and work/industry accidents. As is apparent from Table 4.2, motor vehicle accidents account for approximately half of all injuries in many of the studies. The most notable exceptions to this general trend are studies of urban samples such as the works of Desai et al. (1983) and Whitman, Coonley, and Desai (1984), which are based on studies of Chicago samples; Cooper et al. (1983), who studied a sample drawn from the Bronx; Parkinson et al. (1985) in Winnepeg; and the urban China study conducted by Wang et al. (1986). It is reasonable to conclude that, because of the fewer number of high speed roads in urban areas and the greater tendency to rely on public transportation that is available there, fewer people are injured in the course of road accidents. (It is interesting to note, however, that the occurrence of assaults and interpersonal violence in urban areas of the United States compensates for the reduction in the incidence of traffic accidents in those regions. See Table 4.2.)

Of the motor vehicle accidents, motorcycles account for an inordinate number of injuries and death (Kraus et al., 1984). In fact, Parkinson et al. (1985) estimate the accident rate among motorcyclists to be 4.3 times that for other motor vehicle operators. While they constitute only 3.6% of the registered vehicles in Ontario, California, motorcycles were the mode of transportation being used by 48% of those who succumbed to their injuries resulting from road traffic accidents. In other words, motorcyclists are both more likely to be head injured and more likely to die as a result of their injuries than are drivers of other vehicles.

Falls are the second leading cause of head trauma, accounting for approximately 28% of those injuries reported in the epidemiological literature and occurring quite frequently among the very young and the elderly (see Figure 4.1). Falls tend to be followed by assaults (16%) and injuries resulting from sports and recreational activities (7%).

Assaults predominate among the poor and unemployed and account for the majority of head injuries in urban settings (Barber & Webster, 1974; Cooper et al., 1983; Kerr, Kay, & Lassman, 1971; Parkinson et al., 1985). Pediatric assault victims have also been found to live in more congested areas, are from the lower socioeconomic strata, and tend to have unemployed or emotionally disturbed parents (Klonoff, 1971). In one urban sample, the assailant was known to the victim in approximately 45% of those cases; in another 4%, the perpetrator was a police officer (Desai et al., 1983). In the Olmstead County sample, those assaults that entailed gunshot wounds to the head were by and large suicide attempts (82%). Accidents accounted for another 12% of those gunshot wounds and homicides, 6% (Annegers et al., 1980). This contrasts with the information provided by the New York State Department of Health's Bureau of Biostatistics, which reported that fatal injuries from firearms in New York State were the result of homicides in 65% of all cases, suicides in 31%, and were accidental in only 2% (Axelrod, 1986).

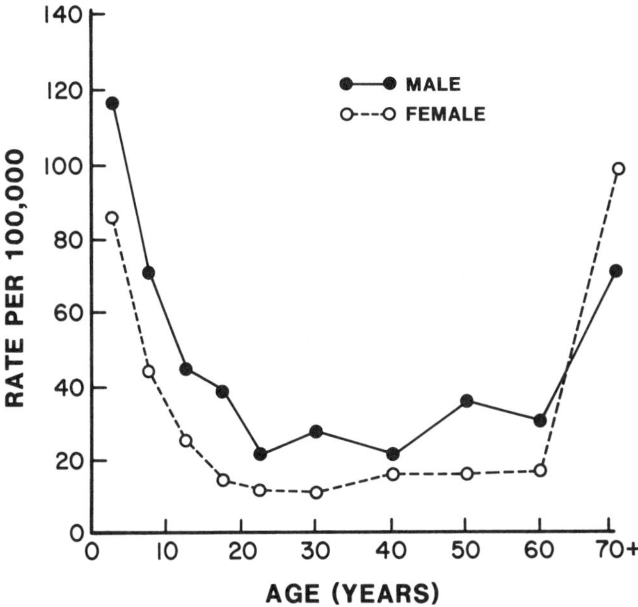

Figure 4.1. Age and gender specific incidence rates for brain injuries resulting from falls. *Note.* Adapted from "The Incidence of Acute Brain Injury and Serious Impairment in a Defined Population" by J.F. Kraus, M.A. Black, N. Hessol, P. Ley, W. Rokaw, C. Sullivan, S. Bowers, S. Knowlton, & L. Marshall, 1981, *American Journal of Epidemiology,* 119, p. 195. Reprinted by permission.

One study includes a more in-depth investigation of the specific causes of head injuries resulting from sports and recreational activities. Annegers et al. (1980) report that horseback riding accounts for 21% of those accidents. Horseback riding is followed by football (19%), sledding and tobogganing (13%), baseball and softball (10%), ice hockey (9%), skating (6%), basketball (4%), swimming and diving (3%), gym class activities (2%), golf (2%), and skiing (1%). Certainly, to some extent, the relative frequencies of injuries from these various recreational activities are location-dependent and do not generalize to other geographic areas.

CORRELATES OF TRAUMATIC BRAIN INJURY

Age, gender, socioeconomic status, and other demographic variables correlate with the incidence of head trauma in general. In many cases, the relationship between these variables and the rate of traumatic brain injury has been demonstrated and replicated numerous times, suggesting that, rather than being unique to any given sample, those findings are extremely reliable and merit further study.

Age

There is ample evidence that head injuries resulting from the spectrum of causes are not distributed randomly across the age range but, rather, are more likely to occur at given ages than others. There is some suggestion that a peak of incidence occurs very early in life, from ages 1 to 5 (Fife et al., 1986; Frankowski, 1986; Kraus et al., 1984; Wang et al., 1986), although this has not always been found to be the case (Klauber et al., 1981). Epidemiologic studies have repeatedly shown a second, more pronounced peak of closed head injuries during the period from midadolescence to the midtwenties. About this, there is little question; the consistency with which this finding has been reported is striking (Anderson et al., 1983; Annegers et al., 1980; Edna, 1987; Field, 1976; Fife et al., 1986; Frankowski, 1986; Jagger et al., 1984; Klauber et al., 1981; Kraus, 1978, 1980; Kraus et al., 1984; Levin, Benton, & Grossman, 1982; Parkinson et al., 1985; Simpson et al., 1981). A third peak occurs later in life, after approximately age 65, although this is typically significantly lower than the second and has not been as reliably demonstrated as that which occurs earlier.

Those periods of increased incidence early and late in life are largely the result of falls, which occur more frequently among those groups (Annegers et al., 1980; Cooper et al., 1983; Desai et al., 1983; Edna, 1987; Fife et al., 1986; Frankowski, 1986; Jagger et al., 1984; Klauber et al., 1981; Kraus et al., 1984; Parkinson et al., 1985). In fact, falls were the mode of injury in 73% of all head injured patients younger than 5 and older than 64 in one sample (Fife et al., 1986).

There is also evidence that the very young and the elderly are particularly vulnerable pedestrians (Steadman & Graham, 1970). By one estimate, motor vehicle/pedestrian accidents accounted for approximately half of the injuries to those younger than 9 and older than 70 years of age (Parkinson et al., 1985). In contrast, the leading causes of head trauma among the young adult subsample are typically motor vehicle accidents and assaults (Annegers et al., 1980; Cooper et al., 1983; Fife et al., 1986; Klauber et al., 1981; Kraus et al., 1984; Parkinson et al., 1985; Steadman & Graham, 1970). (See Figure 4.2.)

Age is also related to the length of stay in the hospital recovering from head injury, with older patients tending to require longer hospitalizations. Edna (1987) reported that the median hospital stay for patients aged 65 or older was 4.7 days in contrast to 2.1 days for subjects aged 25–44 (see Figure 4.3). In another study, stays lasting a week or longer constituted approximately 20% of hospitalizations for those aged 34 or younger, while 56% of people aged 65 and older required a week or more to recover from their injuries (Fife et al., 1986).

In addition to increased incidence, head trauma tends to have more severe ramifications for elderly individuals. For example, the percentage of

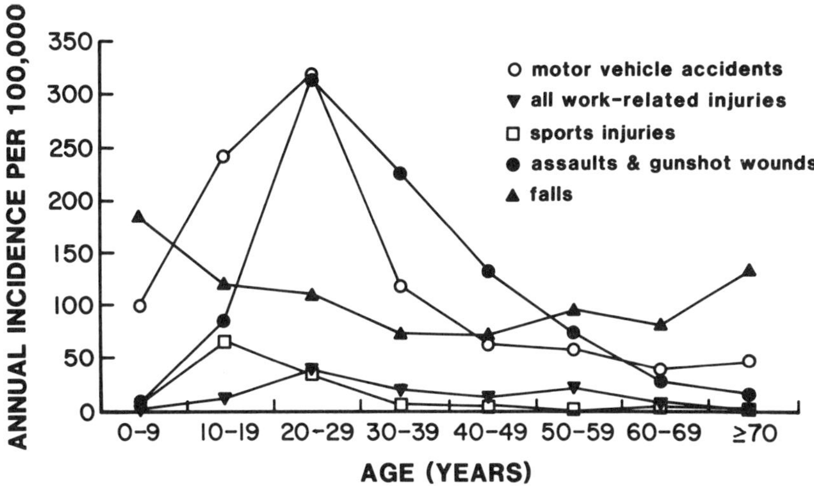

Figure 4.2. Age and etiology specific incidence rates for brain injuries. *Note.* Adapted from "Head Injuries: A Prospective, Computerized Study" by D. Parkinson, S. Stephenson, & S. Phillips, 1985, *Canadian Journal of Surgery, 28,* p. 80. Reprinted by permission.

head injury victims who are unable to return home is directly correlated with age (see Figure 4.4). The older the patients, the less likely they will be able to care for themselves at home in the postinjury period (Fife et al., 1986). The reason for this relationship is not necessarily straightforward. The greater need for nursing home care among elderly closed head injury survivors may be the result of their inability to recover from their brain trauma (or other injuries that occurred at the time of their accidents). A second possibility is that their head traumas may compound other medical conditions that predate their injuries. Still another possible explanation is that the elderly often lack the home support that may enable younger patients to return home (Fife et al., 1986).

Similarly, the percentage of patients dying from their head traumas increases with age (Jennett & MacMillan, 1981; Klauber et al., 1981; Overgaard et al., 1973), although, according to Annegers et al. (1980), this higher mortality rate is in part the result of a greater number of successful suicides among the elderly. Whereas only 3.1% of subjects aged 25–44 succumbed as a result of their injuries, 9.1% of those aged 65 and above died due to their trauma (Edna, 1987). Figure 4.3 presents this information in graph form.

This receives further support from Jennett and Teasdale (1981), who reviewed 668 cases collected by the International Coma Data Bank. The percentage of patients who were dead or remained in a vegetative state following their injuries increased with age, to nearly 100% of those over the

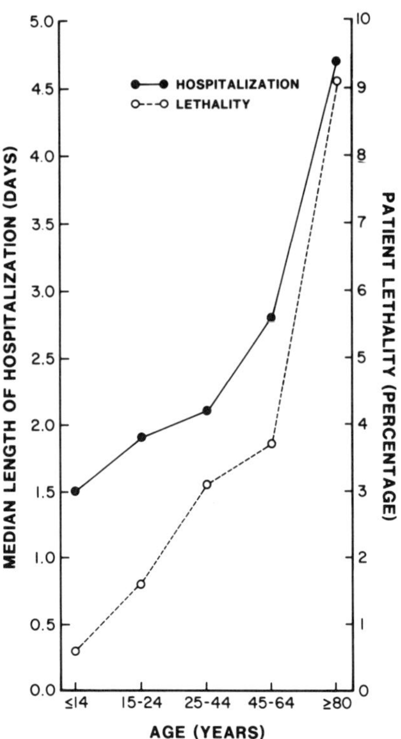

Figure 4.3. Duration of hospitalization and lethality of head injury by age. *Note.* Adapted from "Head Injuries Admitted to Hospital: Epidemiology, Risk Factors and Long Term Outcome" by T.H. Edna, 1987, *Journal of the Oslo City Hospitals, 37,* p. 107. Reprinted by permission.

age of 75. Conversely, younger patients were found to be more likely to have a better outcome (see Figure 4.5).

Gender

As is apparent in Table 4.1, research has repeatedly demonstrated that head injured victims are predominantly male. The male to female ratios of various studies range from 1.62:1 to 3.84:1 and reveal that males constitute 61.8% to 79.3% of head trauma samples. This overrepresentation of males among epidemiologic studies is all the more compelling in light of the fact that most research has found that males are at greater risk for head injuries resulting from the full range of etiologies (Fife et al., 1986; Goldstein & Levin, 1987; Kraus et al., 1984; Kraus, Fife, & Conroy, 1987) and across virtually the entire age range (Cooper et al., 1983; Fife et al., 1986; Frankowski, 1986; Jagger et al., 1984; Klauber et al., 1981; Kraus et al., 1984). (See Figure 4.6.)

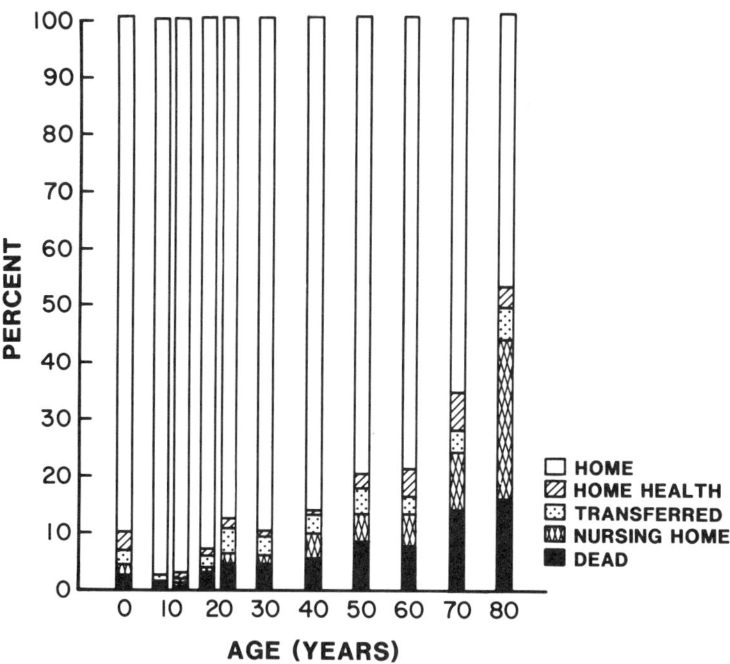

Figure 4.4. Disposition following hospitalization for head injury by age. *Note.* Adapted from "Incidence and Outcome of Hospital-Treated Head Injury in Rhode Island" by D. Fife, G. Faich, W. Hollinshead, & W. Boynton, 1986, *American Journal of Public Health, 76,* p. 776. Reprinted by permission.

The male-female ratio is as high as 3–4:1 during middle adolescence and early adulthood due to the high numbers of young males who are injured by assaults and motor vehicle accidents (Cooper et al., 1983; Klauber et al., 1981; Steadman & Graham, 1970). In fact, by some estimates, relative to females, males are more frequently involved in motorcycle accidents (which occur primarily during this age period) by a ratio of 6.75:1 (Kraus et al., 1984) or 7.2:1 (Klauber et al., 1981). Also, males injured in the course of athletics, sports, and recreational events outnumber females by a ratio of 6:1 by one estimate (Kraus et al., 1984). Some exceptions to this rather consistent pattern have been reported and deserve mention.

One of the most apparent of those exceptions is seen in the case of pedestrians and passengers of automobiles, where females have been found to outnumber males in ratios of 1.16:1 and 1.93:1, respectively (Parkinson et al., 1985). Another exception pertains to injuries occurring later in life. The number of females among elderly victims has been found to surpass that of males in some samples (Fife et al., 1986; Chowdhary, 1978). This is pre-

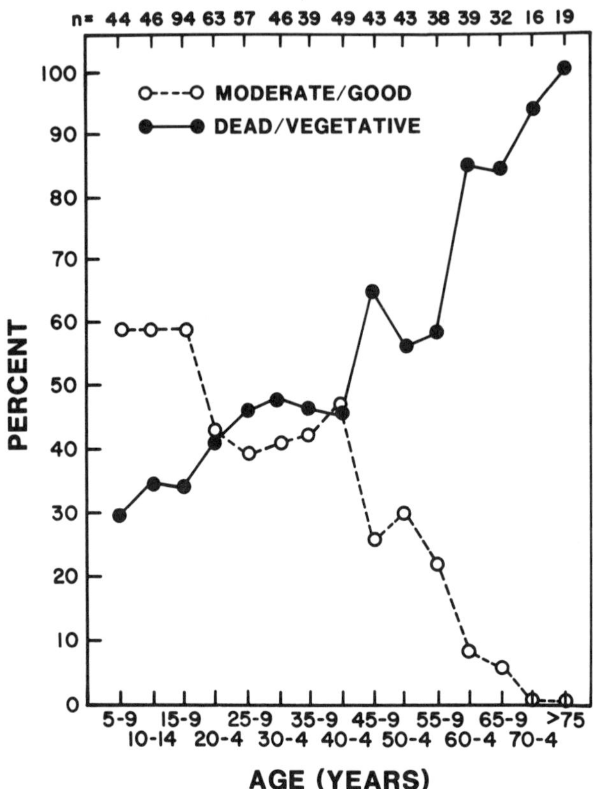

Figure 4.5. Outcome of severe head injury by age, based on data from the International Coma Data Bank. *Note.* Adapted from *Management of Head Injuries (p. 321)* by B. Jennett & G. Teasdale, 1981, Philadelphia: F.A. Davis. Reprinted by permission.

sumably due to females' greater likelihood to survive to those ages and, consequently, greatly outnumber males in the general population. However, it bears repeating that this has been suggested only by selected studies. Other studies have actually found that the increased male-female ratio extends beyond age 60 (Klauber et al., 1981). The male-female ratio is also less dramatic during the early years of life, when girls are as likely as boys to be injured due to falls and child abuse/assault (Fife et al., 1986; Jagger et al., 1984; Kraus et al., 1984).

In addition to their greater incidence of head injury, males tend to incur more severe trauma (Annegers, 1983; Goldstein & Levin, 1987; Klauber et al., 1981) and are more likely to succumb to their injuries than females (Jennett & MacMillan, 1981; Klauber et al., 1981). Male fatalities have been found to outnumber those of females by a margin of 2.6:1 to as high as 4:1 (Klauber et al., 1981; Kraus et al., 1984; Moyes, 1980; Parkinson et al., 1985; Simpson et al., 1981). This finding, too, is consistent across all etiologies (Simpson et al., 1981). Fife et al. (1986) found that, of those patients aged 55 or older who failed to return home after hospitalization, males were more likely than females to expire (53% vs. 35%) rather than be discharged to chronic care facilities (47% vs. 65%).

Alcohol Consumption

The consumption of alcohol is perhaps "the most firmly established" of all the predisposing factors of head injury (Frankowski, 1986). It has been estimated that a third to more than a half of all head injuries occur after alcohol consumption (Barber & Webster, 1974; Desai et al., 1983; Edna, 1987; Parkinson et al., 1985; Ring et al., 1986). Most research has suggested that approximately one half of all motor vehicle accidents occur following alcohol intake. Kraus et al. (1987), in their investigation of head injury resulting from bicycle accidents, report that, even among bicyclists aged 16 or older, alcohol intoxication is apparent in more than half of all victims.

The role of alcohol is somewhat more prominent in the case of assaults, having been implicated in 59% to 84% of head injuries resulting from interpersonal violence (Desai et al., 1983; Edna, 1987; Parkinson et al., 1985), although it has been pointed out that that percentage is not significantly different from the overall percentage of accidents in which alcohol was involved (Desai et al., 1983). Table 4.3 summarizes the percentage of brain traumatic accidents in which alcohol consumption was evident as reported in eight different studies.

Alcohol intoxication is more commonly a factor in head injuries among adult males than females. Alcohol has been implicated in 29% to 73% of accidents involving men but only 10% to 27% of those involving women (Edna, 1987; Field, 1976; Parkinson et al., 1985). Intoxication is more frequently uncovered among victims of accidents occurring at night and on weekends (Edna, 1987). Parkinson et al. (1985) reported that, while welfare recipients and the unemployed make up less than 11% of the population, they account for 79.6% of all head injuries involving drugs or alcohol. Not surprisingly, then, chronic alcoholics are overrepresented among closed head injured patients, accounting for as much as 25% to 66% of some samples (Barber & Webster, 1974; Field, 1976).

In an effort to further illuminate the relationship between chronic alcoholism and head trauma, Alterman and Tarter (1985) differentiated their sample of 76 alcoholics into those with a family history of alcoholism (FH+) and those without (FH–). They note that FH+ alcoholics tend to start

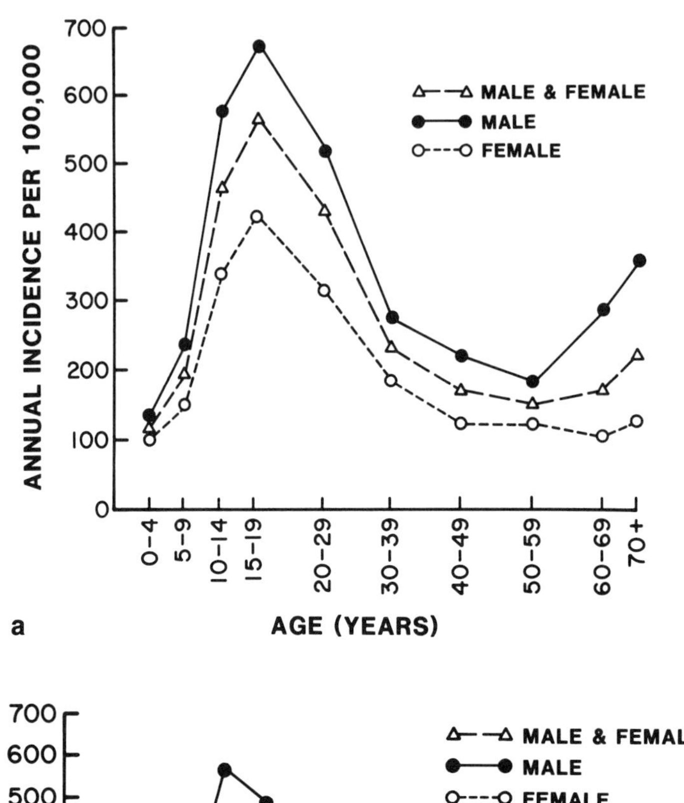

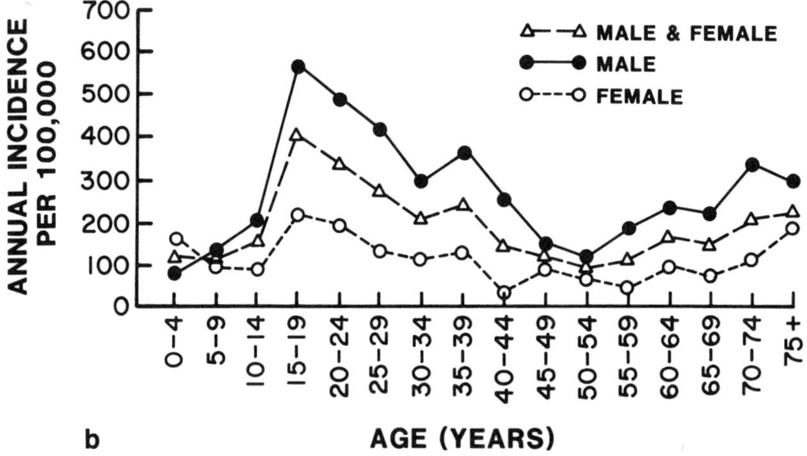

Figure 4.6. (this page and facing page) Age and gender specific incidence rates for four samples. Note the consistency of the relationship between age and gender to head injury incidence across these studies despite the fact that each is based on a separate sample. *Note.* **a)** Adapted from "The Epidemiology of Head Injury: A Prospective Study of an Entire Community—San Diego County, California, 1978" by M.R. Klauber, E. Barrett-Connor, L.F. Marshall, & S.A. Bowers, 1981, *American Journal of Epidemiology, 113,* p. 502. Reprinted by permission. **b)** Adapted from "Epidemiologic Features of Head Injury in a Predominantly

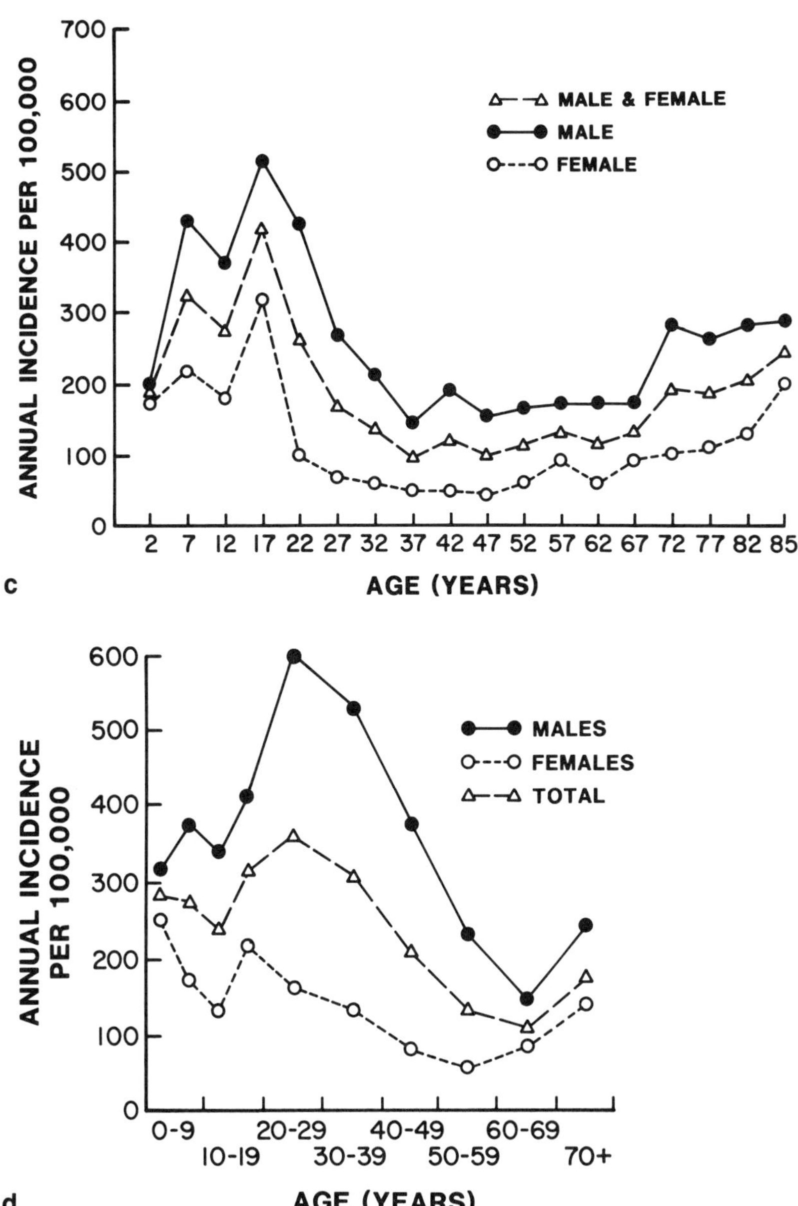

Rural Population" by J. Jagger, J.I. Levine, J. Jane, & R.W. Rimel, 1984, *Journal of Trauma, 24,* p. 41. Reprinted by permission. **c)** Adapted from "Head Injuries Admitted to Hospital: Epidemiology, Risk Factors and Long Term Outcome" by T.H. Edna, *1987, Journal of the Oslo City Hospitals, 37,* p. 105. Reprinted by permission. **d)** Adapted from "The Epidemiology of Head Injury in the Bronx" by K.D. Cooper, K. Tabaddor, W.A. Hauser, K. Shulman, C. Feiner, & P. R. Factor, 1983, *Neuroepidemiology, 2,* p. 76. Reprinted by permission.

TABLE 4.3
Percentage of Accidents in Which Alcohol was a Predisposing Factor

Study	MVA	Assault	Overall
Barber et al. (1974)	—	—	52.0
Desai et al. (1983)	—	59.0	54.0
Edna (1987)[1]	20.0	84.0	32.0
Parkinson et al. (1985)[2]	—	76.0	45.6
Ring et al. (1986)	44.0	—	—
Simpson et al. (1981)[3]	44.0	—	33.0
Jennett et al. (1981)	>60.0	—	—
Klonoff et al. (1969)	—	—	13.0

[1]also reported involvement of alcohol in 52% of domestic accidents and 45% of pedestrian accidents

[2]also reported involvement of alcohol in 39.4% of sports injuries.

[3]also reported involvement of alcohol in 39% of suicides and 27% of accidental falls

drinking at a younger age (McKenna & Pickens, 1981) and tend to become more severely addicted than FH– alcoholics (Fitzgerald & Mulford, 1981). Also, FH+ alcoholics are characterized by greater cognitive deficits and are more likely to have shown signs of hyperactivity and minimal brain dysfunction during childhood (Alterman, Petrarulo, Tarter, & McGowan, 1982; Schaeffer, Parsons, & Yohman, 1984).

It was determined that 60% of the FH+ alcoholics had suffered head trauma (with loss of consciousness of at least 5 minutes on one occasion, loss of consciousness on at least two occasions, or loss of consciousness requiring hospitalization) as compared to only 35% of the FH– alcoholics. The explanation for this finding is not clear; it has been reported that children of alcoholics are more likely to be hyperactive, manifest a conduct or antisocial personality disorder (Alterman et al., 1982), or to be the victims of physical abuse from their parents (Tarter, Hegedus, Goldstein, Shelly, & Alterman, 1984). Any of these conditions inflates the risk of trauma among those offspring and may contribute to the group differences noted by Alterman and Tarter (1985).

Certainly, it is irrefutable that alcohol consumption plays a prominent role in the etiology of head injuries. Yet the number of accidents in which alcohol intake is a factor likely has been underestimated in the epidemiological research because testing is not uniformly performed. Following an accident, altered consciousness is often assumed to be a symptom of the delirium resulting from the head injury rather than possible alcohol intoxication, and testing is not done for that reason (Parkinson et al., 1985). Furthermore, alcohol intoxication may contribute to the brain injury either directly, by compounding the central nervous system damage (Flamm et al., 1977), or indirectly, by rendering the patient more difficult to evaluate, thereby reducing the likelihood that intracranial complications will be recognized and treated (Edna, 1987), or by predisposing the patient to still another head injury. Sims (1985) speculated that, because closed head injury results in a reduced tolerance for alcohol, head trauma patients who continue to drink will be all the more likely to be intoxicated and, consequently, predisposed to additional injury.

The abuse of other substances in addition to alcohol has also been implicated in the etiology of head trauma. Barber and Webster (1974), after reviewing 150 cases of head injury among an urban sample, reported that five of their patients had been heroin addicts and were intoxicated at the time of their accidents and that two others under the influence of barbiturates sustained their injuries as the result of falls. Cigarette smoking was attributed a causal role in two motor vehicle accidents in that series when it was reported that one accident occurred as the driver was lighting his cigarette and another accident took place as the smoker exhaled a cloud of smoke.

Race

There is mixed information regarding the relationship between race and closed head injury. Anderson et al. (1983) failed to uncover any noteworthy difference in the rate of new cases of head trauma between whites and nonwhites. Others, however, have reported a preponderance of nonwhites in their samples, but several neglect to provide any information on the racial composition of the population from which those samples were drawn. Desai et al. (1983) found that 77.6% of their subjects at Cook County Hospital in Illinois were black, 9.2% were Latino, and 13.2% were white. Whitman, Coonley, and Desai (1984) found the incidence rate among blacks to be approximately twice that for whites in Evanston, Illinois. In their sample from the Bronx, Cooper et al. (1983) found a similar albeit less dramatic pattern, with blacks having an age-adjusted rate of 277.5/100,000; Hispanics, 261.9/100,000, and whites, 209.2/100,000. They concluded that the higher rates among blacks and Hispanics are primarily attributable to the greater rate of trauma as a result of assaults in young males of those groups. This pattern of incidence closely parallels the finding of Jagger et al. (1984), who report an incidence rate of 288/100,000 for nonwhites and 194/100,000 for whites, indicating that nonwhites are approximately 49% more likely to suffer injury than whites.

Employment/Socioeconomic Status

Some research has suggested that there is no significant relationship between socioeconomic status and hospitalization for head injury (Steadman & Graham, 1970) or that those with the fewest completed years of education have the lowest rate of trauma (Kraus, 1978). However, many researchers have concluded that hospitalization rates are *inversely* related to socioeconomic status (Kerr et al., 1971; Selecki, Hou, & Ness, 1968).

Fife et al. (1986) found that incidence rates among subjects in the lowest decile of median income were twice those for individuals in the highest decile. Consistent with this, Desai et al. (1983) found that 70% of their urban patients had annual incomes below $6,000, while only 5% earned more than $20,000. By one estimate, nearly half of the victims injured by assaults were among the lowest socioeconomic level (Kerr et al., 1971). Barber and Webster (1974) observed the same pattern in their urban setting: Fifty-two percent of their subjects were unemployed, leading them to conclude that, in urban hospitals, head injury patients typically come from the lowest socioeconomic strata of society. This is also mirrored by the work of Parkinson et al. (1985), who noted that welfare recipients and the unemployed were overrepresented among victims. Although they constituted only 1% of the population in Winnepeg, welfare recipients made up more than 29% of their head injured sample and were involved in nearly 75% of the fights and falls causing head injury. The unemployed accounted for 18.3% of that head injured sample but only 10% of the general population. Together, then, these two groups accounted for 47.5% of all cases, but only11% of the catchment population. The other 52.5% of head trauma patients in that series were divided among the following socioeconomic/employment groups: unskilled workers (11.7%), skilled workers (6.9%), laborers (6.8%), housewives/husbands (6.4%), clerical workers (3.8%), self-employed (2.8%), professionals (1.7%), semiskilled workers (1.6%), farmers (1.1%), and managers (0.7%). The remaining 9% had been admitted without information regarding their employment status.

Psychological Disorders, Delinquency, and Previous Head Trauma

There is some evidence to suggest that the incidence of head injury is related to neurosis and other psychological disorders (Jennett, 1972; Servadei et al., 1985). In his review of that evidence, Sims (1985) contends that personal problems and disturbed social relationships, life stressors, psychological disorders, and the abuse of alcohol and psychopharmacological agents have been associated with brain injuries or the accidents that may cause them. Selzer and Vinokur (1975), in an effort to identify those drivers who are at greater risk for having motor vehicle accidents, found an association between the occurrence of major life events, increased subjective stress, and road accidents. Connolly (1981) also found that men having accidents while alone tend to have experienced an excess of major life events in the 6 months prior to their accidents. In their work comparing taxi drivers prone to accidents to those who are not, Tilman and Hobbs (1949) report that accident prone cabbies are more likely to have divorced parents, a history of truancy and disciplinary problems in school, poor work records including being fired, going AWOL while in the armed services, or sexual promiscuity. Kerr et al. (1971), after comparing the base rate of divorce in the population to that among their head injured patients, report a fourfold increase of divorce among their subjects relative to the expected rate.

Guilford (1973) reports that motor vehicle accidents were highly correlated to accidents in the home. He argues that the incidence of accidents in general was related to emotional instability, hypochondriasis, and anxiety as well as the feeling of a lack of self-reliance and a need for freedom. As further evidence of the association between emotional disturbance and automobile accidents, MacDonald (1964) found that psychiatric disorders were 30 times more prevalent among drivers suffering fatal injuries than the general population. Furthermore, drivers involved in single-car accidents have been found to manifest significantly more psychopathology than drivers involved in multiple-car accidents (Schmitt, Perlin, Fisher, & Shaffer, 1972). Figure 4.7 presents a schematic showing the interrelationships among neurosis, accident proneness, and head injury.

Jamieson and Kelly (1973) report that, relative to noninjured individuals, adult head trauma patients tend to be young and have histories of antisocial behavior, a higher incidence of disturbance of family life, and a higher incidence of domestic and industrial accidents. This finding led Sims (1985) to speculate that head injuries may actually *precipitate* accident proneness. To the extent that head trauma results in impaired coordination and clumsiness or a loss of confidence in activities requiring coordination, victims may be at greater risk for incurring additional injury (see also Goethe & Levin, 1986). Sims points out that, following head injury, children frequently show "restless overactivity" and explosive emotional outbursts, which in turn may predispose them to additional injuries. Similarly, boxers suffering from *pugilistica dementia* (the so-called "punch drunk" syndrome) often manifest a chronic amnestic condition, progressive cognitive deterioration, impaired coordination, morbid jealousy and rage reactions, and, as a result, are more likely to suffer further injuries than someone without that pattern of behavioral disturbance (Johnson, 1969).

This notion receives some additional support from the work of Lewis and Shannock (1977), which involved the study of delinquent and nondelinquent children. The medical histories of the participants were reviewed, and the delinquent subjects were found to be more likely to have hospital contacts

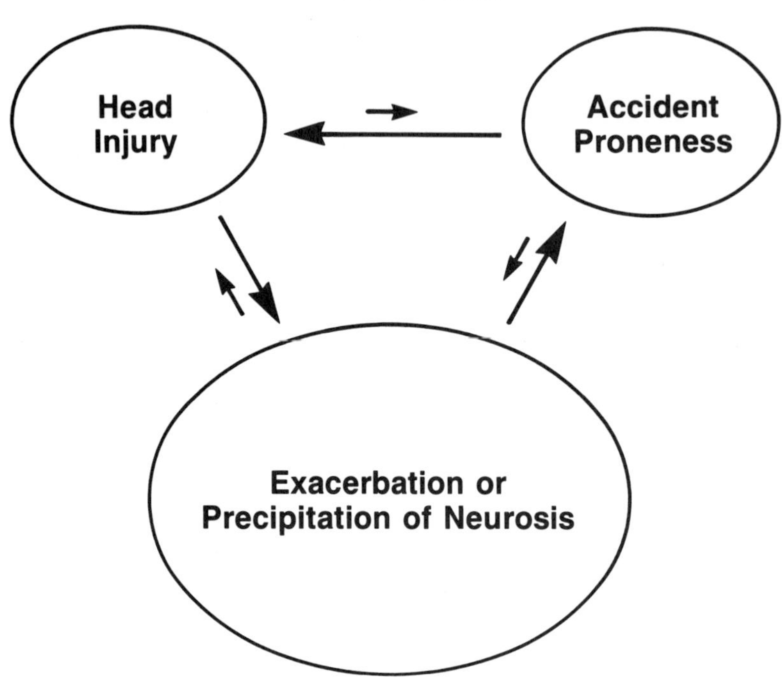

Figure 4.7. The interrelationships among neurosis, accident proneness, and head injury. Each of the links is most accurately considered as bi-directional, so that each factor in the triad is both a precipitant and an effect. *Note.* Adapted from "Head Injury, Neurosis and Accident Proneness" by ACP Sims, 1985, *Advances in Psychosomatic Medicine, 13,* p. 59. Reprinted by permission.

prior to 4 years of age and later, between the ages of 14 and 16. The authors conclude that early accidents and injuries may have contributed to dysfunction of the central nervous system, thereby exacerbating the children's impulsivity and social adaptability. Similarly, Barnes and O'Gorman (1978) report that delinquent boys aged 10 to 16 are nearly twice as likely as nondelinquents to have a history of significant head injury with loss of consciousness and admission to the hospital for more than 48 hours.

Irrespective of the reason, the risk of head trauma appears to be greater among those already injured. In contrast to earlier research that failed to uncover such a relationship (Jamison & Kaye, 1974; Klonoff, 1971; Partington, 1960), Annegers (1983) found that head injured boys are twice as likely to suffer additional injuries as those who are not head injured. A subgroup making up 4.6% of the subjects studied by Parkinson et al. (1985) had a history of prior trauma. This suggests that the risk of subsequent injury among head trauma survivors is considerable, as they constitute only approximately 0.8%

of the population at any given time (see Prevalence, above). Annegers et al. (1980) investigated this relationship more closely and determined that, for the group of subjects having suffered one head injury, the incidence rate triples; following a second injury, that rate increases to eight times the rate within the general population. They also uncovered an age-dependent relationship, with subsequent injuries being more likely to occur among those victims aged 25 and older. The incidence rate doubles for those under 14 years of age, triples for those aged 15 through 24, and continues to increase until, for people aged 25 or more, the incidence rate is five times the anticipated rate. They hypothesize that alcohol consumption may well play a role in the higher incidence among older head trauma survivors.

In addition to being more accident prone, this group is more likely to suffer more severe injuries, as subsequent trauma appears to have an additive effect (Gronwall & Wrightson, 1975; Rutherford, 1977). In support of this notion, Edna (1987) found an increased tendency for late complaints (e.g., headaches, memory problems, dizziness, irritability, insomnia, depression, and anxiety) among head trauma "repeaters" relative to those victims with only one injury.

Learning Disabilities

Some research has linked the presence of learning disabilities (LD), poor academic performance, and/or the behavioral problems associated with learning impairments to the incidence of head injury (Haas, Cope, & Hall, 1987; Rutter, 1981). Craft, Shaw, and Cartlidge (1972) uncovered a higher incidence of premorbid hyperactivity and behavioral problems in the histories of head injured children relative to their classmates, but later research suggests that a history of developmental problems and poor academic performance is primarily limited to males (Klonoff & Paris, 1974). Fuld and Fisher, in 1977, found that only three head injured children in their sample of 18 had average or better academic histories.

In their attempt to offer an explanation for the relationship between learning difficulties and closed head injury, Haas et al. (1987) note that LD students frequently have diminished attention spans, are highly distractible, have limited frustration tolerance, and are impulsive or show poor judgment. They speculate that such behavioral deficits may predispose children with LD to injury, as they are unable to accurately anticipate situations that entail risk and to plan accordingly. Similarly, "perceptual-motor deficits, figure-ground confusion, difficulty with spatial relationships and cognitive impairment persisting into adulthood may compromise one's ability to process information correctly, or to respond in a precise, calculated manner" (p. 54). Furthermore, to the extent that children so affected are stigmatized and feel rejected, isolated, and inferior to their peers due to their academic failure, they are at greater risk for developing the antisocial behavior (rebelliousness and sociopathy) or for turning to alcohol or other drugs that often predispose one to accidents resulting in physical injury.

In fact, the relationship between head injury and learning disability may be confounded to a significant extent by the association of delinquency and LD; a number of researchers have noted a high rate of learning difficulties among juvenile delinquents (e.g., Bachara & Zaba, 1978; Berman & Siegal, 1976; Duling, Eddy, & Risko, 1970). Also, delinquents often have poor peer relationships and defective interpersonal cognitive problem-solving ability as adults (Eyre, Rounsaville, & Kleber, 1982), are impulsive and distractible, and, in fact, may manifest any of a variety of psychiatric disturbances (e.g., Mendelson, Johnson, & Stewart, 1971; Morrison, 1979; Weiner, 1980; Weiss, Minde, Werry, Douglas, & Nemeth, 1971; Wood, Reimherr, Wender, & Johson, 1976). Haas et al. (1987) speculate that traumatic brain injured patients are typically characterized by poor academic achievement prior to their injuries. Among their sample of 64 patients having suffered a severe traumatic brain injury, nearly half (42.2%) showed poor academic achievement or had been labeled as learning disabled *premorbidly.* This suggests that individuals with learning difficulties are at much higher risk for closed head injuries than those without such problems.

Temporal Fluctuations

Clearly, some individuals are at greater risk than others for incurring a head injury; victims are not randomly distributed with regard to age, gender, premorbid personality characteristics, and so forth. Similarly, head injuries are not randomly distributed with regard to the time at which they occur. A number of investigations have uncovered marked hourly, daily, monthly, and seasonal variations.

Hourly Variations. Not surprisingly, head trauma occurs more frequently during those hours when people are most physically active. Accordingly, the peak hours for injury span from late afternoon/early evening to early morning. The actual hours of highest incidence vary across studies largely as a result of the means by which the day is divided into time periods. Parkinson et al. (1985) report that the majority of such injuries occur from approximately 3:00 p.m. until 3:00 a.m. Klonoff and Thompson (1969) found that 65% of patients admitted to the hospital and 70% of those seen in the emergency room were injured between 5:00 p.m. and 9:00 a.m. Children are naturally most vulnerable from the time that school ends until they go to bed in the early evening (Levin et al., 1982). Conversely, the fewest injuries occurred between the hours of 6:00 a.m. and 8:00 a.m. (Parkinson et al., 1985).

There is some variability with regard to the time at which various types of accidents occur. After dividing the day into 3-hour periods, Jagger et al. (1984) report that motor vehicle accidents occur most frequently between 6:00 p.m. and 9:00 p.m., and they are less likely to occur between 3:00 a.m. and 6:00 a.m. Less than 3% of those accidents transpire between 9:00 a.m. and noon. In the case of falls, the peak occurrence is observed between noon and 6:00 p.m. Assaults tend to occur with greater frequency in the evening hours, between 6:00 p.m. and 12:00 a.m., with the peak frequency occurring between 9:00 p.m. and midnight. Desai et al. (1983) report that only 1.4% of the assault cases of their sample took place between midnight and 6:00 a.m., suggesting that the risk of incurring such an injury does not steadily increase as the night wears on.

Daily Variations. The evidence overwhelmingly indicates that head injuries occur with greater frequency on the weekends (Anderson et al., 1983; Edna, 1987; Galbraith, Murray, Patel, & Knill-Jones, 1976; Kalsbeek et al., 1980; Klauber et al., 1981), with peaks occurring on either Friday (Edna, 1987) or Saturday (Klonoff & Thompson, 1969; Parkinson et al., 1985), depending upon the sample studied. In fact, Jagger et al. (1984) report that 41.4% of head injuries recorded in their study occurred over the 48-hour period from Saturday through Sunday (just 28.5% of the week). This is also reflected, albeit to a slightly lesser extent, in the data provided by Klonoff and Thompson (1969), which indicate that 33.6% of those head trauma patients seen in the emergency room and 34.7% of those admitted to hospital were injured over the weekend, with Saturday accounting for 20.5% and 19.9% of the emergency room and hospitalized groups, respectively. Conversely, head injuries appear to occur most infrequently on Mondays (Parkinson et al., 1985).

Monthly and Seasonal Variations. Monthly and seasonal variations appear to depend largely upon the location of the sample being studied. The weather and, not coincidentally, the monthly/seasonal rate of head injuries in San Diego County are rather stable (Klauber et al., 1981). However, most research in geographic locales where weather is more variable has suggested that seasonal variations do affect the incidence of brain trauma and that people are particularly prone to head injury requiring hospitalization during the spring and/or summer months, from April through September (Cooper et al., 1983; Edna, 1987; Jagger et al., 1984; Klauber et al., 1981; Klonoff & Thompson, 1969; Parkinson et al., 1985).

Klauber et al. (1981) found that, in San Diego in May 1978, accidents occurred more frequently than the expected rate in a number of categories: motorcycle accidents were up 80%; bicycle accidents, 55%; fights and assaults, 54%; and falls, 23%. In Minnesota, north central Virginia, and

Norway, bicycle, motorcycle, and car accidents occurred with greater frequency slightly later in the year, during the summer (Annegers et al., 1980; Edna, 1987; Jagger et al., 1984).

While the sun and warmth of spring and summer herald more activity and a concomitant increase in head trauma, in Minnesota, Winnepeg, central Virginia, and even Southern California, winter ushers in a lull, with particular drops in motor vehicle accidents and assaults (Annegers et al., 1980; Jagger et al., 1984; Klauber et al., 1981; Parkinson et al., 1985), although some researchers have noted an increase in the number of falls during those months (Annegers et al., 1980; Jagger et al., 1984). The presence of snow and ice in many of those locations might well account for the increase in falls during that period, although such an explanation makes the relative drop in motor vehicle accidents somewhat puzzling. Epidemiologic studies indicate that, despite more hazardous road conditions in the winter, fewer drivers than expected suffer head injuries, suggesting that operators of motor vehicles are more judicious in their handling of their vehicles. Also contributing to this seasonal pattern is the relative absence of bicycles and motorcycles on the road during that time.

Secular Trends. Only one study has spanned a sufficient period of time to allow for meaningful data regarding the trend of head injury over the past 40 years. Annegers et al. (1980) report that, from 1935 to 1974, head trauma rates increased for both males and females, with particular changes noted in the rate of minor head injuries. "Moderate," "severe," and fatal injuries have remained rather stable during that period of time. The authors speculate that the Great Depression and World War II likely limited travel and recreation and that people were relatively reluctant to seek medical care during that era, thus resulting in artificially suppressed incidence rates during those years.

Regional Variations

There appears to be little variation across geographic regions of the United States with regard to the incidence of head injury (Anderson & McLaurin, 1980; Anderson et al., 1983; Annegers & Kurland, 1979). Annegers and Kurland (1979) quote earlier findings revealing an annual incidence rate of 1.9% in the Northeast, 1.8% in the North Central United States, 1.5% in the West, and 1.3% in the South. However, as Fife et al. (1986) point out, most studies that have attempted to uncover such variations have not taken into consideration population density. They report that the rate of hospitalization for head trauma in Rhode Island increases as population density increases; those in urban settings are more vulnerable that those in rural areas. This is in contrast to data from Australia, where life in rural portions of the country is linked to a significantly higher mortality rate than metropolitan life.

Simpson et al. (1981) point out that the only neurosurgical units in New South Wales are found on the east coast, in Sydney and Newcastle, where 72% of the population resides. The remaining 28% of the population living in the country are overrepresented among the fatalities of head trauma, as they accounted for 39% of those deaths. In South Australia, 41% of the casualties are nonurban residents who, as in New South Wales, accounted for only 28% of the total population of the state. The availability of neurosurgical services in Adelaide is credited for the lower incidence of death from head injury there. Conversely, the difficulty in placing telephone calls to request transport to medical facilities and delays in ambulance service to rural areas likely contribute to the higher fatality rate among rural victims.

PREVENTIVE MEASURES

Incidence and prevalence data are maximally useful when they are used to guide efforts to reduce the risk and severity of head injury in the population. As pointed out by Fife et al. (1986), "Head injury is not simply a random event; it is related to living circumstances and behavior, and therefore, reducing its incidence by appropriate alterations of the social and physical environment may be possible" (p. 778). Identifying those most likely to suffer head trauma and the etiologies that are responsible for those injuries has the potential to fuel efforts to develop countermeasures and encourage legislative mandates that can potentially limit the number and severity of accidents resulting in closed head injury.

Frankowski (1986) divides preventive efforts into primary, secondary, and tertiary countermeasures. Primary measures are those that identify people at risk and seek to prevent the incidents that result in trauma. Several such countermeasures have already been implemented with promising results. Reducing the speed limit from 65 to 55 mph on the country's major highways saved an estimated 5,000 to 10,000 lives in 1977–1978 alone (Kraus, 1978). Alterations in automotive design and highway systems and programs aimed at getting intoxicated drivers off of the road are all examples of other primary countermeasures (Frankowski, 1986). Along these lines, Jagger et al. (1984) recommended a postponement of the licensing of teenage drivers by raising the legal driving age or, curiously, by limiting access to school driver education programs. Such programming has been associated with the premature licensure of adolescents without a concomitant improvement in safe driving ability that it has been presumed to foster (Insurance Institute for Highway Safety, 1980). The installation of window guards to prevent children from falling has saved a number of young children (Spiegel & Lindaman, 1977). The development and use of design modifications such as low-impact surface materials in playgrounds (Fisher, Harris, VanBuren, & DeMaio, 1980) and stair railings, stair treads, and lighting in nursing homes (Axelrod, 1986) would help to limit injuries resulting from falls among the young and elderly.

Secondary systems, which are intended to mediate the agent of the injury, include the compulsory use of restraining systems in automobiles. Many writers have endorsed such notions (Fife et al., 1986; Hawthorne, 1978; Klauber et al., 1981; Ring et al., 1986). The fact that seatbelts were worn by only 4% of those aged 10–39 (who accounted for approximately 75% of all motor vehicle accident victims in one sample) suggests the need for passive restraint systems such as automatic seatbelts and airbags (Jagger et al., 1984). As a direct result of similar efforts, child passenger laws have been enacted in many states and have been attributed with having diminished the death rate of children under the age of 5 (Decker, Dewey, Hutcheson, & Schaffner, 1984). The mandatory use of helmets by motorcyclists and bicyclists as well as equestrians, boxers, and other high-risk athletes (Axelrod, 1986) is another example of a secondary measure.

Tertiary countermeasures are those directed at altering the environment in which the injury occurs and come into play only after the accident has taken place. Examples include improving the transportation of head injured individuals to medical care facilities (Ring et al., 1986) and the development and strategic placement of emergency medical services and rehabilitation centers in order to allow for prompt care to minimize the consequences of injury (Frankowski, 1986). Another tertiary measure involves the specialized training of clinical personnel. Such training would enable personnel to more efficiently identify likely sequelae of various types of injuries and would improve their ability to treat them when they arise (Goldstein & Levin, 1987).

SUMMARY AND CONCLUSIONS

Traumatic brain injury now constitutes a major health problem. Its causes and the factors that correlate with its occurrence deserve continuing study. Identifying those agents most responsible for accidents resulting in head trauma and the populations that are most at risk provides some direction for the development of measures to prevent injuries or lessen their severity.

Approximately one-half of those injuries result from motor vehicle accidents, and another 25% are the consequence of falls. Males and adolescents and young adults are particularly vulnerable and tend to suffer more severe injuries. Alcohol consumption and other substance abuse play a prominent role in the occurrence of accidents. Those individuals with a history of psychiatric/psychological disturbance, marital discord and divorce, juvenile delinquency, learning disability, or previous head injury are overrepresented among victims. Some evidence suggests that nonwhites, individuals within the lower socioeconomic levels, and those living in congested urban areas are more accident prone than others. Accident rates increase in direct proportion to activity level, with peaks typically noted during the spring and summer months, on weekends, and from the early afternoon to early morning hours. A number of preventive measures directed at certain accident types among specific populations have been implemented with promising results, while others have been proposed or are in the developmental stages.

REFERENCES

Alterman, A.I., & Tarter, R.E. (1985). Relationship between familial alcoholism and head injury. *Journal of Studies on Alcohol, 46*, 256–258.

Alterman, A.I., Petrarulo, E.W., Tarter, R.E., & McGowan, J.R. (1982). Hyperactivity and alcoholism: Familial and behavioral correlates. *Addictive Behavior, 7*, 413–421.

Anderson, D.W., & McLaurin, R.L. (Eds.). (1980). The National Head and Spinal Cord Injury Survey. *Journal of Neurosurgery* (Suppl.), S1–S43.

Anderson, D.W., Miller, J.D., & Kalsbeek, W.D. (1983). Findings from a major U.S. survey of persons hospitalized with head injuries. *Public Health Reports, 98*, 475–478.

Annegers, J.F. (1983). The epidemiology of head trauma in children. In K. Shapiro (Ed.), *Pediatric head trauma* (pp. 1–10). Mount Kisco, NY: Futura.

Annegers, J.F., Grabow, J.D., Kurland, L.T., & Laws, E.R. (1980). The incidence, causes, and secular trends of head trauma in Olmstead County, Minnesota, 1935–1974. *Neurology, 30*, 921–919.

Annegers, J.F., & Kurland, L.T. (1979). The epidemiology of central nervous system trauma. In L. Odom (Ed.), *Central nervous system trauma research status report.* Washington, DC: National Institutes of Health.

Axelrod, D. (1986). *Head injury in New York State: A report to Governor Cuomo and the Legislature.* New York State Department of Health, Office of Health System Management, Division of Health Care Standards and Surveillance, pp. 6–27.

Bachara, G., & Zaba, J. (1978). Learning disabilities and juvenile delinquency. *Journal of Learning Disabilities, 11*, 242–245.

Barber, J.B., & Webster, J.C. (1974). Head injuries: Review of 150 cases. *Journal of the National Medical Association, 66*, 201–204.

Barnes, T., & O'Gorman, N. (1978). Some medical and social features of delinquent boys. *Journal of the Irish Medical Association, 71*, 19–20.

Berman, A., & Seigal, A. (1976). A neurophysiological approach to etiology, prevention, and treatment of juvenile delinquency. In Davis, A. (Ed.), *Child personality and psychopathology: Current topics* (Vol. 3). New York: John Wiley.

Chowdhary, U.M. (1978). Comparative epidemiology of head injuries in developed and developing countries. *Journal of the Irish Medical Association,*

71, 617–620.

Connolly, J. (1981). Accident proneness. *British Journal of Hospital Medicine, 26*, 470–481.

Cooper, K.D., Tabaddor, K., Hauser, W.A., Schulman, K., Feiner, C., & Factor, P.R. (1983). The epidemiology of head injury in the Bronx. *Neuroepidemiology, 2*, 70–88.

Craft, A.W., Shaw, D.A., & Cartlidge, N.E. (1972). Head injuries in children. *British Medical Journal, 4*, 200–203.

Decker, M.D., Hutcheson, R.H., & Schaffner, W. (1984). The use and efficacy of child restraint devices. *The Journal of the American Medical Association, 252*, 2571–2575.

Desai, B.T., Whitman, S., Coonley-Hoganson, R., Coleman, T.E., Gabriel, G., & Dell, J. (1983). Urban head injury: A clinical series. *Journal of the National Medical Association, 75*, 875–881.

Duling, F., Eddy, S., & Risko, V. (1970). *Learning disabilities of juvenile delinquents.* Morgantown, WV: Department of Educational Services, R.F. Kennedy Youth Center.

Edna, T.H. (1983). Risk factors in traumatic head injury. *Acta Neurochirurgica, 69*, 15–21.

Edna, T.H. (1987). Head injuries admitted to hospital: Epidemiology, risk factors and long term outcome. *Journal of the Oslo City Hospitals, 37*, 101–116.

Eyre, S.L., Rounsaville, B.J., & Kleber, H.D. (1982). History of childhood hyperactivity in a clinic population of opiate addicts. *Journal of Nervous and Mental Disease, 170*, 522–529.

Field, J.H. (1976). *Epidemiology of head injury in England and Wales: With particular application to rehabilitation* (pp. 1–109). Leicester, England: Willsons.

Fife, D., Faich, G., Hollinshead, W., & Boynton, W. (1986). Incidence and outcome of hospital-treated head injury in Rhode Island. *American Journal of Public Health, 76*, 773–778.

Fisher, I., Harris, V.G., VanBuren, J.Q., & DeMaio, A. (1980). Assessment of a pilot child playground injury prevention project in New York State. *American Journal of Public Health, 70*, 1000–1002.

Fitzgerald, J., & Mulford, H.A. (1981). Alcoholics in the family? *International Journal of Addiction, 16*, 349–357.

Flamm, E.S., Demopoulos, H.B., Seligman, M.L., Tomasula, J.J., DeCrestico, V., & Ransohoff, J. (1977). Ethanol potentiation of central nervous system trauma. *Journal of Neurosurgery, 46*, 328–335.

Frankowski, R.F. (1986). Descriptive epidemiologic studies of head injury in the United States: 1974–1984. *Advances in Psychosomatic Medicine, 16*, 153–172.

Freedman, L.S., Saunders, M.P., & Briggs, M. (1986). Analysis of the head injuries admitted to the Oxford Regional Neurosurgical Unit 1980–1982. *Injury, 17*, 113–116.

Fuld, P.A., & Fisher, P. (1977). Recovery of intellectual ability after closed head injury. *Developmental Medicine and Child Neurology, 19*, 495–502.

Galbraith, S., Murray, W.R., Patel, A.R., & Knill-Jones, R. (1976). The relationship between alcohol and head injury and its effect on the conscious level. *British Journal of Surgery, 63*, 128–130.

Goethe, K.E., & Levin, H.S. (1986). Neuropsychological consequences of head injury in children. In R.E. Tarter & G. Goldstein (Eds.), *Advances in clinical neuropsychology* (Vol 3, pp. 213–242). New York: Plenum Press.

Goldstein, F.C., & Levin, H.S. (1987). Epidemiology of pediatric closed head injury: Incidence, clinical characteristics, and risk factors. *Journal of Learning Disabilities, 20*, 518–525.

Gronwall, D., & Wrightson, P. (1975). Cumulative effect of concussion. *Lancet, 2*, 995–997.

Guilford, J.S. (1973). Prediction of accidents in a standardised home environment. *Journal of Applied Psychology, 57*, 306–313.

Haas, J.F., Cope, D.N., & Hall, K. (1987). Premorbid prevalence of poor academic performance in severe head injury. *Journal of Neurology, Neurosurgery and Psychiatry, 50*, 52–56.

Hawthorne, V.M. (1978). Epidemiology of head injuries. *Scottish Medical Journal, 23*, 92.

Insurance Institute for Highway Safety. (1980). High school driver education promoting early licensure. *NHTSA Status Report, 15*, 9.

Jagger, J., Levine, J.I., Jane, J., & Rimel, R.W. (1984). Epidemiologic features of head injury in a predominantly rural population. *Journal of Trauma, 24*, 40–44.

Jamieson, K.G., & Kelly, D. (1973). Crash helmets reduce head injuries. *Medical Journal of Australia, ii*, 806–809.

Jamison, D.L., & Kaye, H.H. (1974). Accidental head injury in children. *Archives of Disease in Childhood, 49*, 376–381.

Jane, J.A., & Rimel, R.W. (1982). Prognosis in head injury. *Clinical Neurosurgery, 29*, 346–352.

Jennett, B. (1972). Head injuries in children. *Developmental Medicine and Child Neurology, 14*, 137–147.

Jennett, B., & MacMillan, R. (1981). Epidemiology of head injury. *British Medical Journal, 282*, 101–104.

Jennett, B., & Teasdale, G. (1981). *Management of head injuries*. Philadelphia: F.A. Davis.

Jennett, B., Teasdale, G., Braakman, R., Minderhoud, J., & Knill-Jones, R. (1976). Predicting outcome in individual patients after severe head injury. *Lancet, 1*, 1031–1034.

Johnson, J. (1969). Organic psychosyndromes due to boxing. *British Journal of Psychiatry, 115*, 45–53.

Kalsbeek, W., McLaurin, R., Harris, B., & Miller, J. (1980). The National Head and Spinal Cord Injury Survey: Major findings. *Journal of Neurosurgery, 53*, S19–S31.

Kerr, T.A., Kay, D.W.K., & Lassman, L.P. (1971). Characteristics of patients, type of accident, and mortality in a consecutive series of head injuries admitted to a neurosurgical unit. *British Journal of Preventive and Social Medicine, 25*, 179–185.

Klauber, M.R., Barrett-Connor, E., Marshall, L.F., & Bowers, S.A. (1981). The epidemiology of head injury: A prospective study of an entire community—San Diego County, California, 1978. *American Journal of Epidemiology, 113*, 500–509.

Klonoff, H. (1971). Head injuries in children: Predisposing factors, accident conditions, accident proneness and sequelae. *American Journal of Public Health, 61*, 2405–2417.

Klonoff, H., & Paris, R. (1974). Immediate, short-term and residual effects of acute head injuries in children: Neuropsychological and neurological correlates. In R.M. Reitan & L.A. Davison (Eds.), *Clinical neuropsychology: Current status and applications* (pp. 179–210). New York: John Wiley.

Klonoff, H. & Thompson, G.B. (1969). Epidemiology of head injuries in adults: A pilot study. *Canadian Medical Association Journal, 100*, 235–241.

Kraus, J.F. (1978). Epidemiologic features of head and spinal cord injury. *Advances in Neurology, 19*, 261–278.

Kraus, J.F. (1980). Injury to the head and

spinal cord: The epidemiological relevance of the medical literature published from 1960 to 1978. *Journal of Neurosurgery* (Suppl.), *53*, 3–10.

Kraus, J.F., Black, M.A., Hessol, N., Ley, P., Rokaw, W., Sullivan, C., Bowers, S., Knowlton, S., & Marshall, L. (1984). The incidence of acute brain injury and serious impairment in a defined population. *American Journal of Epidemiology, 119*, 186–201.

Kraus, J.F., Fife, D., & Conroy, C. (1987). Incidence, severity and outcomes of brain injuries involving bicycles. *American Journal of Public Health, 77*, 76–78.

Kurtzke, J.F. (1982). The current neurologic burden of illness and injury in the United States. *Neurology, 32*, 1207–1214.

Levin, H.S., Benton, A.L., & Grossman, R.G. (1982). *Neurobehavioral consequences of closed head injury* (pp. 49–62). New York: Oxford University Press.

Lewis, D.O., & Shannock, S.S. (1977). Medical histories of delinquent and non-delinquent children: An epidemiologic study. *Journal of Psychiatry, 134*, 1020–1025.

MacDonald, J.M. (1964). Suicide and homicide by automobile. *Journal of American Psychiatry, 121*, 366–370.

McKenna, T., & Pickens, R. (1981). Alcoholic children of alcoholics. *Journal of Studies on Alcohol, 42*, 1021–1029.

Mendelson, W., Johnson, N., & Stewart, M. (1971). Hyperactive children as teenagers: A follow-up study. *Journal of Nervous and Mental Disease, 153*, 273–279.

Morrison, J.R. (1979). Diagnosis of adult psychiatric patients with childhood hyperactivity. *American Journal of Psychiatry, 136*, 955–958.

Moyes, C.D. (1980). Epidemiology of serious head injuries in childhood. *Child Care Health Development, 6*, 1–6.

Overgaard, J., Hvid-Hansen, O., Land, A.M., Pedersen, K.K., Christehsen, S., Haase, J., Hein, O., & Tweed, W.A. (1973). Prognosis after head injury based on early clinical examination. *Lancet, ii*, 631–635.

Parkinson, D., Stephenson, S., & Phillips, S. (1985). Head injuries: A prospective, computerized study. *Canadian Journal of Surgery, 28*, 79–83.

Partington, M.W. (1960). The importance of accident proneness in the aetiology of head injuries in childhood. *Archives of Disease in Childhood, 35*, 215–223.

Rimel, R.W., Giordani, B., & Barth, J.T. (1981). Disability caused by minor head injury. *Neurosurgery, 9*, 221–228.

Ring, I.T., Berry, G., Dan, N.G., Kwok, B., Mandryk, J.A., North, J.B., Selecki, B.R., Sewell, M.F., Simpson, D.A., Stening, W.A., & Vanderfield, G.K. (1986). Epidemiology and clinical outcomes of neurotrauma in New South Wales. *Australia New Zealand Journal of Surgery, 56*, 557–566.

Rutherford, W.H. (1977). Sequelae of concussion caused by minor head injuries. *Lancet, 1*, 1–4.

Rutter, M. (1981). Psychological sequelae of brain damage in children. *American Journal of Psychiatry, 138*, 1535–1544.

Schaeffer, K.W., Parsons, O.A., & Yohman, J.R. (1984). Neuropsychological differences between male familial and nonfamilial alcoholics and nonalcoholics. *Alcoholism: Clinical and Experimental Research, 8*, 347–351.

Schmitt, C.W., Perlin, S., Fisher, R.S., & Shaffer, J.W. (1972). Characteristics of drivers involved in single car accidents—A comparative study. *Archives of General Psychiatry, 27*,

800–803.

Schoenberg, B. (1978). Neurological epidemiology: Principles and clinical applications. In *Advances in Neurology* (Vol. 19). New York: Raven Press.

Selecki, B.R., Hoy, R.J., & Ness, P. (1968). Neurotraumatic admissions to a teaching hospital: A retrospective survey. Part 2. Head injuries. *Medical Journal of Australia, 1,* 851–855.

Selzer, M.L., & Vinokur, A. (1975). Role of life events in accident causation. *Mental Health Society, 2,* 36–54.

Servadei, F., Bastianelli, S., Naccarato, 18 G., Staffa, G., Morganti, C., & Gaist, G. (1985). Epidemiology and sequelae of head injury in San Marino Republic. *Journal of Neurosurgical Sciences, 29,* 297–303.

Simpson, D., Antonio, J.D., North, J.B., Ring, I.T., Selecki, B.R., & Sewell, M.F. (1981). Fatal injuries of the head and spine: Epidemiological studies in New South Wales and South Australia. *The Medical Journal of Australia, 2,* 660–664.

Sims, A.C.P. (1985). Head injury, neurosis and accident proneness. *Advances in Psychosomatic Medicine, 13,* 49–70.

Spiegel, C.N., & Lindaman, F.C. (1977). Children can't fly: A program to prevent childhood morbidity and mortality from window falls. *American Journal of Public Health, 67,* 1143–1147.

Steadman, J.H., & Graham, J.G. (1970). Head injuries: An analysis and follow-up study. *Proceedings of the Royal Society of Medicine, 63,* 3–8.

Symonds, C. (1962). Concussion and its sequelae. *Lancet, i,* 1–5.

Tarter, R.E., Hegedus, A.M., Goldstein, G., Shelly, C., & Alterman, A.I. (1984). Adolescent sons of alcoholics: Neuropsychological and personality characteristics. *Alcoholism: Clinical and Experimental Research, 8,* 216–222.

Tilman, W.A., & Hobbs, L.E. (1949). The accident prone automobile driver. *American Journal of Psychiatry, 106,* 321.

Wang, C., Schoenberg, B.S., Li, S., Yang, Y., Cheng, X., & Bolis, C.L. (1986). Brain injury due to head trauma: Epidemiology in urban areas of the People's Republic of China. *Archives of Neurology, 43,* 570–572.

Weiner, J. (1980). A theoretical model of the acquisition of peer relationships of learning disabled children. *Journal of Learning Disabilities, 13,* 42–47.

Weiss, G., Minde, K., Werry, J.S., Douglas, V., & Nemeth, E. (1971). Studies on the hyperactive child. *Archives of General Psychiatry, 24,* 409–414.

Whitman, S., Coonley-Hoganson, R., & Desai, B.T. (1984). Comparative head trauma experience in two socioeconomically different Chicago-area communities: A population study. *American Journal of Epidemiology, 119,* 570–580.

Wood, D.R., Reimherr, F.W., Wender, P.H., & Johson, G.E. (1976). Diagnosis and treatment of minimal brain dysfunction in adults. *Archives of General Psychiatry, 33,* 1453–1460.

PART II

ASSESSMENT ISSUES

5

Neuropsychological Assessment of Traumatic Brain Injury in Children

LINDA EWING-COBBS

JACK M. FLETCHER

Despite the high mortality and morbidity of pediatric closed head injury (CHI) (Annegers, 1983), few systematic, carefully controlled studies assessing neurobehavioral recovery in children have been completed. The development of educational programs geared toward remediation of residual deficits has been limited, reflecting in part the paucity of information regarding neuropsychological sequelae of head injury in children. In this chapter, we briefly discuss posttraumatic sequelae and models of neuropsychological assessment. Implications of the neuropsychological evaluation for education programming for head injured children are addressed.

Preparation of this manuscript was supported in part by the National Institute for Neurological and Communicative Disorders and Stroke. Grant NS-21889, Neurobehavioral Outcome of Head Injury in Children.

NEUROBEHAVIORAL SEQUELAE

Recent investigations of recovery from CHI have identified a wide range of alterations in cognitive and behavioral functioning. Since these studies have been reviewed in detail elsewhere (Fletcher & Levin, 1987; Levin, Benton, & Grossman, 1982), only a brief review of intellectual, motor, memory, language, academic, and behavioral sequelae will be provided to illustrate the need for broad-based neuropsychological evaluation.

The criteria used to define a severe CHI differ across studies. Severe CHI is commonly defined by a Glasgow Coma Scale (GCS) (Teasdale & Jennett, 1974) score of 8 or less on hospital admission. This corresponds to a lack of eye opening, failure to respond to commands, and an inability to verbalize. Posttraumatic amnesia, characterized by confusion and an inability to consolidate information about ongoing events in memory, is also used as a criterion for severe CHI if it persists for 1 week. In addition, coma persisting for at least 24 hours is suggestive of severe head injury.

Intelligence

A variety of studies have shown persistent declines in intelligence test scores following severe CHI in children. Levin and Eisenberg (1979) reported that intelligence scores in the low average range occurred frequently in children rendered comatose for at least 24 hours. Studies employing the Wechsler Intelligence Scale for Children–Revised indicated more severe and persistent Performance IQ deficits as compared with Verbal IQ deficits in children sustaining severe head injury producing posttraumatic amnesia for at least 1 week (Chadwick, Rutter, Brown, Schaffner, & Traub, 1981) or a GCS score of 7 or less (Winogron, Knights, & Bawden, 1984). The dissociation between the verbal and performance IQ is probably related to the different response requirements of the scales. Although the verbal subtests generally require retrieval and use of overlearned information, the performance subtests emphasize speed, motor dexterity, and problem-solving skills (Fletcher, Ewing-Cobbs, McLaughlin, & Levin, 1985). It is unclear whether IQ scores eventually return to preinjury levels. Comparison of posttraumatic IQ scores with premorbid estimates of intellectual functioning suggests that only a partial intellectual recovery is attained by most severely injured children (Levin & Eisenberg, 1979; Richardson, 1963).

Visual-Motor

Difficulties with visual perceptual and visual motor functions occur frequently following pediatric CHI. Levin and Eisenberg (1979) identified visual and spatial impairment, characterized by difficulty constructing three dimensional block designs and copying geometric figures, in nearly one-third of patients with CHI. Bawden, Knights, and Winogron (1985) reported that severely injured children were more impaired than children with mild or moderate injuries on highly speeded tasks 1 year postinjury. Severity group differences were not apparent on visual motor tasks with reduced requirements for speeded performance.

Attention and Memory

Although the capacity to consolidate and retrieve information is obviously crucial for academic success, relatively few studies have evaluated posttraumatic attentional and memory functions. The most systematic investigations of memory functions were performed by Levin and colleagues (Levin & Eisenberg, 1979; Levin, Eisenberg, Wigg, & Kobayashi, 1982). Memory impairment was the most common cognitive deficit identified within 6 months following pediatric CHI; nearly one-half of children with injuries of varying severity exhibited verbal memory deficits. By 1 year postinjury, severely injured children continued to have difficulty retrieving newly learned verbal information from long-term storage. In addition, performance on a measure of visual recognition memory was characterized by greater difficulty inhibiting responses during continuous recall, which is often associated with attentional problems on vigilance and continuous performance tasks. Similar to this latter finding, Chadwick, Rutter, Schaffner, and Shrout (1981) reported impaired performance 4 months postinjury on a continuous performance task assessing sustained attention. However, by 1 year after the injury, performance of severely injured children did not differ from that of controls. Differences in the results obtained by Levin and Chadwick may reflect differences in procedures for determining injury severity as well as the assessments of neuropsychological outcome.

Language

Despite the importance of language functions for academic performance, few studies have emphasized posttraumatic language abilities. Even subtle language processing deficiencies may adversely affect scholastic performance (Ewing-Cobbs, Fletcher, Levin, & Landry, 1985). During the acute stage of recovery, difficulties have been identified in naming, oral fluency, and auditory comprehension of complex sentences (Chadwick, Rutter, Brown, Schaffner, & Traub, 1981; Chadwick, Rutter, Schaffner, & Shrout, 1981; Gaidolfi & Vignolo, 1980; Levin & Eisenberg, 1979). In comparison to mild

CHI, injury producing impaired consciousness for at least 1 day and/or CT scan abnormalities was associated with reduced performance on composite measures of naming, expressive, and written language functions. Specific areas of difficulty included visual confrontation naming, verbal associative fluency, writing to dictation, and writing to copy (Ewing-Cobbs, Levin, Eisenberg, & Fletcher, in press).

School Achievement

Alterations in academic abilities are commonly observed following CHI. Despite the importance of academic skills for the child's adaptive functioning, few investigators have examined the type and severity of posttraumatic academic difficulties. During the initial stages of recovery, arithmetic skills appear to be the most vulnerable to disruption. In addition to computational deficiencies, these findings may reflect difficulty focusing and sustaining attention and difficulty independently organizing work. Levin and Benton (1986) identified significant reductions in arithmetic scores 6 months postinjury in comparison with both preinjury and postinjury reading scores. Schaffner, Bijur, Chadwick, and Rutter (1980) retrospectively evaluated reading ability at least 2 years following CHI producing depressed skull fractures. Fifty-five percent of the children were reading 1 or more years below chronological age level; 33% performed at least 2 years below expected levels. Klonoff, Low, and Clark (1977) reported that 26% of children less than 9 years of age at injury had either failed a grade or been placed in resource classes. Twenty-one percent of the older children received special placements. These rates are strikingly high considering the generally mild injuries in this sample. Other studies have confirmed that a high proportion of children require special classroom placement following CHI (Brink, Garrett, Hale, Woo-Sam, & Nickel, 1970; Fuld & Fisher, 1977).

Behavior

Although the severity of closed head injury is directly related to residual cognitive difficulties, the relationship between injury severity and psychosocial adjustment appears to be more complex. In the prospective research of Brown, Chadwick, Schaffner, and Traub (1981), children with mild or severe CHI were matched on a variety of social and demographic variables with children sustaining orthopedic injuries. Parent and teacher interviews and personality questionnaires were administered at the time of injury and 4 months, 1 year, and 2 years postinjury. The rates of new psychiatric disorders arising after the injury were unchanged following mild CHI or orthopedic injury. In contrast, nearly half of the severely injured children developed new psychiatric disorders. By 2 years postinjury, the rate of behavioral disturbance was nearly three times higher in the severe injury group than in controls. Despite impressive improvement in cognitive functions, behavioral disturbances persisted throughout the follow-up period. Behavioral problems commonly reflected preinjury behavior; pre-existing difficulties were exacerbated after the injury. There was no single homogeneous pattern of disrupted behavior following CHI with the exception of a tendency toward socially uninhibited behavior following severe CHI. Adverse social circumstances in the preinjury environment were also related to the presence of behavioral disturbances after severe closed head injury.

Summary

The wide range of neurobehavioral sequelae following head injury in children underscores the need for broad-based assessment of abilities. Neuropsychological assessment is crucial for maximizing adjustment to academic environments since even subtle changes in cognitive processing abilities may profoundly affect school performance. Reduction in intelligence scores may reflect changes in skills involving abstract reasoning, psychomotor speed, language usage, or sequencing. Difficulties in visual, motor, and visual-motor functions may lead to educational problems involving graphomotor activities such as writing and copying. Moreover, such difficulties often provide highly visible evidence to children for changes in their abilities. Attention and memory deficits clearly have major implications for the child's adjustment to the classroom. Although previously acquired information is frequently unaffected, learning and retaining new information may be quite disrupted. This often necessitates significant changes in the curriculum as well as modifications of child and family expectations for performance.

Additionally, difficulties in higher order processing, such as generalizing from one situation to another, independently organizing work, and reduced rate of information processing, may also affect academic adjustment. Since changes in emotional and behavioral functioning interact with alterations in cognitive functioning, family issues and the child's adjustment must be addressed. Assessment of these factors and provision of appropriate cognitive and behavioral interventions at home and at school may markedly facilitate the head injured child's adjustment.

NEUROPSYCHOLOGICAL ASSESSMENT

Neuropsychological approaches to the assessment of children are currently of great interest to practitioners in many disciplines. Neuropsychological assessment is generally viewed as the administration and interpretation of a set of psychometric tests measuring a broad range of specific cognitive abilities required for success at school and in the community. Test results are interpreted in accordance with (1) the psychometric properties of the tests and (2) additional factors such as motivational and emotional concerns that influence the child's performance. Inferences regarding central nervous system dysfunction are commonly made based on neuropsychological test findings. However, since brain-behavior relationships are less well established in children than in adults (Rutter, 1981), caution is required in interpretation of test data. Evaluation of head injured children should emphasize a description of the child's capabilities rather than issues related to localization. This is especially true because of the widespread, generally diffuse effects of CHI. Even when focal injury is present, localization of behavioral sequelae may be imprecise. For example, Ewing-Cobbs et al. (in press) and Levin, Grossman, and Kelly (1976) found that linguistic difficulties were nonspecific and did not vary consistently with the laterality of focal cerebral involvement following CHI. Independent of inferences regarding the integrity of central nervous system functions, neuropsychological assessment should generate information leading to a remedial plan addressing both cognitive and behavioral components of functioning (Rourke, Fisk, & Strang, 1986).

Approaches to Assessment

Several approaches to neuropsychological assessment can be identified. Neuropsychological batteries, traditional ability measures, and experimental cognitive tests have been used to evaluate children. For example, Rourke et al. (1986) supplement the Halstead-Reitan battery with other tests of language, attention, and memory. Other neuropsychologists, such as Wilson (1986), use traditional tests evaluating intelligence, language, and perceptual abilities as integral parts of the neuropsychological evaluation. Finally, a third approach more explicitly emphasizes assessment of specific cognitive abilities. Measures of cognitive functions from the literature on experimental child psychology are used clinically. To illustrate, Taylor, Fletcher, and Satz (1984) and Dennis (1985) use experimental measures of language, memory, and attentional functions derived from contemporary cognitive theories to clarify the nature of ability structures.

All three approaches have contributed to the expanding knowledge base on the neurobehavioral correlates of various childhood disorders. Although practitioners use different tests, the principles, goals, and methods of interpretation are quite similar. First, in each approach, psychometric tests are administered to help define the nature of the problem (e.g., intellectual, learning, attentional, language, or motor disability). Second, each approach uses other measures of cognitive skills that are correlated with the disorder. For example, head injured children often have difficulty learning and retaining new information. An attempt would be made to define the exact nature of any memory deficiencies in the context of other cognitive skills. Third, an assessment is made of environmental variables that might affect the child's test performance and habilitation potential. A child who is inattentive, unmotivated, or easily frustrated may not display true potential on psychometric tests. Cultural variables clearly influence performance on intelligence tests and have similar effects on performance on other cognitive tasks.

Fourth, information from these three levels of analysis is integrated with biological and medical data regarding central nervous system integrity. Fifth, a remedial plan is developed based on the results of the assessment. This plan will typically highlight areas for intervention, describe methods for remediation, and, if necessary, identify potential agents of intervention (e.g., special education).

Assessment Model

Figure 5.1 depicts the various levels of analysis that are common to neuropsychological assessment of children (Taylor et al., 1984). This model divides the assessment process into four components. (1) The *manifest disabilities* represent the problems leading to the assessment (e.g., school-based problems, language difficulties, problems with conduct). Assessing the manifest disability requires interviews of the child, parent, and teacher, developmental and medical histories, behavioral observation, and psychometric assessment. (2) *Basic competencies* are core skills (memory, attention, language) that correlate with the manifest disability. These skills are assessed with neuropsychological tests. (3) *Moderator variables* are social, environmental, and motivational factors that influence the covariation of the manifest disability and basic competencies. These variables impact the child's ability to cope and adjust to the presenting disorder. (4) *Biological indices* represent neurologic influences on the relationship of manifest disabilities and basic competencies. The lesion of an aphasic child, severity of a closed head injury, and family history of learning disability are examples of biological variables that would influence ability development.

The four components in Figure 5.1 can be represented as three levels of analysis. At the first level, the neuropsychologist attempts to understand the relationship between the presenting problems (Manifest Disabilities) and a set of core skills (Basic Competencies). At the second level of analysis, the influence of external factors (Moderator Variables) on the interaction of the manifest disabilities and basic competencies is considered. Children rarely develop problems that are unrelated to the environment or internal variables

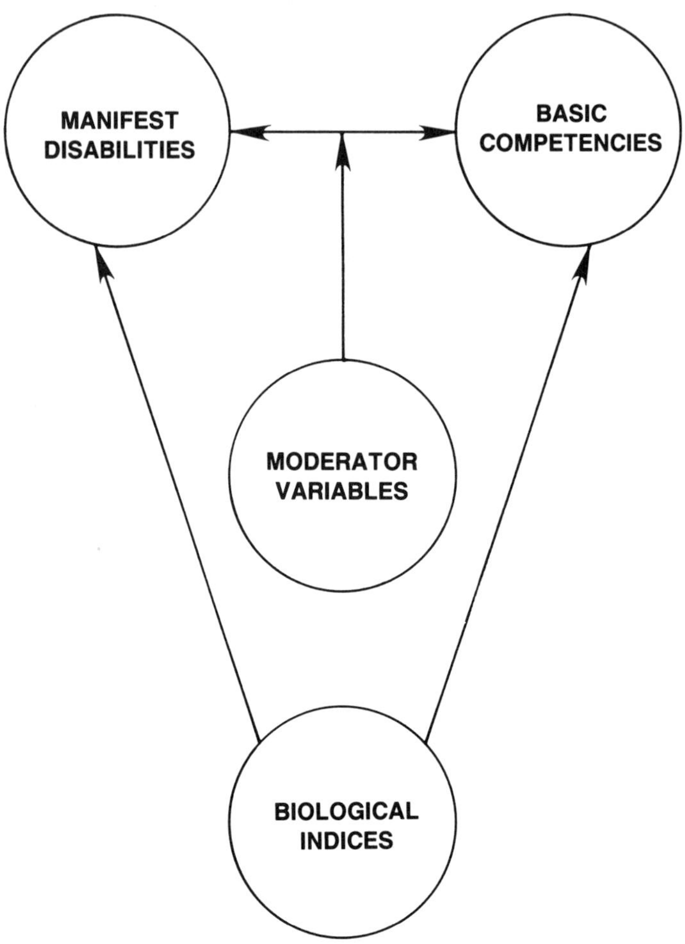

Figure 5.1. Interrelationships among components of neuropsychological assessment.

such as attitude and motivation. At the third level, attempts are made to relate the influence of central nervous system variables to the manifest disabilities, basic competencies, and moderator variables. We assume that the biological indices influence behavior. The goal is to determine the degree to which the influence is apparent in the child's ability structure. The analysis of the nature of the presenting problems begins at the level of behavior and proceeds into a more biological level. The purpose is to understand the relationship of these four components at behavioral and biological levels of analysis, not to make simplistic inferences concerning central nervous system (CNS) status

(Fletcher & Taylor, 1984). In the next section, we will apply this general approach to the assessment of pediatric CHI.

Assessment of Posttraumatic Sequelae

Neuropsychological assessment of the sequelae of head injury may serve several purposes. Assessment during the subacute stages of recovery provides a baseline level of performance that permits subsequent estimation of the degree of recovery at different time intervals. Periodic evaluations that identify changing patterns of strengths and weaknesses are useful for monitoring the efficacy of rehabilitation efforts. Neuropsychological assessment may also address the appropriateness of intervention strategies at different stages in the recovery process.

Intelligence and Academic Tests. Since IQ tests are well standardized and assess a variety of verbal and perceptual abilities, they provide a means of estimating general mental functions. Assessment of intellectual function following CHI is often required for determination of eligibility for special educational placement. Disruption of cognitive and motor abilities is sometimes not sufficient for placement of children in special education. Eligibility guidelines are often extrapolated from those designed for non-brain-injured children with learning disabilities to include traumatically injured children. Guidelines for resource room placement based on criteria for learning disabilities typically require intellectual function to be above the mentally deficient range; academic achievement scores must be at least one standard deviation below IQ scores. Consequently, IQ tests may be required if placement recommendations are to be accepted by an educational institution. Unfortunately, tests such as the WISC-R are frequently overemphasized with brain injured children and may lead to inappropriate decisions concerning placement in special education (Fletcher, in press).

Intelligence tests are often sensitive to the behavioral effects of brain injury. However, these procedures do not evaluate all aspects of a child's cognitive functioning. For example, the WISC-R provides a limited and largely indirect assessment of memory and attentional skills, which are frequently impaired in head injured children. Therefore, it is not surprising that the use of IQ tests with brain injured children is often unfair and may prevent entry into necessary special education classes. Indeed, children with severe CHI often show a reduction in IQ scores after injury; recovery appears to be incomplete in most cases (Chadwick, Rutter, Brown, Schaffner, & Traub, 1981; Chadwick, Rutter, Schaffner, & Shrout, 1981; Levin & Eisenberg, 1979). If the child is evaluated shortly after injury, the IQ scores will be reduced, and the needed discrepancy between IQ and academic achievement scores will not be established. Basic academic skills in reading and spelling are often not immediately affected by head injury (Levin & Benton, 1986). Reading problems often emerge several years after injury, reflecting the cumulative influences of the child's subtle learning deficiencies (Schaffner et al., 1980). Consequently, achievement test scores will be inflated estimates of the child's ability to function in a regular classroom and will prevent qualification for services (Ewing-Cobbs et al., 1986). As this example illustrates, results of IQ tests may be useful with brain injured children. However, they may yield a biased view of the child's abilities, thereby affecting placement and intervention.

Since intelligence tests are generally well standardized and measure a variety of cognitive skills, most child neuropsychologists include IQ tests in their evaluations. However, IQ tests are often overemphasized, reflecting current legislation and a tendency to use the tests for purposes for which they were not designed and for which they may not be well suited. For many diagnosticians, the definitions of learning disability embodied in P.L. 94-142 are not adequate because IQ and achievement tests do not measure a sufficiently broad range of skills. Educational programming for a head injured child requires much broader assessment of a variety of potentially impaired skills. This emphasis is one of the basic differences between psychoeducational and neuropsychological evaluations.

Neuropsychological Tests. The specific tests used by neuropsychologists vary considerably across settings. The common element in different test batteries is the attempt to measure a variety of skills in several key areas. To illustrate, Table 5.1 outlines the tests used by Rourke et al. (1986), while Table 5.2 summarizes tests used by Fletcher (1987). Although a brief description of measurement characteristics is provided, more specific descriptions should be obtained from the primary sources.

Both tables divide the tests into major areas. Rourke et al. (1986) emphasize tests of tactile-perceptual, visual-perceptual, language, problem-solving, motor, and "other" skills. Like Rourke et al. (1986), Fletcher (1987) administers tests of language, visual-perceptual, somatosensory (tactile), and motoric skills. While Rourke et al. (1986) also include measures of problem solving and concept formation, Fletcher (1987) emphasizes memory, learning, and attentional skills. Additional overlap between test batteries is evident; Rourke et al (1986) have tasks in the "other" category with memory and attentional components (Tactual Performance Test, Underlining Test). The commonality between batteries is the broad range of abilities measured and the nature of the constructs identified as important. The tests in Tables 5.1 and 5.2 have normative information allowing extrapolation to children and the elderly. It is not assumed that the measurement characteristics and usefulness of the tests are the same for children and adults. It is often misleading to simply take

TABLE 5.1
Modified Version of the Halstead-Reitan Neuropsychological Test Battery for Children

I. Tactile-perceptual
  1. Reitan-Klove Tactile-Perceptual and Tactile-Forms Recognition Test
    a. Tactile Imperception and Suppression
    b. Finger Agnosia
    c. Fingertip Number-Writing Perception (9–15 yrs.)
       Fingertip Symbol-Writing Recognition (5–8 yrs.)
    d. Coin Recognition (9–15 yrs.)
       Tactile-Forms Recognition (5–8 yrs.)

II. Visual-perceptual
  1. Reitan-Klove Visual-Perceptual Tests
  2. Target Test
  3. Construction Dyspraxia Items, Halstead-Wepman Aphasia Screening Test
  4. WISC-R Picture Completion, Picture Arrangement, Block Design, Object Assembly subtests
  5. Trail Making Test for Children, Part A (9–15 yrs.)
  6. Color Form Test (5–8 yrs.)
  7. Progressive Figures
  8. Individual Performance Test (5–8 yrs.)
    a. Matching Figures
    b. Star Drawing
    c. Matching V's
    d. Concentric Squares Drawing

III. Auditory-perceptual and language-related
  1. Reitan-Klove Auditory-Perceptual Test
  2. Seashore Rhythm Test (9–15 yrs.)
  3. Auditory Closure Test
  4. Auditory Analysis Test
  5. Peabody Picture Vocabulary Test
  6. Speech-Sounds Perception Test
  7. Sentence Memory Test
  8. Verbal Fluency Test
  9. WISC-R Information, Comprehension, Similarities, Vocabulary, Digit Span subtests
  10. Aphasoid Items, Aphasia Screening Test

IV. Problem solving, concept information, reasoning
  1. Halstead Category Test
  2. Children's Word-Finding Test
  3. WISC-R Arithmetic subtest
  4. Matching Pictures Test (5–8 yrs.)

V. Motor and psychomotor
  1. Reitan-Klove Lateral Dominance Examination
  2. Dynamometer
  3. Finger Tapping Test
  4. Foot Tapping Test
  5. Klove-Matthews Motor Steadiness Battery
    a. Maze Coordination Test
    b. Static Steadiness Test
    c. Grooved Pegboard Test

VI. Other
  1. Underlining Test
  2. WISC-R Coding Subtest
  3. Tactual Performance Test
  4. Trail Making Test for Children, Part B (9–15 yrs.)

TABLE 5.2
Neuropsychological Assessment Procedures for Evaluation of Basic Competencies

Construct	Test	Operation
I. Language		
	1. Word Fluency	Retrieval of words to letters
	2. Rapid Naming	Naming of common pictured items
	3. Auditory Analysis	Breaking words into phonological segments
	4. Token Test	Comprehension of sentences
	5. Peabody Picture Vocabulary Test	Comprehension of single words
II. Visual-Spatial and Constructional		
	1. Beery Visual-Motor Integration	Copying of geometric figures
	2. Recognition-Discrimination	Matching of geometric figures
	3. 3-D Block Construction	Construction of 3-dimensional block arrays
III. Somatosensory		
	1. Stereognosis Test	Lateralized haptic processing of sandpaper figures
IV. Motor-Sequential		
	1. Finger Tapping	Lateralized fine motor speed: tapping key
	2. Grooved Pegboard	Lateralized fine motor Motor speed and dexterity: peg insertion
	3. Trail Making Test	Sequential motor speed: number and number/letter connection
V. Memory and Learning		
	1. Paragraph Recall	Memory for passages
	2. Continuous Recognition Memory Test	Recognition of previously presented pictures
	3. Verbal Selective Reminding	Word list learning
	4. Nonverbal Selective Reminding	Memory for dot locations
VI. Attention		
	1. Continuous Performance Test	Selection of target stimuli from sequentially presented stream of stimuli

tests developed for adults and apply them to children (or the elderly) without considering task difficulty and differences in measurement characteristics (Fletcher & Taylor, 1984).

Behavioral Assessment. Due to the high incidence and persistence of behavior problems secondary to CHI, assessment of adaptive behavior and behavioral functioning is important for generation of appropriate intervention strategies. Estimation of the child's preinjury level of functioning in these areas is invaluable for documenting areas of strength and difficulty as well as monitoring recovery. The Vineland Adaptive Behavior Scales (Sparrow, Balla, & Cicchetti, 1984) permits assessment of habitual, everyday behavior through a semistructured parental interview. A standardized composite score, as well as standard scores and age equivalents for performance in each of the domains, is generated. The communication domain evaluates performance in receptive, expressive, and written language. Daily living skills involving personal, domestic, and community activities are assessed. To determine the level of functioning in the socialization domain, interpersonal relationships, the use of play and leisure time, and coping skills are addressed. Fine and gross motor coordination is evaluated in children under 6. Since the neuropsychological evaluation often provides an assessment of a child's optimal postinjury performance, assessment of everyday competencies is valuable for determining the level of functioning in a variety of areas.

Although a clinical interview is recommended, the interview may be supplemented with behavior checklists. The Child Behavior Checklist (Achenbach & Edelbrock, 1983) evaluates social competence and the severity of behavior problems in children ages 4 through 16. Based on factor analytic studies, behavior problems are divided into separate scales, such as Somatic Complaints, Depressed, Schizoid, Social Withdrawal, Obsessive, Aggressive, Sex Problems, and Hyperactive. In addition, separate standard scores are provided for internalizing and externalizing dimensions. However, the Child Behavior Checklist may be less sensitive than other measures to posttraumatic behavioral difficulties (Fletcher, Ewing-Cobbs, Miner, Levin, & Eisenberg, in press).

The Personality Inventory for Children (Wirt, Lachar, Klinedinst, & Seat, 1977) is an empirically constructed parental checklist that provides personality descriptions of children ages 6 to 16. Three validity scales are included to identify response sets and tendencies for parents to be defensive about their child's behavior. The Adjustment scale attempts to identify children needing psychological evaluation and serves as a general measure of poor psychological adjustment. The 12 clinical scales are Achievement, Intellectual Screening, Development, Somatic Concern, Depression, Family Relations, Delinquency, Withdrawal, Anxiety, Psychosis, Hyperactivity, and

Social Skills. The Personality Inventory for Children appears to be a promising instrument for characterizing behavioral sequelae of head injury (Rourke et al., 1986).

Limitations of the Neuropsychological Evaluation. Despite the broad range of abilities assessed in a neuropsychological evaluation, results may be misleading if findings are not interpreted cautiously. Since previously learned information is often less affected by cerebral trauma, assessment focusing on overlearned abilities such as reading may underestimate the severity of information processing difficulties. These difficulties may be apparent on tests involving abilities such as attention and the acquisition of new information. Most evaluations provide estimates of a child's optimal, rather than typical, level of functioning. If this factor is not accounted for, predictions of the child's functional abilities at school and in the community may be quite inflated.

As noted by Baxter, Cohen, and Ylvisaker (1985), the formal testing situation may minimize posttraumatic cognitive deficiencies. For example, difficulties with attention and concentration may be minimized by the structured nature of the testing situation, quiet environment, and one-on-one interaction. Moreover, the highly organized nature of the testing situation may partially compensate for difficulty initiating, sequencing, inhibiting, and monitoring behavior. While head injured children often have difficulty learning, retaining, and applying new concepts over several days or weeks, the neuropsychological evaluation typically assesses learning and retention over vastly shorter time periods. Generalization of concepts or skills to new situations is rarely evaluated. In addition, demands for quantity and rate of information processing are usually reduced in the testing situation in comparison to the classroom setting. These factors limit the accuracy of prediction of functional abilities. Through integration of information from the neuropsychological evaluation, behavioral assessment, parental interview, and teacher report, determination of the child's level of functioning can be made more accurately.

Application to Head Injury

Neuropsychologists are commonly asked to evaluate children who have sustained traumatic injuries to the brain. Manifest disabilities typically involve difficulty learning in school accompanied by conduct problems at home and/or at school. Basic competency deficits vary across individual children. Deficits occur more frequently on measures of performance-based intelligence; speeded motor abilities (e.g., rate of finger tapping); subtle aspects of language (e.g., naming); and memory and attention. Moderator variables involve the availability of rehabilitation resources in the school and the community, the child's response to the injury (e.g., depression), and the family's finances and capacity for dealing with an injured child (Fletcher, 1987).

Head injury provides an example of how to evaluate biological indices in neuropsychological assessment (Fletcher & Levin, 1987). An evaluation of injury data should include an analysis of the nature and impact of the injury (i.e., etiology). For example, it is possible to fracture the skull without sustaining a significant brain injury, depending on the severity of the impact and the nature of the injury. Impact forces may differ according to the angle and speed with which the head impacts objects, leading to different central nervous system effects. Primary pathophysiological effects of head trauma include both multifocal and generalized injury due to stretching of axonal fibers upon impact (Adams, Mitchell, Graham, & Doyle, 1977). Edema, hemorrhagic contusions, and hematomas may produce mass effects. A host of potential secondary pathophysiological effects require careful evaluation. Head injury is associated with multiple complications, including ischemic hypoxia, increased intracranial pressure, and shock. An evaluation of the child's condition would include review of Glasgow Coma Scale scores, clinical neurological status, duration of posttraumatic amnesia, and coma duration. Serial review of recovery in the intensive care unit, along with cerebral imaging procedures, will help elucidate the influence of secondary effects as well as late changes (e.g., ventricular dilation, degeneration of white matter) that occur with head injury and potentially influence behavior.

The value of reviewing injury data has been demonstrated in several studies correlating indices of head injury with specific measures of cognitive development obtained after injury. These studies show that injury severity is the overriding predictor of the degree of recovery. Variables related to severity of injury, including coma duration, GCS scores, and length of posttraumatic amnesia, are most consistently associated with recovery. The presence of brain stem abnormalities, including oculomotor and oculocephalic signs, is associated with poorer outcome on global ratings of recovery focusing on mortality and general quality of life. The locus of focal injury documented through cerebral tomography has not been consistently related to the type of neurobehavioral deficits observed (Ewing-Cobbs et al., in press; Levin et al., 1976). However, focal injury may have specific effects on the child's recovery.

This example illustrates the need to consider neurologic sources of variation in completing neuropsychological assessments of children, particularly if actual brain injury is involved. The task of the neuropsychologist is to establish behavioral and cognitive consequences of the injury and address the relationship of the injury and environment to recovery. Treatment recommendations depend on the nature of basic competency deficits, moderator variables, and habilitation options.

To illustrate the types of neuropsychological sequelae we commonly observe, two case studies are presented.

Case 1

A girl of 3 years and 8 months was immediately rendered unconscious when she sustained a severe CHI in a motor vehicle accident on February 9, 1984. Examination on hospital admission revealed no eye opening, no vocalization, and withdrawal from painful stimuli (GCS scores = 6). Pupils were equal, round, and reactive to light. Five days after the injury, she was able to follow one-stage commands. Speech was produced 13 days postinjury. At discharge, a right hemiparesis involving the upper and lower extremities, as well as the face, was present. Her gait was ataxic.

A CT scan obtained on the day of admission revealed a hemorrhagic contusion in the left basal ganglia, multiple punctate lesions in the pons, two small hemorrhagic contusions in the right temporal lobe, and a linear fracture of the left mastoid. Follow-up scans obtained 5 days and 2 weeks postinjury indicated resolution of the focal abnormalities previously visualized. However, mild to moderate diffuse cerebral atrophy accompanied by ventricular enlargement was present.

A baseline neuropsychological evaluation was performed 50 days after the injury following resolution of posttraumatic amnesia. On the Stanford-Binet Intelligence Scale (Terman & Merrill, 1972), she obtained an IQ score of 92, which is in the lower portion of the average range of functioning. Consistent with the basal ganglia hemorrhage, the main area of difficulty was apparent on tasks requiring fine motor coordination. Although incoordination of all extremities was observed, motor difficulties were most prominent on the right side. Speech was dysarthric and was characterized by effortful, halting utterances. She performed at a higher level on tasks requiring visual perception and abstract reasoning than on language-based tasks. Further evaluation of language functions using the Sequenced Inventory of Communication Development (Hedrick, Prather, & Tobin, 1974) indicated that receptive language functions were at or above age-appropriate levels. Expressive language functions were generally at expected levels for her age. However, decreased imitation of nonspeech sounds and difficulty repeating words were noted. The majority of her spontaneous utterances were average in terms of length and syntactic complexity. The remaining utterances were slightly simplified. For example, parts of speech such as adjectives and conjunctions were used infrequently.

A parental interview indicated that she was functioning above her age level prior to the injury. Because of the excellent adjustment of the child and family members to the sequelae of the injury, intervention emphasized motor and language rehabilitation as opposed to psychological intervention. She was enrolled in an early childhood education program through the public school system for provision of speech, occupational, and physical therapies. Additional motor intervention was provided.

One year postinjury, an IQ equivalent of 98 was obtained on the McCarthy Scales of Children's Abilities (McCarthy, 1972). Her performance was in the average range on verbal, perceptual-performance, quantitative, and memory scales. Motor performance was in the low average range; difficulties were most evident on tasks requiring coordination of the upper extremities. Coordination of the lower extremities was reduced by poor balance secondary to the hemiparesis. Although improvement was noted, speech remained dysarthric and was characterized by articulation difficulties; speech was occasionally explosive in nature. Visual discrimination, visual motor integration, and verbal memory were intact. Assessment of adaptive behavior revealed that her habitual level of functioning was age appropriate in communication, family living skill, and socialization domains. Motor functions continued to be below expected levels. Parental report indicated mild difficulties in the areas of attention and concentration, activity level, attention-seeking behavior, and impulsivity. Her behavior at home and at school was judged to be within normal limits for her age. We recommended that she continue attending both the early childhood education program and physical therapy. Considering the severity of the injury, the extent of neurobehavioral recovery was remarkable. In addition, since scaled scores either improved or remained the same, she was continuing to acquire new skills and information at an appropriate rate in comparison to other children.

Three years following the injury, the manifest disability involved school achievement. Continued improvement was observed in basic competency areas involving verbal, quantitative, and memory functions. Her General Cognitive Index on the McCarthy was 106, indicating functioning within the upper portion of the average range. Motor skills remained in the low average range; difficulties with speed, coordination, and balance on the right side persisted. Neuropsychological evaluation revealed performance at or above age-appropriate levels in visual perception, visual motor integration, verbal memory, nonverbal memory, and visual attention. Academic achievement scores from the Wide Range Achievement Test (Jastak & Jastak, 1978) were uniformly in the high average to superior range. Her adaptive behavior continued to be appropriate. Despite her excellent recovery and well-developed academic abilities, she had difficulty keeping up in a regular first grade classroom due to slowed motoric and information processing rates. Although intellectual and academic scores indicated average to above average abilities, these scores clearly overestimated her ability to function in a classroom setting. The school instituted curriculum modifications to reduce the amount of written assignments. We recommended speech-language therapy with an emphasis on the development of written language skills.

Case 2

A 14-year-old boy was involved in a high speed motor vehicle accident on March 9, 1983. Neurologic examination on hospital admission revealed an absence of eye opening and verbalization; application of noxious stimulation produced withdrawal of the extremities (GCS = 6). Spontaneous eye opening and vocalization were initially observed 8 days postinjury. The boy was able to follow commands 15 days after the injury.

A CT scan obtained on the day of admission was within normal limits. A repeat scan 12 days postinjury was consistent with moderate ventriculomegaly, with most prominent enlargement of the right lateral ventricle.

Following discharge from an inpatient rehabilitation facility, a neuropsychological evaluation was completed on July 7, 1983. Performance on estimates of intellectual functioning was in the average range. Memory for verbal and spatial material was well below age level. Receptive language skills were within normal limits. However, expressive language was characterized by decreased fluency accompanied by mild word retrieval difficulties. Visuomotor skills were significantly impaired, and fine motor coordination was reduced bilaterally. Assessment of academic skills revealed age-appropriate reading and spelling. Computational arithmetic was grossly impaired. Referral was made for outpatient cognitive retraining and resource placement upon resumption of school.

Considerable recovery was apparent by 1 year postinjury. Performance during the evaluation was reduced by impulsivity, which was characterized by poor planning and organization. Intellectual function recovered to the high average range. Although memory for spatial material was at age-appropriate levels, persistent deficits were apparent in the retrieval of verbal information from long-term storage. Performance on linguistic measures was within normal limits except for mild word retrieval difficulties. Considerable improvement was observed on measures of academic achievement. Reading and spelling were in the normal range while computational arithmetic was one standard deviation below expected levels. His current academic placement was on the lower track of a tiered system. Parental report disclosed persistent difficulties with concentration, fatigue, feelings of inferiority, social judgment, and school achievement.

Comparison of these findings with premorbid estimates of cognitive abilities suggested that a significant decline in most skill areas was present 1 year following the accident. The Standard Achievement Test had been administered several weeks prior to the injury. In comparison with national norms, the composite battery total was at the 75th percentile. Even though performance in many skill areas had recovered to the normal range, this represents significant residual impairment when viewed within the context of premorbid capabilities.

Three years postinjury, the manifest disabilities were poor school achievement and affective disturbance. Mild improvements were present in fine motor coordination, verbal memory, and word retrieval. Other basic competencies were basically unchanged from previous levels. Standard scores on academic achievement tests remained comparable, indicating age-appropriate development in basic academic areas. However, he failed all classes except one even though he remained in the lower tier placement and worked with a private tutor. His parents had requested that he remain in this placement although resource placement had been recommended. Even though adaptive behavior was age appropriate, he exhibited difficulty with concentration, withdrawal, depression, impulse control, and oppositional behavior. Referral for supportive psychotherapy was recommended to address issues related to self-esteem and mood.

CONCLUSION

The case samples illustrate the levels of analysis underlying the neuropsychological assessment of pediatric CHI. The initial evaluation occurs shortly after the injury, following resolution of posttraumatic amnesia. Serial evaluations are completed because of the dynamic nature of recovery and the child's changing needs. The assessment begins with the identification of manifest disabilities and relates these disabilities to a set of core skills and external variables. The assessment of moderator variables is crucial and often determines the success of any intervention plans. There is an attempt to relate these levels of analysis to parameters of the injury, but the primary goal is to establish a remedial plan for the child. This plan will change, but will serve as a focal point of subsequent evaluations. The limitations of P.L. 94-142 necessitate a careful liaison with public school officials. Advocacy efforts are sometimes necessary to establish eligibility and procure necessary services for the child. Given the level of information at the public school level concerning head injury, these efforts, which are facilitated by the neuropsychological assessment, are essential to the long-term habilitation of the head injured child.

REFERENCES

Achenbach, T.M., & Edelbrock, C. (1983). *Manual for the child behavior checklist.* New York: Queen City Printers.

Adams, J.H., Mitchell, D.E., Graham, D.I., & Doyle, D. (1977). Diffuse brain damage of the immediate impact type. *Brain, 100,* 489–502.

Annegers, J.F. (1983). The epidemiology of head trauma in children. In K. Shapiro (Ed.), *Pediatric head trauma* (pp. 1–10). Mount Kisco, NY: Futura.

Bowden, H.N., Knights, R., & Winogron, H.W. (1985). Speeded performance following head injury in children. *Journal of Clinical and Experimental Neuropsychology, 7,* 39–54.

Baxter, R., Cohen, S.B., & Ylvisaker, M. (1985). Comprehensive cognitive assessment. In M. Ylvisaker (Ed.), *Head injury rehabilitation: Children and adolescents* (pp. 219–246). San Diego: College Hill.

Brink, J.D., Garrett, A.L., Hale, W.R., Woo-Sam, J., & Nickel, V.L. (1970). Recovery of motor and intellectual function in children sustaining severe head injuries. *Developmental Medicine and Child Neurology, 12,* 565–571.

Brown, G., Chadwick, O., Schaffner, D., Rutter, M., & Traub, M. (1981). A prospective study of children with head injuries: III. Psychiatric sequelae. *Psychological Medicine, 11,* 63–78.

Chadwick, O., Rutter, M., Brown, G., Schaffner, D., & Traub, M. (1981). A prospective study of children with head injuries: II. Cognitive sequelae. *Psychological Medicine, 11,* 49–61.

Chadwick, O., Rutter, M., Schaffner, D., & Shrout, P.E. (1981). A prospective study of children with head injuries: IV. Specific cognitive deficits. *Journal of Clinical Neuropsychology, 3,* 101–120.

Dennis, M. (1985). Intelligence after early brain injury I: Predicting IQ scores from medical variables. *Journal of Clinical and Experimental Neuropsychology, 7,* 526–554.

Ewing-Cobbs, L., Fletcher, J.M., & Levin, H.S. (1986). Neurobehavioral sequelae following head injury in children: Educational implications. *Journal of Head Trauma Rehabilitation, 1,* 57–65.

Ewing-Cobbs, L., Fletcher, J.M., Levin, H.S., & Landry, S.H. (1985). Language disorders after pediatric head injury. In J.K. Darby (Ed.), *Speech and language evaluation in neurology: Childhood disorders* (pp. 97–112). Orlando, FL: Grune & Stratton.

Ewing-Cobbs, L., Levin, H.S., Eisenberg, H.M., & Fletcher, J.M. (in press). Language functions following closed head injury in children and adolescents. *Journal of Clinical and Experimental Neuropsychology.*

Fletcher, J.M. (1987). Brain injured children. In L. Terdal & E. Marsh (Eds.), *Behavioral assessment of childhood disorders* (2nd ed.). New York: Guilford.

Fletcher, J.M., Ewing-Cobbs, L., Miner, M.E., Levin, H.S., & Eisenberg, H.M. (in press). Adaptive behavior deficits following closed head injury in children. In M.E. Miner & K.A. Wagner (Eds.), *Neurotrauma 3.* Boston: Butterworths.

Fletcher, J.M., Ewing-Cobbs, L., McLaughlin, E.J., & Levin, H.S. (1985). Cognitive and psychosocial sequelae of head injury in children:

Implications for assessment and management. In B.F. Brooks (Ed.), *The injured child* (pp. 30–39). Austin: University of Texas Press.

Fletcher, J.M., & Levin, H.S. (1987). Neurobehavioral effects of brain injury in children. In D. Routh (Ed.), *Handbook of pediatric psychology.* New York: Guilford.

Fletcher, J.M., & Taylor, H.G. (1984). Neuropsychological approaches to children: Towards a developmental neuropsychology. *Journal of Clinical Neuropsychology, 6,* 24–37.

Fuld, P.A., & Fisher, P. (1977). Recovery of intellectual ability after closed head injury. *Developmental Medicine and Child Neurology, 19,* 495–502.

Gaidolfi, E., & Vignolo, L.A. (1980). Closed head injuries of school aged children: Neuropsychological sequelae in early adulthood. *Italian Journal of Neurological Sciences, 1,* 65–73.

Hedrick, D.L., Prather, E.M., & Tobin, A.R. (1974). *Sequenced inventory of communication development examiner's manual.* Seattle: University of Washington Press.

Jastak, J.F., & Jastak, S. (1978). *The Wide Range Achievement Test manual of instructions.* Wilmington, DE: Jastak Associates.

Klonoff, H., Low, M.D., & Clark, C. (1977). Head injuries in children: A prospective five year follow-up. *Journal of Neurology, Neurosurgery, and Psychiatry, 40,* 1211–1219.

Levin, H.S., & Benton, A.L. (1986). Developmental and acquired dyscalculia in children. In I. Flemhig & L. Sterns (Eds.), *Child development and learning behavior* (pp. 317–322). Stuttgart, West Germany: Gustav Fischer.

Levin, H.S., Benton, A.L., & Grossman, R.G. (1982). *Neurobehavioral consequences of closed head injury.* New York: Oxford.

Levin, H.S., & Eisenberg, H.M. (1979). Neuropsychological impairment after closed head injury in children and adolescents. *Journal of Pediatric Psychology, 4,* 389–402.

Levin, H.S., Eisenberg, H.M., Wigg, N.R., & Kobayashi, K. (1982). Memory and intellectual ability after head injury in children and adolescents. *Neurosurgery, 11,* 668–673.

Levin, H.S., Grossman, R.G., & Kelly, P.J. (1976). Aphasic disorder in patients with closed head injury. *Journal of Neurology, Neurosurgery, and Psychiatry, 39,* 1062–1070.

McCarthy, D. (1972). *McCarthy scales of children's abilities.* New York: Psychological Corp.

Richardson, F. (1963). Some effects of severe head injury. A follow-up study of children and adolescents after protracted coma. *Developmental Medicine and Child Neurology, 5,* 471–482.

Rourke, B.P., Fisk, J., & Strang, J.D. (1986). *Neuropsychological assessment of children: A treatment-oriented approach.* New York: Guilford.

Rutter, M. (1981). Psychological sequelae of brain damage in children. *American Journal of Psychiatry, 138,* 1533–1544.

Schaffner, D., Bijur, P., Chadwick, O., & Rutter, M. (1980). Head injury and later reading disability. *Journal of the American Academy of Child Psychiatry, 19,* 592–610.

Sparrow, S.S., Balla, D.A., & Cicchetti, D.V. (1984). *Vineland adaptive behavior scales survey form manual.* Circle Pines, MN: American Guidance Service.

Taylor, H.G., Fletcher, J.M., & Satz, P. (1984). Neuropsychological assessment of children. In G. Goldstein & M. Hersen (Eds.), *Handbook of psychological assessment* (pp. 211–234). New York: Wiley.

Teasdale, G., & Jennett, B. (1974). Assessment of coma and impaired consciousness: A practical scale. *Lancet, 2*, 81–84.

Terman, L.M., & Merrill, M.A., (1972). *Stanford-Binet intelligence scale manual for the third revision.* Boston: Houghton Mifflin.

Wilson, B. (1986). Neuropsychological assessment of pre-school children. In S. Filskov & T.J. Boll (Eds.), *Handbook of clinical neuropsychology*. New York: Wiley.

Winogron, H.W., Knights, R.M., & Bawden, H.N. (1984). Neuropsychological deficits following head injury in children. *Journal of Clinical Neuropsychology, 6*, 269–286.

Wirt, R.D., Lachar, D., Klinedinst, J.K., & Seat, P.D. (1977). *Multidimensional description of child personality: A manual for the personality inventory for children.* Los Angeles: Western Psychological Services.

6

Neuropsychological Assessment of Traumatic Brain Injury in Adults

C. MUNRO CULLUM

JULIA KUCK

RONALD M. RUFF

Traumatic Brain Injury (TBI) represents one of the more common etiologies of acquired cerebral damage, particularly among younger adults (Jennett & Teasdale, 1981; Rimel & Jane, 1983; also see Chapter 3 by Goldstein & Levin, this volume). Neuropsychological deficits commonly accompany TBI, and vary among individuals depending on a host of factors, including the nature of damage (e.g., closed vs. open head injury), the primary cerebral systems involved, the extent and severity of damage, and additional complicating neuromedical variables (e.g., coma duration and the presence of hematoma). In addition, intraindividual premorbid variables such as cognitive strengths and weaknesses, personality traits, and psychosocial resources also serve as mediators in the neurobehavioral sequelae of TBI. Despite the multiplicity of factors that contribute to post-TBI status, there are a number of neuropsychological deficits that tend to be commonly observed following TBI in adults. Table 6.1 lists some of the biopsychosocial sequelae that may be observed following TBI.

TABLE 6.1
Major Common Residuals Secondary to Traumatic Brain Injury

Physical	Mental	Emotional	Psychosocial
Motor Ranging from paralysis or hemiparesis to gait disturbances, reduced motor speed, and coordination.	*Attention* Ranging from altered consciousness, disorientation to hemi-inattention and distractibility.	*Irritability* Ranging from mild to severe agitation and frustration to anger and overt hostility.	*Isolation* Ranging from loss of family, divorce, to loss of friends at school or work and feelings of alienation.
Vision Ranging from blindness to visual field cuts to double vision.	*Memory* Ranging from global amnesia, varying degrees of post-traumatic amnesia to anterograde memory difficulty. May involve the processing of verbal and/or nonverbal material.	*Emotional Lability* Ranging from mood swings to alternating pessimism/optimism and silliness.	*Dependence* Ranging from 24-hr. supervision to need to rely on others for assistance in activities of daily living.
Audition Ranging from deafness to reduced hearing acuity.	*Language/Communication* Ranging from dysarthria, aphasia to anomia or subtle communication deficits.	*Depression* Ranging from suicidal ideation, loss of hope, feelings of helplessness to sadness and grief. May be long-lasting or brief.	*Status Change* Ranging from loss of vocational identity and financial loss to need to rely on state support.
Olfaction Ranging from total to partial loss of smell.			

TABLE 6.1 (cont.)

Physical	Mental	Emotional	Psychosocial
Hypersensitivity Ranging from total or partial changes in noise, light, and heat tolerance.	*Visuospatial* Ranging from disorientation to lack of spatial mapping ability and nonverbal cognitive deficits.	*Denial* Ranging from anosognosia to impaired understanding of mental and emotional dysfunction.	*Sexual Adjustment* Ranging from disinhibition or hypersexuality to insensitivity or indifference to others and/or decreased libido.
Seizure Disorder Ranging in severity and frequency, often limited to early recovery stages.	*Problem Solving* Ranging from general intellectual deficits, poor judgment, decreased abstraction to perseverative tendencies, concreteness, and problems shifting cognitive sets.	*Paranoia* Ranging from loss of trust in others to increased suspiciousness or overt paranoia.	*Drug and Alcohol Use* Ranging from infrequent to frequent use for self-medication; often decreased tolerance due to TBI effects and/or medications.
Headache Ranging from consistent to occasional pain.		*Anxiety* Ranging from generalized stress disorder to episodic anxiety.	
Energy Level Ranging from anergia to increased fatigue and reduction of energy toward end of day.	*Initiation* Ranging from impulsiveness to indecisiveness to anergia.		

The goal of this chapter is to address some of the key issues in the neuropsychological evaluation of the adult TBI patient and to provide an overview of the deficits commonly seen in association with TBI. We begin with a discussion of the role of neuropsychological assessment as an important component in the comprehensive multidisciplinary evaluation of the TBI patient. Following a brief discussion of various approaches to neuropsychological assessment, an overview is presented of those areas of cognitive functioning that require careful evaluation, along with representative findings in the TBI literature. A subsequent section addresses the special considerations in the neuropsychological assessment of TBI, and finally, we outline some of the limitations and challenges faced by neuropsychology in the assessment of TBI, which serves to conclude what can only be a limited overview of such a complex, multifaceted topic.

THE ROLE OF NEUROPSYCHOLOGICAL ASSESSMENT IN TBI

As part of a multidisciplinary evaluation of TBI, comprehensive neuropsychological assessment provides one of the most sensitive measures of cerebral functional status. Although focal and/or generalized neurostructural findings (most commonly ventricular dilation, cortical atrophy, edema, and sometimes focal contusions or hemorrhage) may be observed on CT or MRI, persistent cognitive deficits can occur in patients in the absence of detectable neuroradiological findings (Bigler, 1987). Such deficits may be a result of trauma-induced neurophysiological changes and/or microscopic changes in brain tissue (particularly in the white matter) that fall below the resolution of current neuroimaging techniques (e.g., see Genarelli, Adams, & Thibault, 1982; Kwentus, Hart, Peck, & Kornstein, 1985).

Whereas the utility of the comprehensive neuropsychological evaluation in the acute phase following moderate to severe TBI may be limited (e.g., due to patients' level of consciousness and their ability/willingness to cooperate), neuropsychological assessment of cognitive functions in post-TBI patients can not only yield information important regarding the patient's current level of functioning, but also provide baseline data that can be compared with later follow-up evaluations. In this way, the *nature and degree* of recovery of various abilities over time can be psychometrically assessed and clearly documented. The adoption of a comprehensive approach to neuropsychological assessment furthermore allows for a multidimensional characterization not only of an individual's deficits, but also of his or her strengths. In addition, information from such an assessment can be useful to not only the rehabilitation team, but also to patients and their families. Clinically, for example, it can be both informative and therapeutic for a patient to know that 3 months postinjury he or she was functioning at the 5th percentile in a particular area of ability in comparison to peers, and now, 8 months later, is at the 25th percentile.

In order for a neuropsychological (NP) evaluation to be comprehensive, the test results must incorporate historical information, neuromedical findings, and behavioral observations from clinical interviews as well as during testing. These latter sources of data can be critical in evaluating a patient's performance, since many factors (e.g., motivation, fatigue, psychiatric status, and ability to cooperate) can have a major impact on test results. In addition, although often given too little attention in practice, the comprehensive NP evaluation should include an assessment of patients' emotional status and psychological adjustment (see Chapter 17 by Lezak & O'Brien and Chapter 9 by McGuire & Sylvester, this volume). Information from these various sources is then integrated into the interpretation of the test results to produce an overall neurobehavioral characterization of patients' brain-behavior deficits as well as strengths. These data augment patient information gathered by other disciplines (e.g., neurology, neurosurgery, psychiatry and speech, occupational, and physical therapy) and thus serve as an important component in the multidisciplinary approach to TBI assessment and treatment. Table 6.2 summarizes some of the primary functions of NP assessment in TBI.

The Referral Question

The primary aim of the neuropsychological evaluation is to be sensitive to the clinical and/or research questions that prompt the referral. Therefore, the neuropsychologist needs to be aware "why" this specific patient was referred, then determine "what" the unique needs are. In the following section, a number of key issues relevant to the referral process are discussed.

Most referring clinicians are interested in having the neuropsychologist provide documentation of the patient's level of cognitive functioning beyond the general level of information provided by bedside mental status examinations and instruments such as the Glasgow Coma Scale (Teasdale & Jennett, 1974), the Galveston Orientation and Amnesia Test (GOAT; Levin, O'Donnell, & Grossman, 1979), and the Mini-Mental State Examination (Folstein, Folstein, & McHugh, 1975). To even begin to depict the range of human cognitive abilities requires the evaluation of an array of functions and, accordingly, the generation of a comprehensive neuropsychological patient profile. As part of any neuropsychological examination, it is imperative that the evaluation not only focus on deficits, but also determine relative areas of strength for each patient. Preferably, a functionally based multidimensional profile should be established that is based on sound psychometric classifications (i.e., including T or Z scores and/or percentile ranks which readily allow

TABLE 6.2
Functions of Neuropsychological Assessment in TBI

Assess presence, severity, and nature of cognitive dysfunction.
Establish baseline characterization of neurobehavioral strengths and weaknesses.
Make treatment recommendations.
Outline likely prognosis.
Provide postevaluation feedback.
Consult with cognitive remediation team and/or psychotherapist (individual, marital, and/or family) where indicated.
Evaluate cognitive recovery over time.

for comparison with normative samples of individuals of similar age, sex, and educational backgrounds). Only from a profile of relative strengths and weaknesses across an array of NP domains can information be provided about potential compensatory strategies that may be available to the patient. For example, if a patient has a severe nonverbal memory deficit and the potential for additional recovery appears low, that patient might be encouraged to utilize verbal cues to help compensate for his or her nonverbal memory problem.

Prognosis

Information from the NP evaluation is frequently requested to help establish a likely prognosis, since the aggressiveness and focus of the treatment program may depend on the potential for recovery. All too often, global indices such as intelligence test scores are used to presumably (yet inadequately) gauge the severity of a patient's deficits, and it is up to the neuropsychologist to prevent misinterpretation of such data and to provide information that more accurately depicts a patient's post-TBI status. It also is the neuropsychologist's responsibility to educate referral sources as to what questions can and should be asked regarding patients' cognitive abilities. In the case of TBI, the question regarding a patient's recovery over time is often asked, and therefore follow-up assessments are frequently needed. In repeat evaluations, "baseline" test results are compared with later assessments, thereby allowing for a detailed analysis of functional changes over time. In this manner the neuropsychologist can address not only basic referral questions pertaining to the presence and severity of deficits, but also the pattern of recovery of function over time. Some interpretive difficulty can arise in this area, however, since practice effects of repeated tests can contribute to increases in performance over time. The use of alternate test forms can help address this issue, although such forms are not available for the majority of NP tests. Thus it is up to the neuropsychologist to partial out the likely effects of practice from recovery of function per se.

With regard to prognosis, we still are at a primitive level of actuarial prediction of specific long-term TBI sequelae. If we consider the most basic outcome as being survival following TBI, however, we know from a variety of studies that a patient with severe TBI (Glasgow Coma Scale score below 8) has a 50% to 70% chance of survival (Levin, Benton, & Grossman, 1982, p. 64). Defining what constitutes good or poor outcome has also varied across investigators, although the Glasgow Outcome Scale (Jennett & Bond, 1975) has been popularly used to describe four levels of recovery, ranging from persistent vegetative state, severe disability, and moderate disability to good recovery. Each of these categories involves a clinical judgment regarding patients' level of physical, cognitive, and social functioning, although these reflect global ratings and do not address more specific areas of functional recovery. Other general areas by which recovery can be defined include return to employment, degree of independence, and social adjustment, although specific operational definitions for each of these can be difficult and may reflect only partial aspects of what we mean by recovery (see Brooks, 1987, for a discussion of the difficulties in defining and measuring recovery from TBI).

As noted, predicting recovery of specific abilities is much more difficult than predicting general outcome, yet it is so often asked about early in the recovery period. Results from NP evaluations completed within a few months following TBI have been shown to be related to test performance at 1 year (Dikmen & Temkin, 1987), although such long-term predictive power is only at a global level and is far from perfect. Comparing the results of serial assessments of TBI patients over time has the additional complicating factor of potential practice effects, which thereby may lead to an overestimation of recovery (Brooks, 1987). Nevertheless, having some basic information regarding patients' current NP status, their age at the time of injury, additional medical complications, and so on, in addition to some notion regarding their premorbid abilities (which will be discussed later), the neuropsychologist can make some prognostic statements with some degree of confidence. For example, if a TBI patient has recovered to the 50th percentile on a measure of vocabulary at 6 months postinjury (and there is good reason to believe that his or her premorbid level of functioning in this area was no greater than this), it is unlikely that much additional improvement in this area will occur.

Large-scale multiple regression studies of TBI patients and demographically similar controls are needed to better address the issue of recovery of specific cognitive abilities.

THEORETICAL AND PRACTICAL CONSIDERATIONS IN NEUROPSYCHOLOGICAL ASSESSMENT

There are a number of popular approaches to neuropsychological assessment of brain function. These approaches often utilize different measures and reflect different clinical and theoretical orientations. A complete review of the multitude of neuropsychological measures in use with TBI patients is well beyond the scope of this chapter, but a brief discussion of some of the more important areas of cerebral functioning that should be assessed in the comprehensive NP evaluation will be presented following a discussion of some major approaches to NP assessment.

As noted, a number of different theoretical and procedural orientations exist among clinical neuropsychologists. For example, many use a standard battery of NP tests in the evaluation of brain injured patients, yet the specific components of such batteries tend to vary across settings. Some occasionally heated debates regarding the "best" tests or batteries of tests occur, yet the important underlying issue is whether the measures used represent valid, reliable indicators of cerebral function. (Also, of course, the background and skills of the neuropsychologist interpreting the test results are of extreme importance!)

Neuropsychological Test Batteries and Normative Data

The more popular batteries of neuropsychological tests generally are composed of standard psychometric measures that have (in some cases) been administered to large samples of non-brain-damaged populations, thereby providing normative data by which to compare the performance of patients with known brain dysfunction. When a patient is evaluated, his or her scores on various measures can then be compared with data from non-brain-injured individuals. Ideally, data from nonneurologic and nonpsychiatric individuals of similar age and educational backgrounds are utilized in this comparison.

"Cutoff" scores which statistically separate brain damaged from non-brain-damaged individuals are commonly used on a number of neuropsychological measures, although the characteristics of the population in whom the cutoff scores were derived must be carefully considered when interpreting an individual's performance. This is a particularly important point with respect to background variables such as age, education level, and in some instances gender, which have been shown to be significantly related to the level of performance on many NP measures (Heaton, Grant, & Matthews, 1986; Parsons & Prigatano, 1978). To illustrate, blindly applying norms and cutoff scores derived from middle class college sophomores to the case of a 65-year-old TBI patient with 5 years of formal education might suggest that the individual has a variety of moderate or even severe cognitive deficits as a result of TBI, when in fact, performance might be within normal limits for someone of that age and educational level. Thus, whereas normative data are critical in the interpretation of NP test results, the sample from which the norms were derived must be considered, and traditional cutoff scores may be inappropriate in some individual cases.

The Standard or Fixed Battery Approach

The standard or fixed battery approach uses a predetermined group of tests that (hopefully) assess a variety of abilities, and the entire battery typically is administered to all patients, regardless of primary presenting complaint or referral question. The number of individual test batteries in use today is potentially as large as the number of different centers using NP measures to assess brain function, although the group of tests developed by Ward Halstead and modified by Ralph Reitan, known as the Halstead-Reitan neuropsychological battery, is still probably the most popular (see Reitan, 1986, for a discussion of the approach and theoretical rationale). In most centers where the Halstead-Reitan battery is used, the battery is supplemented by additional measures, most notably an assessment of general intellectual abilities, academic skills, and, most important, measures of verbal and nonverbal memory, which are absent in the original battery alone. Many clinical and research laboratories have adopted at least some of the HRB measures for use in the assessment of brain injured patients, even when the entire battery is not utilized.

Other standard or fixed batteries of NP tests have been constructed (e.g., probably the second most popular fixed battery being the Luria-Nebraska NP test battery; Golden, Hammeke, & Purisch, 1978), and as noted, a key factor in the composition of such batteries is that a wide range of neuropsychological abilities be assessed to allow for a comprehensive evaluation. Whereas there are no right or wrong NP test batteries in capable hands, measures that are lacking in important theoretical and psychometric properties (i.e., validity and reliability) certainly cannot be recommended.

The standard battery approach has the advantage of obtaining the same test measures on all subjects, thereby facilitating comparison across groups on any of a number of measures. This is particularly important in research settings, since the problem of missing data on various tests (which, e.g., would interfere with statistical analyses) is substantially reduced. (See Lezak, 1983, for further discussion of common test batteries.) In the context of a fixed battery approach, many neuropsychologists use brief screening measures and/or stepdown batteries in those cases where a larger-scale evaluation may not be feasible (e.g., in the severely brain injured patient with limited cognitive resources). The standard battery approach also has the advantage of being readily administered by well-trained technicians, since test selection by the interpreting neuropsychologist typically is not an issue.

The Eclectic or Flexible Battery Approach

In contrast to the use of a standard battery, the eclectic or flexible approach emphasizes the selection of measures based on the presenting problem and may be further modified based on the patient's performance during the evaluation. Other considerations that can be addressed using a flexible approach include the time-cost factor in administering the battery and available clinical resources such as technician support. In addition, intraindividual patient variables such as physical condition, degree of cognitive impairment, attentional capabilities, age, and education level also may help determine which measures are administered. Such an approach has the advantages of allowing for specific test selection and hypothesis testing, and of readily allowing for the addition of new measures as they are developed. The use of varying groups of tests across patients allows full exploration of specific questions or deficits, yet this may make comparison of patient populations difficult, depending on the number of overlapping measures. Currently an enormous array of NP measures (including standard clinical instruments as well as specialized research tools) is available for assessing a wide variety of cognitive abilities. Although we will mention some popular measures that typify the assessment of certain types of abilities, the reader is referred to Lezak (1983) for a comprehensive compendium of popular NP tests.

The Mixed Model Approach

It should be noted that the adoption of an eclectic approach to NP assessment can be incorporated into the context of a standard battery (i.e., allowing for the administration of additional measures depending on the individual case). In such an approach, a standard core group of tests is administered to most or all patients typically within a time frame of 3–4 hours. Additional measures are subsequently added to address specific clinical and/or research questions; for example, Ruff and colleagues have developed such an approach utilizing the San Diego Neuropsychological Test Battery (Baser & Ruff, 1987). As with the flexible approach, this method is most popular in clinical settings wherein comparison of patient groups across the same measures tends to be less critical.

The mixed model approach offers the capacity for individual adaptation while providing basic information about cognitive functioning which is available for all patients assessed. One rationale behind this approach in the case of TBI is to have an assessment available that is relatively brief and appropriate if the patient is in the early phase of recovery. A second reason for utilizing a mixed model approach is based on the likelihood that the patient will need to be evaluated longitudinally. Therefore, if a core group of tests is consistently employed, comparison across measures over time will be possible. This approach also provides the flexibility to administer additional tests that may be necessary before the patient enters a rehabilitation program. For example, if the patient is to participate in a cognitive remediation program, more detailed testing may be required (e.g., in the areas of attention and memory). Like the flexible approach, the mixed model additionally allows for the incorporation of new ideas and techniques. Figure 6.1 depicts a schematic representation of a mixed model approach to NP assessment, with additional testing and rehabilitation modules added when indicated.

AREAS OF COGNITIVE FUNCTIONING THAT SHOULD BE ASSESSED

All neuropsychological evaluations of TBI patients should be comprehensive to the extent that an array of cognitive abilities is assessed. Even brief neuropsychological screening evaluations and mental status examinations should assess multiple areas of cognition. If an assessment is too narrowly focused, significant deficits may be overlooked altogether. Additionally, inadequate assessment of abilities may result in misleading findings, since the efficacy of some cognitive abilities is dependent on the integrity of other processes. To illustrate, dysfunction of basic abilities (e.g., attention/concentration) may result in deficit performance on other, more complex measures, and poor performance on such measures in isolation may occur as a result of a multitude of factors. These issues are of particular importance in the assessment of TBI, since the nature of the damage to the CNS tends to be generalized, even when more focal deficits are present (see Chapter 2 by Bigler, this volume). A comprehensive approach acknowledges the importance of global evaluation across domains in view of the extreme complexity of human cognitive functions.

Administration of tests that tap a variety of abilities also is important from the standpoint of interpreting the overall *pattern* of results (qualitative as well

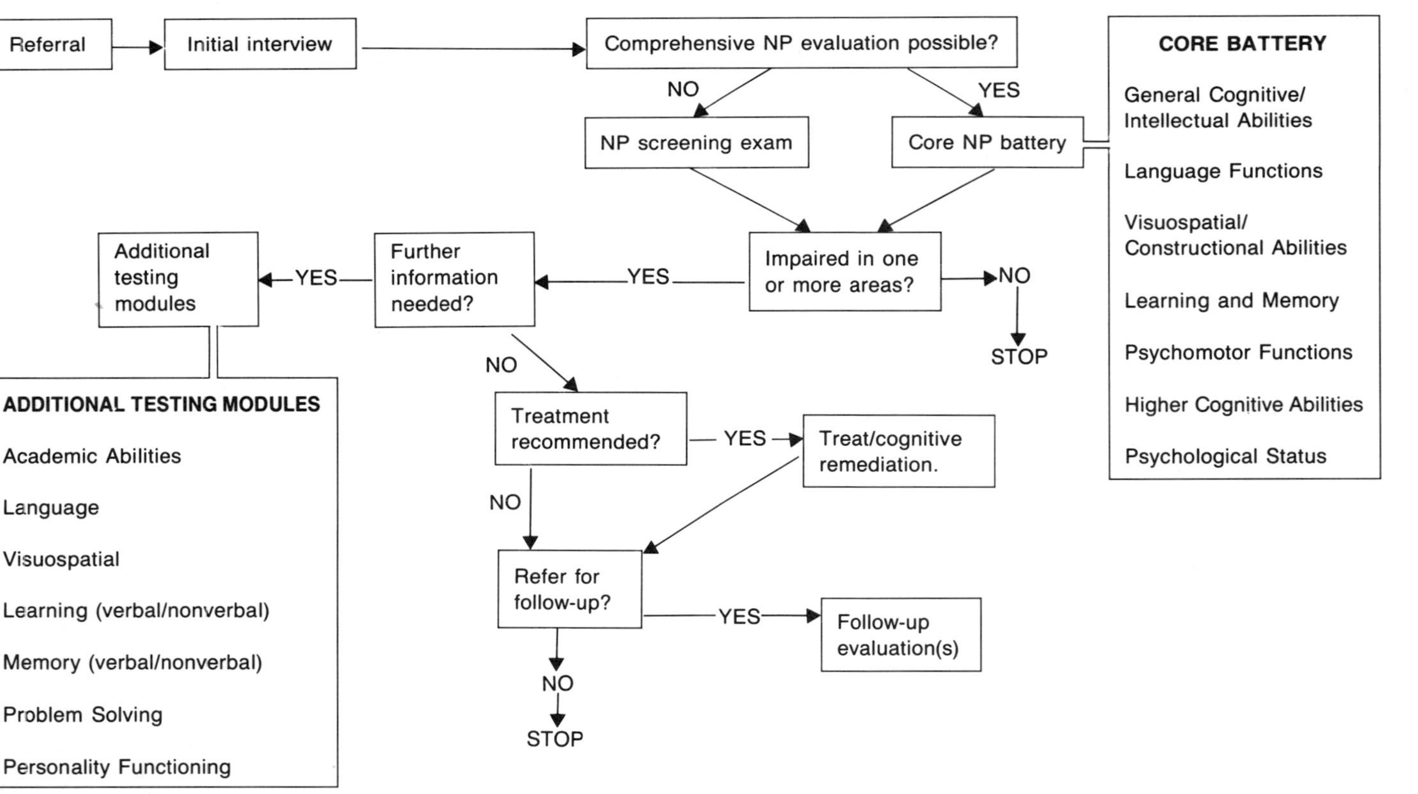

Figure 6.1. Example of mixed model neuropsychological evaluation/treatment approach.

as quantitative), in addition to the *level* of performance on each measure. As a rule, single, unidimensional measures should not be interpreted in isolation, and only with the comparative interpretation of a number of measures can specific conclusions be reached regarding the implications for underlying cerebral dysfunction. When screening evaluations are indicated (e.g., in severely dysfunctional patients), instruments such as the Dementia Rating Scale (Mattis, 1976), commonly used in the assessment of dementia patients, may be useful, since some quantitative measure of a variety of abilities is obtained that can be compared with subsequent evaluations. Such instruments may be inappropriate in the case of mild to moderate TBI, however, because of ceiling effects, and thus the administration of measures more sensitive to subtle cerebral dysfunction is in order. Issues involved in the interpretation of NP test results are discussed in a subsequent section.

Some of the basic areas of cognitive function that should generally be assessed in the TBI patient include general cognitive/intellectual abilities, language, visuospatial and constructional abilities, attention and concentration skills, verbal and nonverbal learning and memory abilities, psychomotor functioning, and higher cognitive abilities (e.g., abstract reasoning, novel problem solving, cognitive flexibility). In the following section, these areas of NP function are addressed briefly, and representative findings from the TBI literature are discussed. It should be noted that any categorical listing of areas of cognitive function is to some degree arbitrary, since many NP measures require a number of similar underlying abilities. A listing of some of the more popular measures in use today along with the functional areas assessed is provided in Table 6.3. For a more comprehensive compendium of NP tests, the reader is referred to Lezak (1983).

I. General Cognitive/Intellectual Abilities

TBI frequently impacts a variety of underlying cerebral functions which may result in lowered intellectual capabilities compared with premorbid abilities. In terms of assessment, the Wechsler Adult Intelligence Scale–Revised (WAIS-R; Wechsler, 1981) IQ scores are commonly used as indices of overall cognitive/intellectual functioning in clinical as well as research settings. Although designed for intellectual assessment per se, the WAIS-R scales have proven to be useful and popular in NP assessment. IQ scores, which provide a global index regarding overall intellectual status, are commonly reported in studies of TBI and can be clinically useful if interpreted appropriately. It is, however, critical that more weight is given to interpreting the individual subtests rather than the overall IQ scores. To further illustrate, specific functional deficits (e.g., visual field cuts, hemi-paresis, attention deficits, etc.) can confound specific NP subtest performances, and thereby lower the

TABLE 6.3
Major Cognitive Functional Areas and Popular NP Measures

Functional Areas	Popular Measures	Reference
I. *General Cognitive/Intellectual Abilities*	Wechsler Adult Intelligence Scale–Revised (WAIS-R)	(Wechsler, 1981)
II. *Language Functions*	Aphasia Screening Test	(Reitan, 1984)
	Boston Diagnostic Aphasia Exam	(Goodglass & Kaplan, 1983)
	Controlled Oral Word Association Test	(Benton & Hamsher, 1976)
	"FAS": Verbal Associative Fluency Test	(Benton, 1968)
	Peabody Individual Achievement Test	(Dunn & Markwardt, 1970)
	Token Test	(Boller & Vignolo, 1966)
	Wide Range Achievement Test–Revised: Spelling and Reading subtests	(Jastak & Jastak, 1984)
III. *Visuospatial/Visuomotor/Visuoconstructional Abilities*	WAIS-R: Block Design, Digit Symbol, Object Assembly	(Wechsler, 1981)
	Trail Making Test	(Reitan & Davison, 1974)
	Boston Parietal Drawings	(Goodglass & Kaplan, 1983)
	Hooper Visual Organization Test	(Hooper, 1958)
	Rey-Osterrieth Complex Figure–Copy	(Lezak, 1983)
	Tactual Performance Test	(Halstead, 1947; Reitan & Davison, 1974)
	Wechsler Memory Scale–Revised (WMS-R): Visual Reproductions–Copy	(Wechsler, 1987)

TABLE 6.3 (cont.)

Functional Areas	Popular Measures	Reference
IV. *Attention/Concentration*	Digit Span (WAIS-R)	(Wechsler, 1981)
	Digit Vigilance	(Lewis & Kupke, 1977)
	The 2 & 7 Test	(Ruff, Evans, & Light, 1986)
	Paced Auditory Serial Addition Test	(Gronwall, 1977)
	Block Span	(Milner, 1971)
	Seashore Rhythm Test	(Reitan & Davison, 1974)
	Speech Sounds Perception Test	(Reitan & Davison, 1974)
	The Stroop Test	(Stroop, 1935)
V. 1) *Learning Ability:*		
A) Verbal Modality	California Verbal Learning Test (CVLT)	(Delis, Kramer, Kaplan, & Ober, 1987)
	Rey Auditory Verbal Learning Test	(Lezak, 1983)
	Story Learning Test	(Heaton, Nelson, Thompson, Burkes, & Franklin, 1985)
	Selective Reminding Test	(Buschke & Fuld, 1974)
	WMS-R: Verbal Paired Associate Learning	(Wechsler, 1987)
B) Nonverbal Modality	WMS-R: Visual Paired Associates	(Wechsler, 1987)
	Visual Learning Test	(Heaton et al., 1985)
	Ruff-Light Trail Learning Test	(Ruff & Light, 1984)

TABLE 6.3 (cont.)

Functional Areas	Popular Measures	Reference
2) *Memory Ability:*		
A) Verbal Modality	CVLT: Delayed & Cued Recall, Recognition	(Delis et al., 1987)
	RAVLT: Recall & Recognition	(Lezak, 1983)
	Wechsler Memory Scale (WMS)	(Wechsler, 1945)
	WMS-R: Verbal subtests	(Wechsler, 1987)
	Story Memory Test	(Heaton et al., 1985)
B) Nonverbal Modality	WMS-R: Nonverbal subtests	(Wechsler, 1987)
	Benton Visual Retention Test	(Benton, 1974)
	Rey-Osterrieth Figure: Recall	(Lezak, 1983)
	Visual Memory Test	(Heaton et al., 1985)
	Tactual Performance Test: Memory & Location	(Reitan & Davison, 1974)
VI. *Motor Functioning*	Finger Tapping Test	(Reitan & Davison, 1974)
	Grip Strength	(Reitan & Davison, 1974)
	Grooved Pegboard	(Klove, 1963)
VII. *Higher Cognitive Functioning*	Category Test	(Reitan & Davison, 1974)
	Wisconsin Card Sorting Test	(Grant & Berg, 1948; Heaton, 1981)
	Figural Fluency Test	(Ruff, Evans, & Marshall, 1986)
	Raven's Progressive Matrices	(Raven, 1960)
	WAIS-R: Similarities	(Wechsler, 1981)
	California Proverb Test	(Delis, Kramer, & Kaplan, 1987)
VIII. *Psychological Status*	Minnesota Multiphasic Personality Inventory (MMPI)	(Hathaway & McKinley, 1967)
	Neurobehavioral Rating Scale	(Levin et al., 1987)

patient's overall IQ scores; it obviously would be erroneous to necessarily interpret this lowered IQ as representing a global reduction of intellectual functioning in such cases.

Even though Verbal and Performance IQ differences may have some implications for the relative lateralization of brain damage in some cases, it is known that in general, the verbal subtests as a group tend to be less sensitive to acquired brain damage in adults (Bigler, Steinman, & Newton, 1981; Russell, 1979). These measures require more overlearned, well-established, or "crystallized" cognitive abilities that are less susceptible to the effects of TBI. On the other hand, the performance subtests as a group represent more fluid types of tasks, requiring adaptive, novel learning abilities that are more readily affected by cerebral dysfunction (Cullum, Steinman, & Bigler, 1984). In any case, it should be noted that general omnibus measures of a patient's cognitive status can be useful in the global characterization of an individual's general abilities, yet such measures alone are entirely inadequate in the assessment of brain injured patients. Significant generalized cerebral damage and/or specific, circumscribed deficits may go undetected without administration of additional NP measures.

Literature Findings. As noted, a general decline in intellectual abilities is common in TBI, particularly when structural brain damage is present (Bigler et al., 1981). Beyond assessing the presence and extent of cognitive deficit, however, the neuropsychologist is often asked about recovery potential. Levin et al. (1982) reviewed 17 studies that examined intellectual recovery following closed head injury. Unfortunately, comparison across studies is difficult because of a number of factors, including different selection/ screening criteria, differential and/or unclear assessment of posttraumatic amnesia (PTA), and varying means of defining TBI severity. Not surprisingly, there nevertheless appears to be a consistent finding of a decrease in intellectual test performance in the early stages of recovery following TBI that is related to the severity of injury. Longer coma and PTA duration and age at the time of injury tend to be associated with lower intellectual test scores in those studies that have examined these factors (Brooks, 1983; Jennett, 1986).

More disagreement is found among investigators examining the longer-term effects of TBI on intellectual processes. It appears that a great deal of intellectual recovery is possible following even severe TBI, although whether individuals return to premorbid levels of functioning remains an issue and is dependent on a host of factors. In Mandleberg and Brooks's (1975) often-cited study of serial WAIS administrations to patients with severe TBI (all had PTA over 4 days; 88% over 7 days), for example, patients demonstrated clearly impaired scores initially, yet their IQ scores improved over time and eventually reached the average range. This recovery was more rapid for Verbal IQ (approximately 1 year) than Performance IQ (approximately 3 years), but nevertheless was suggestive of improved functioning. Such results should by no means be taken to indicate that TBI patients recover to their premorbid level of functioning, however, since the ultimate scores of "recovered" patients (despite possibly being in the average range) may in fact represent a level considerably lower than they would have achieved had they been assessed prior to injury. In addition, the effects of repeated assessment with the same instruments over time may result in exaggerated recovery curves.

The ultimate degree of recovery depends on a number of factors, including TBI severity. Levin and colleagues (Levin, Grossman, Rose, & Teasdale, 1979) investigated long-term posttraumatic outcome in a series of TBI patients and found persistent intellectual deficits in the majority of patients with a history of severe head injury. Furthermore, it was found that the strongest single predictor of persistent NP dysfunction was the presence of early oculovestibular deficit, suggesting the involvement of brain stem as well as cerebral systems. In summary, residual intellectual/cognitive deficit is common following severe TBI, even though some degree of recovery of function is often seen.

II. Language Functions

Language abilities may be affected to various degrees in TBI, depending on the site, extent, and severity of damage. Lesions of the left hemisphere (in most individuals) in particular may affect a number of language functions, and thus a careful assessment of a variety of language abilities is necessary in the TBI patient. The basic language functions that should be assessed to some extent in the comprehensive NP evaluation include comprehension of speech, spontaneous speech, reading comprehension, confrontation naming, verbal fluency, vocabulary skills, repetition, written language, and general conversational abilities. Impairment in basic comprehension ability, for example, may affect the results of most other NP tests, and therefore must be evaluated to some degree.

Literature Findings. Although various disturbances in language function are frequently observed and may persist following TBI (Sarno, 1984), frank residual aphasia appears to be an uncommon sequelae (Heilman, Safran, & Geschwind, 1971). Defective performance on specific tasks such as visual confrontation naming have been found to be common, for example, occurring in 40% of a consecutive series of patients with varying levels of TBI severity in a study by Levin and colleagues (Levin, Grossman, & Kelly, 1976). In terms of the recovery of language functions following TBI, it has been reported that despite wide variability across individuals, aphasia recovery (to the extent that it occurs) largely takes place within 6 to 9 months following injury (Heilman et al., 1971; Newcombe & Fortuny, 1979). Thomsen (1984), however, reported that 84% of 19 initially aphasic TBI patients remained significantly aphasic at 2½ years postinjury, but this dropped to 21% at 10- to 15-year follow up. Dysarthria, on the other hand, showed a strong tendency to persist over time. Levin, Grossman, Sarwar, and Meyers (1981) found that generalized language deficits persisted in patients who sustained severe TBI, but that these deficits were in association with global cognitive impairment. (For further discussion of language and communication disorders in TBI, see Chapter 8 by Marquardt, Stoll, & Sussman, this volume.)

III. Visuospatial, Visuoconstructional, and Visuoperceptual Abilities

This category includes a wide variety of nonverbal skills that may be affected in TBI, particularly when there is damage to right hemisphere systems. Some of the more common abilities in this area include constructional ability, visuospatial problem solving, visuoperceptual abilities, and drawing ability. For a general review of many of these types of deficits, the reader is referred to Benton (1985).

Literature Findings. Although not often a focus of published NP studies of TBI, some degree of visuospatial deficit is not uncommon. Abilities on more nonverbal tasks such as the Performance subtests of the WAIS-R in particular have been shown to be readily affected by TBI, often to a greater extent than their Verbal subtest counterparts (Russell, 1979). As noted above, these measures often represent more novel types of tasks that require fluid as opposed to overlearned, crystallized abilities. The Digit Symbol subtest of the WAIS-R, for example, tends to be highly sensitive to brain dysfunction irrespective of lesion location (Bigler, 1988, p. 47) and relies on a number of visuospatial abilities. Measures of constructional praxis also may be affected by TBI, as nicely illustrated by the cases presented in Bigler (1988, pp. 130–135). Ruff, Evans, and Marshall (1986) found significant deficits on a novel measure of nonverbal fluency analogous to verbal fluency deficits in a group of 35 TBI patients. Studies of facial recognition performance in TBI patients have been few, although Levin, Grossman, & Kelly (1977) found deficient performance in over one-fourth of their sample of TBI patients who had been unconscious for more than a few minutes. Such deficits maybe associated primarily with right hemisphere involvement (e.g., particularly in the case of posterior hematoma), although further investigations of visuospatial and visuoperceptual abilities in TBI appear warranted in patients with and without evidence of right hemisphere damage per se.

IV. Attention/Concentration

Deficits in attention are extremely common in TBI, and such complaints may persist following mild as well as severe injuries (Binder, 1986). Because of the prominent role of these functions in other NP abilities and many daily tasks, assessment of attention/concentration abilities is of key importance in the neuropsychological evaluation of the TBI patient. For example, it is possible that an impaired performance on a measure of verbal recall may be the result of decreased attention per se, when in fact those brain mechanisms primarily involved in recall may be relatively intact. Although basic attentional abilities can be assessed clinically during an interview and during performance of various tasks, some of the more popular measures of attention/concentration abilities include digit repetition (digit span), number or letter cancellation tasks, serial addition tasks, and measures of sustained auditory attention.

Literature Findings. As noted, deficits in attention and concentration following TBI are very commonly reported by patients, although the underlying neural mechanisms are not well understood (Posner, 1987). Attentional deficits vary in severity, and it has been postulated that they may relate to a slowed rate of information processing (Van Zomeren, 1981). Gronwall (1987) reviewed the literature on attention and information processing following TBI and indicated that slowed responding by TBI patients was noted in the majority of studies and tends to be related to TBI severity and time since injury. Thus, many measures requiring sustained attention as a major component ability are likely to show deficits when administered to TBI patients. To further illustrate this point, a number of studies have demonstrated deficits in attentional abilities in patients with mild and moderate TBI (Gronwall & Wrightson, 1981; McMillan & Glucksman, 1987). Several chapters in the excellent text by Levin, Grafman, & Eisenberg (1987) address attention/concentration abilities following TBI, and some innovative experimental assessment methods are discussed.

V. Learning and Memory

Deficits in these processes are exceedingly common following TBI, and because of the extensive literature pertaining to memory processes, deficits, and assessment thereof, only some general topics and common clinical procedures are discussed here. For more thorough reviews, see Schacter and Crovitz (1977); Levin et al. (1982); Brooks (1983), and Squire and Butters (1984). Also see Delis (in press) for an overview of NP assessment of learning and memory abilities.

Verbal Learning and Memory Abilities. These areas represent some of the most common complaints of TBI patients and merit thorough evaluation. In terms of memory abilities, anterograde as well as (albeit to a lesser extent) retrograde amnesic deficits are often seen in association with TBI. Because of the cerebrum's situation within the skull, the frontal and temporal regions of the brain are most susceptible to damage from impact (see Chapter 2 by Bigler, this volume, for details). Thus, since temporal lobe systems include some of the central mechanisms involved in memory processes, some of the abilities that are most likely to be affected involve learning and memory functions regardless of the primary site of damage. Furthermore, because of the basic differential contribution of each temporal lobe to memory functioning (i.e., in general, verbal = left; nonverbal = right), comprehensive assessment of various types of learning and memory abilities is called for.

One of the most popular measures of verbal memory is the paragraph recall task (e.g., as in the Wechsler Memory Scale [Wechsler, 1945] and Wechsler Memory Scale–Revised [Wechsler, 1987]), where a paragraph is read to the patient and immediate recall is assessed. Delayed recall (i.e., typically 20–30 minutes later) of the same material is of critical importance to evaluate, since the severe deficits of amnesic patients in anterograde memory tend to be highlighted following delay periods (Butters et al., 1988). Paragraph learning tasks wherein a paragraph is repeatedly presented to the patient until a criterion level of immediate recall is attained also can be used. The rate of forgetting can then be assessed at a later time with a free recall trial.

In the assessment of verbal learning and memory abilities, word-list learning tasks (i.e., the presentation of a list of related or unrelated words across several trials) are popular and available in various formats. Such measures provide indices regarding immediate recall and the ability to learn over time and also allow for an assessment of delayed recall and recognition abilities. Although less well studied in TBI, the importance of assessing recall versus recognition ability in other diagnostic groups (e.g., cortical vs. subcortical dementias) has been demonstrated (Butters, Wolfe, Granholm, & Martone, 1986). In addition, such assessments provide more detailed information regarding the precise nature of the memory, which may have implications for treatment (e.g., whether a patient is able to benefit from memory cues).

Depending on the instrument used, additional information that can be derived from word-list learning tasks includes assessment of the primacy-recency effect (i.e., whether patients passively echo back the last few words of the list, thereby suggesting a more shallow learning), knowledge of the types of strategies used in recalling target stimuli (e.g., whether the patient is using higher-order organizational strategies vs. less efficient serial recall methods), sensitivity to proactive interference, and an assessment of error types (e.g., perseverations and intrusions). Careful analysis of these types of information may have further important implications for rehabilitation strategies.

Paired associate learning tasks also are popular in assessing TBI patients and have proven to be highly sensitive to TBI-induced deficits and neuropathological changes (Cullum & Bigler, 1986). In this paradigm,word pairs are presented to patients, and their task is to learn which words go together. Typically, several trials are given, and a delayed recall or recognition trial also can be administered. It should be noted that many clinical and experimental verbal learning tools exist, and only a few of the more popular clinical measures are listed in Table 6.3.

Nonverbal Learning and Memory Abilities. As with verbal learning and memory, nonverbal or visuospatial memory abilities are often affected by TBI, particularly when there is involvement of right temporal lobe systems. It should be noted that few, if any, "nonverbal" measures are exclusively nonverbal in nature, insofar as most or all of the commonly used figures can be verbally encoded to some degree (e.g., a red square, rectangle, or circular figure), and thus do not represent "pure" measures of nonverbal memory abilities. The formats of various measures differ, but one common practice is to present the visual stimuli (typically geometric figures) for a specified period (e.g., 10 seconds). Then, upon removal of the stimuli, the patient is asked to reproduce the figure(s) from memory. Delayed recall should then be similarly assessed, typically after 20–30 minutes. This format can be applied to both nonverbal learning and memory abilities. Nonverbal learning tasks are less commonly encountered in clinical practice, but may include trial-learning tasks, where the examiner consecutively taps a series of blocks or targets, and afterwards the patient is asked to replicate the examiner's sequence (in the same or reverse order). A trials-to-criterion learning approach also may be implemented with nonverbal stimuli, as with verbal material. Another paradigm involves nonverbal paired associate learning, wherein the patient is presented with pairs of figures and/or colors across several trials, then a single item is presented and the patient is asked to indicate which of an array of items was paired with it. Some of the more common nonverbal learning and memory measures also are presented in Table 6.3.

Literature Findings. As noted, there is an extensive literature on memory deficits following TBI, and far too little room in this chapter to provide a detailed overview. Memory deficits nevertheless are common following TBI and in fact may be a major factor in some patients' lack of cognitive recovery (Ryan & Ruff, 1988). During the PTA period itself (which is a common feature of TBI), patients appear confused and disoriented, although relatively little is known about the efficacy of memory function during that time. The longer the duration of PTA (i.e., over 1 week), however, the greater likelihood of residual memory deficit (Bond, 1986). Deficits in recall for verbal and nonverbal material are among the most common NP deficits of TBI patients, with the severity of verbal versus nonverbal memory impairment depending to some extent on the degree of involvement of left or right temporal lobe structures, respectively. For detailed reviews of the literature on memory function following TBI, the reader is referred to the appropriate chapters in Levin et al. (1982,1987) and Brooks (1983), and to Schacter and Crovitz (1977).

VI. Psychomotor/Visuomotor Functioning

TBI, particularly when specifically involving motor cortex regions, may affect motor abilities, even in the absence of an obvious physical impairment such as a hemi- or paraplegia. Many perceptuomotor tasks involve a variety of cognitive abilities, in addition to the motor components. Measures of fine motor speed, dexterity, and simple strength often are included in comprehensive NP evaluations and are particularly important in assessing TBI because of the typically diffuse nature of cerebral involvement. Knowledge about patients' simple motor and psychomotor abilities can have major implications for rehabilitation and job placement endeavors.

Literature Findings. Psychomotor slowing is a common consequence of TBI, as noted in simple and complex reaction time studies cited above in the attention section. Focal cerebral lesions in particular (e.g., hematoma, cerebral contusion) may impair motor functions to varying degrees, depending on the primary site of damage and the underlying systems involved. Regarding long-term functioning, a recent study by Klonoff, Costa, and Snow (1986) found that motor slowing, as assessed by the finger tapping test (Reitan & Davison, 1974) and Visual Continuous Reaction Time (Van Zomeren, 1981), was significantly related to patient-rated quality of life 2–4 years postinjury.

VII. Higher Cognitive Functioning

Measures of abstract reasoning and complex problem solving are often affected in TBI, since these measures frequently are among the most sensitive to cerebral dysfunction. Such tasks require conceptual reasoning and planning abilities for successful completion, in addition to the integrity of basic executive functions. These measures generally involve the integration of a number of more basic cognitive abilities on which they depend, and disruption to any component function or functions may result in significant deficits. In addition, deficits in higher cognitive functions can occur in the face of relatively normal performance on other more basic tasks, with dysfunction occurring only at the highest integrative levels (see Table 6.3 for a sample of some of the more common measures that may be considered in this group of abilities).

Literature Findings. As noted, NP measures in this category represent complex cognitive tasks that typically involve the integration of a number of abilities. One of the more popular measures is the Category Test from the Halstead-Reitan battery (Halstead, 1947; Reitan & Davison, 1974), and this measure has proven to be the single most sensitive indicator of brain dysfunction in that battery of tests (Jarvis & Barth, 1985). This is a complex measure requiring conceptual reasoning, abstraction, and novel problem solving skills, and poor performance may result from disruption of a number of abilities and/or lower-level cognitive functions. Dikmen, Reitan, and Temkin (1983) reported that impaired Category Test performance was consistently found in a series of 27 patients following mild to severe TBI and that some recovery of function on this as well as simpler measures was observed over time. Another popular clinical measure is the Wisconsin Card Sorting Test (Grant & Berg, 1948; Heaton, 1981). This task is a measure of perseveration and cognitive flexibility and has been shown to be particularly sensitive to lesions of the frontal lobes (Milner, 1964; Robinson, Heaton, Lehman, & Stilson, 1980), although diffuse damage may result in impaired performance. Other measures of abstraction and reasoning include proverb interpretation and similarities tasks, which often are impaired in TBI, as responses tend to be concrete with more severe injuries (Lezak, 1983, p. 252).

Head injured patients are also frequently impaired in their fluency for both verbal and nonverbal information processing. In a recent study comparing severe and moderate TBI patients, Ruff, Evans, and Marshall (1986) found greater impairment associated with the level of severity on both verbal and nonverbal fluency tests.

VIII. Emotional Functioning

Emotional disturbance following TBI is common, and may in fact have a more significant impact on the patient and family than the cognitive deficits that may be present (Lezak, 1978). Therefore, assessment of the emotional status of TBI patients can be of critical importance but is often given too little attention in the NP evaluation. Symptoms of depression and anxiety are frequently seen following moderate to severe TBI (Cullum & Bigler, 1988) and, when present, merit appropriate intervention (see Chapter 17 by Lezak & O'Brien and Chapter 9 by McGuire & Sylvester, this volume). Psychological disturbance following TBI may represent a reaction to acquired deficits and limitations posed by TBI, and also may be directly related to damage to those cerebral systems subserving emotional functions (see Cullum, 1989). Factors important in the development of emotional disturbance following TBI include the primary site of damage and time since onset of the disorder. Although the use of emotional assessment tools (or at least the interpretation of results) must be modified in application to brain damaged populations (Cullum, 1989; Cullum & Bigler, 1988; Lezak, 1983, p. 612), some common assessment instruments in this area include the Minnesota Multiphasic Personality Inventory (MMPI; Hathaway & McKinley, 1967) and the Symptom Checklist (SCL-90; Derogatis, Lipman, Rickels, Uhlenhuth, & Covi, 1974) for self-ratings, and the Neurobehavioral Rating Scale of Levin et al. (1987), a modification of the Brief Psychiatric Rating Scale (Overall & Gorham, 1962) for observer-rated indices of emotional status. Other useful ratings for post-TBI patients include the Katz Adjustment Scale (Katz & Lyerly, 1963), which provides for patient's and relatives' assessments of the patient's psychosocial functioning.

SPECIAL CONSIDERATIONS OF NEUROPSYCHOLOGICAL ASSESSMENT IN TBI

In addition to the major topics in assessment of TBI individuals, there are several areas of assessment that require special consideration. These are overviewed in the following sections.

Interpretation of Neuropsychological Results

As mentioned earlier, one of the main purposes of the comprehensive NP evaluation is to assess and quantify patients' individual strengths and weaknesses across an array of NP abilities. Careful examination of the specific raw and scaled (transformed into the same metric, when possible) scores derived from various measures are critical in assessing a patient's level of performance in different areas. Such an analysis not only attempts to address whether cerebral dysfunction is present, but also provides a multidimensional index regarding the degree of current impairment. Important information can also be derived by examination of the *process* by which individuals arrive at solutions or fail tasks. In addition to patients' overall scores on measures, the types of errors that are made should be examined, since the same score on any given measure can be obtained for many different reasons. These data often serve as a basis for making prognostic inferences, which was discussed earlier.

Premorbid Functioning and Risk Factors

The importance of appropriate normative NP data was discussed in an earlier section, but this point cannot be overstated. Comparison of test results from non-brain-damaged individuals of similar age, education, and (in the case of some measures) gender is critical to allow for appropriate interpretation. Another related issue is the extreme importance of obtaining a careful history and, in particular, knowledge of preexisting conditions that may have bearing on interpretation of NP results. For example, whether the TBI patient had a history of learning difficulties, prior neurological damage, or substance abuse would be essential knowledge in the interpretation of current NP findings. In such cases, it may be difficult to ascribe certain observed deficits entirely to a recent TBI, since preexisting conditions may in fact contribute heavily to the current dysfunction. Careful evaluation of the current pattern of NP deficits in the context of the severity and nature of injury and the presence of premorbid risk factors, however, should allow for a reasonable estimate to be made of the contribution of TBI effects in many cases.

Interviews with family members can also be invaluable in the interpretation of NP results, since they can provide additional information regarding the patient's premorbid functioning. This is relevant not only in terms of cognitive and everyday functional abilities, but also with regard to personality, since the now disinhibited, inappropriate TBI patient we have just evaluated (and made mention of the obvious frontal lobe involvement secondary to TBI) may have been that way before the injury.

Estimation of premorbid NP abilities is most helpful in evaluating current status, and since quantitative premorbid NP data are almost universally absent (although some cognitive test results are occasionally available, for example, military entrance examination scores, school achievement test scores, etc.), we are left with clinical-experiential estimates of premorbid functioning. Reasonable assessments can be made, however, based on knowledge of the patient's age, educational level and academic performance, gender, previous occupational status, and socioeconomic and sociocultural background. Various procedures for quantitative estimates of premorbid intellectual functioning have been derived (e.g., Barona, Reynolds, & Chastain, 1984; Karzmark, Heaton, Grant, & Matthews, 1985), although similar quantitative estimates of specific NP abilities such as premorbid memory functioning are much more problematic. It should be noted that, despite even the best statistical formulae and historical data, precise estimations of individual premorbid function are rarely possible, and, in general, this type of estimation is best made using good clinical experience and judgment by the neuropsychologist.

Posttest Consultation

It is important that the neuropsychologist communicate the results of the examination in a clear and timely fashion to the referring clinician and, when desired, directly to the patient and his or her family. In this regard, a pretest questionnaire where patients estimate their own cognitive strengths and weaknesses is often helpful. Once patients have made a subjective rating of their cognitive abilities, a comparison can be made with the actual neuropsychological performances. Such a comparison addresses both subjective underestimation and overestimation of abilities by providing an objective evaluation of actual abilities. Along these lines, self-rating scales geared toward both cognitive abilities as well as activities of daily living can be useful (e.g., Heaton, Chelune, & Lehman, 1981).

In general, the aim of the posttest consultation is to establish a bridge from the neuropsychological test findings to the patient's current status and everyday abilities. It is critical that everyday behavioral/task examples are sought that will help to communicate the specific neuropsychological findings. This will help to avoid technical jargon and make the feedback understandable and useful to patients and their families. In addition, this will provide the neuropsychologist with a better feel for the impact of NP deficits observed on formal testing of the patient's everyday functioning. Recommendations more directly related to the patient's daily activities and hobbies also can be made in this context. Finally, since many TBI patients suffer from memory difficulties, a brief list of strengths and weaknesses will help to structure the conversation and provide some information patients can refer to at their own leisure.

Cognitive Remediation Issues

With regard to treatment issues, it is often difficult for the neuropsychologist to provide specific recommendations regarding the precise nature of treatment that should be employed for optimal progress. In time, this area will be advanced, as the field of cognitive remediation provides us with more definitive empirical data (see Chapter 12 by Prigatano, this volume). Despite the lack of well-validated treatments for most NP deficits, however, recommendations regarding how patients might improve their functional capacity certainly can be made with the knowledge of a patient's strengths and weaknesses. For example, shortening treatment sessions to minimize fatigue and maximize learning might be an important recommendation for an acute patient, while presenting new information in brief, repeatable bits might be an important recommendation for a patient with a memory deficit. The goal of neuropsychological recommendations then would be to make general statements regarding appropriate helpful strategies in addition to statements about the nature of the cognitive deficits. In a recent pilot study with moderate and severe TBI patients, the former appeared to profit from memory training techniques to a significantly greater degree than the more severely amnesic patients (Ryan & Ruff, 1988). Therefore, it is also critical that neuropsychologists evaluate what type of patient will more likely benefit from a specific treatment mode. Recommendations for adjunctive individual and/or family therapy in some cases also can be very useful.

LIMITATIONS AND CHALLENGES TO NEUROPSYCHOLOGY IN TBI

1. Good normative data on many tests are lacking, although a number of centers are working to remediate this deficiency. Many NP measures include data pertaining to "normative" samples in their instruction manuals, yet these samples typically are small and do not allow for adjustment based on varying age and education levels. A major current deficiency in the NP literature is the almost total lack of adequate normative data for older individuals, despite the fact that age is such an important factor in interpreting NP test results.

2. There is a need for the development of alternate forms of many NP measures. Currently only a handful of tests have alternate forms, and the actual interchangeability of these forms (e.g., in terms of degree of difficulty and psychometric properties) in some cases is questionable. The availability of alternate forms of tests would help reduce practice effects in serial evaluations, although rigorous standardization of such measures would be needed.

3. The difficulties in estimating premorbid abilities were discussed earlier, and currently only general intellectual level estimates have been looked at in the literature.

4. Prediction of long-term NP outcome regarding specific abilities represents a major challenge to NP, as does the prediction of *rates* of functional recovery. The combined use of neurological, neuropsychological, and neuroimaging (e.g., MRI, PET) methods may lead to more accurate predictions about various abilities following TBI.

5. There is a need for the use of standard indices regarding injury severity in research. Although several useful indices are currently available regarding coma duration and PTA (e.g., Glasgow Coma Scale, GOAT), such measures unfortunately are not consistently reported in research studies.

6. There is a strong need for large-scale studies of cognitive remediation programs targeted to specific abilities (see Chapter 12 by Prigatano). Although this area is faced with a myriad of methodological difficulties, it will be

particularly important to include appropriate control groups in such investigations to clearly demonstrate that remediation effects extend beyond what can be expected on the basis of spontaneous recovery alone.

7. The question regarding the ecological validity of NP results in TBI patients is well taken and deserves systematic study. Although we often make general statements regarding patients' abilities to perform certain daily or work-related tasks, this issue has actually received too little scientific attention. As Newcombe (1987) discusses, there are always a number of exceptions to our everyday functioning predictions based on NP results. This can be illustrated by those patients who score in the impaired range on our clinical memory tests yet continue to function adequately at home and even on the job in some instances. Such cases underscore the value of carefully gathering information from patients and significant others regarding the patient's day-to-day functioning, in addition to NP data alone.

SUMMARY

Neuropsychological assessment provides important information regarding patients' functional status following TBI which should be utilized in conjunction with data from other allied professions. Although comprehensive NP assessment of current cognitive status is critical in terms of evaluating an individual's deficits and strengths, our ability to predict long-term recovery of specific functions is at a most rudimentary level. In addition, relatively little is known with respect to the nature of the recovery process—that is, how and at what *rate* the recovery of various abilities occurs from a qualitative as well as quantitative perspective. Nevertheless, it is argued that a comprehensive approach to NP evaluation of TBI sequelae be adopted, and that neuropsychologists be sensitive to developments in other fields such as cognitive psychology and neuroscience in order to incorporate potentially useful techniques in the development of new NP assessment and remediation procedures. The need for large-scale normative data bases and alternate forms of NP measures is clear, as is a more thorough understanding of how NP test results relate to patients' functioning at home and at work. Although many important studies and observations of the TBI population have been conducted in the past decade, many fundamental questions remain unanswered. It is likely that neuropsychological assessment, in conjunction with modern neuroimaging techniques, will continue to provide important insights into the cerebral processes affected by TBI. However, it merits considering that the refinement of our diagnostic procedures will only gain greater clinical significance from the patient's standpoint if efficacious treatment methods are developed that will clearly help patients to achieve optimal functioning levels in their everyday lives.

REFERENCES

Barona, A., Reynolds, C.R., & Chastain, R. (1984). A demographically based index of premorbid intelligence for the WAIS-R. *Journal of Consulting and Clinical Psychology, 52,* 885–887.

Baser, C.A., & Ruff, R.M. (1987). Construct validity of the San Diego Neuropsychological Test battery. *Archives of Clinical Neuropsychology, 2,* 13–32.

Benton, A.L. (1968). Differential behavioral effects in frontal lobe disease. *Neuropsychologia, 6,* 53–60.

Benton, A.L. (1974). *The revised visual retention test* (4th ed.). New York: Psychological Corp.

Benton, A.L. (1985). Visuoperceptual, visuospatial, and visuoconstructional disorders. In K.M. Heilman & E. Valenstein (Eds.), *Clinical neuropsychology* (pp. 151–185). New York: Oxford University Press.

Benton, A.L., & Hamsher, K. deS. (1976). *Multilingual aphasia examination.* Iowa City: University of Iowa.

Bigler, E.D. (1987). Neuropathology of acquired cerebral trauma. *Journal of Learning Disabilities, 20,* 458–473.

Bigler, E.D. (1988). *Diagnostic clinical neuropsychology* (rev. ed.). Austin: University of Texas Press.

Bigler, E.D., Steinman, D.R., & Newton, J.S. (1981). Clinical assessment of cognitive deficit in neurologic disorder. II, Cerebral trauma. *Clinical Neuropsychology, 3,* 13–18.

Binder, L.M. (1986). Persisting symptoms after mild head injury: A review of the postconcussive syndrome. *Journal of Clinical and Experimental Neuropsychology, 8,* 323–346.

Boller, F., & Vignolo, L.A. (1966). Latent sensory aphasia in hemisphere-damaged patients: An experimental study with the Token Test. *Brain, 89,* 815–831.

Bond, M.R. (1986). Neurobehavioral sequelae of closed head injury. In I. Grant & K.M. Adams (Eds.), *Neuropsychological assessment of neuropsychiatric disorders* (pp. 347–373). New York: Oxford University Press.

Brooks, D.N. (1983). Disorders of memory. In M. Rosenthal, E.R. Griffith, M.R. Bond, & J.D. Miller (Eds.), *Rehabilitation of the head injured adult* (pp. 185–196). Philadelphia: F.A. Davis.

Brooks, D.N. (1987). Measuring neuropsychological and functional recovery. In H.S. Levin, J. Grafman, & H.M. Eisenberg (Eds.), *Neurobehavioral recovery from head injury* (pp. 57–72). New York: Oxford University Press.

Buschke, H., & Fuld, P.A. (1974). Evaluating storage, retention, and retrieval in disordered memory and learning. *Neurology, 11,* 1019–1025.

Butters, N., Salmon, D.P., Cullum, C.M., Cairns, P., Tröster, A.I., Jacobs, D., Moss, M., & Cermak, L.S. (1988). Differentiation of amnesic and demented patients with the Wechsler Memory Scale–Revised. *The Clinical Neuropsychologist, 2,* 133–148.

Butters, N., Wolfe, J., Granholm, E.; & Martone, M. (1986). An assessment of verbal recall, recognition and fluency in patients with Huntington's disease. *Cortex, 22,* 11–32.

Cullum, C.M. (1989). Cerebral imaging and emotional correlates. In E.D. Bigler, R.A. Yeo, & E. Turkheimer (Eds.), *Neuropsychological function and brain imaging.* New York: Plenum Press.

Cullum, C.M., & Bigler, E.D. (1986). Ventricle size, cortical atrophy, and the relationship with neuropsychological status in closed head injury. *Journal of Clinical and Experimental Neuropsychology, 8*, 437–452.

Cullum, C.M., & Bigler, E.D. (1988). Short-form MMPI findings in patients with predominantly lateralized cerebral dysfunction: Neuropsychological and computerized axial tomography-derived parameters. *Journal of Nervous and Mental Disease, 176*, 332–342.

Cullum, C.M., Steinman, D.R., & Bigler, E.D. (1984). Relationship between fluid and crystallized cognitive functions using Category Test and WAIS scores. *International Journal of Clinical Neuropsychology, 6*, 172–174.

Delis, D.C. (in press). Neuropsychological assessment of learning and memory. In F. Boller & J. Grafman (Eds.), *Handbook of neuropsychology.* Amsterdam: Elsevier.

Delis, D.C., Kramer, J.H., & Kaplan, E. (1987). *The California proverb test.* Unpublished neuropsychological test.

Delis, D.C., Kramer, J.H., Kaplan, E., & Ober, B.A. (1987). *California verbal learning test manual.* New York: Psychological Corp.

Derogatis, L.R., Lipman, R.S., Rickels, K., Uhlenhuth, E.H., & Covi, L. (1974). The symptom distress check list: A measure of primary symptom dimensions. In P. Pichot (Ed.), *Psychological measurement: Modern problems in pharmacopsychiatry.* Basel, Switzerland: S. Karger.

Dikmen, S., Reitan, R.M., & Temkin, N. (1983). Neuropsychological recovery in head injury. *Archives of Neurology, 40*, 333–338.

Dikmen, S., & Temkin, N. (1987). Determination of the effects of head injury and recovery in behavioral research. In H.S. Levin, J. Grafman, & H.M. Eisenberg (Eds.), *Neurobehavioral recovery from head injury* (pp. 73–87). New York: Oxford University Press.

Dunn, L.M., & Markwardt, F.C., Jr. (1970). *Peabody individual achievement test manual.* Circle Pines, MN: American Guidance Service.

Folstein, M.F., Folstein, S.E., & McHugh, P.R. (1975). Mini-mental state: A practical method for grading the mental state of patients for the clinician. *Journal of Psychiatric Research, 12*, 189–198.

Genarelli, T.A., Adams, J.H., & Thibault, L.B. (1982). Diffuse axonal injury and traumatic coma in the primate. *Annals of Neurology, 12*, 564–574.

Golden, C.J., Hammeke, T.A., & Purisch, A.D. (1978). Diagnostic validity of a standardized neuropsychological battery derived from Luria's Neuropsychological Tests. *Journal of Consulting and Clinical Psychology, 46*, 1258–1265.

Goodglass, H., & Kaplan, E. (1983). *The assessment of aphasia and related disorders* (2nd ed.). Philadelphia: Lea & Febiger.

Grant, D.A., & Berg, E.A. (1948). A behavioral analysis of degree of reinforcement and ease of shifting to new responses in a Weigl-type card-sorting problem. *Journal of Experimental Psychology, 38*, 404–411.

Gronwall, D.M.A. (1977). Paced auditory serial-addition task: A measure of recovery from concussion. *Perceptual and Motor Skills, 44*, 367–373.

Gronwall, D. (1987). Advances in the assessment of attention and information processing after head injury. In H.S. Levin, J. Grafman, & H.M. Eisenberg (Eds.), *Neurobehavioral recovery from head injury* (pp. 355–371). New York: Oxford University Press.

Gronwall, D., & Wrightson, P. (1981). Memory and information processing capacity after minor head injury. *Journal of Neurology, Neurosurgery, and Psychiatry, 44*, 889–895.

Halstead, W.C. (1947). *Brain and intelligence.* Chicago: University of Chicago Press.

Hathaway, S.R., & McKinley, J.C. (1967). *The Minnesota multiphasic personality inventory manual.* New York: Psychological Corp.

Heaton, R.K. (1981). *A manual for the Wisconsin card sorting test.* Odessa, FL: Psychological Assessment Resources.

Heaton, R.K., Chelune, G.J., & Lehman, R.A.W. (1981). *Relation of neuropsychological and personality test results to patients' complaints of disability.* Unpublished manuscript, University of Colorado Health Sciences Center, Denver.

Heaton, R.K., Grant, I., & Matthews, C.G. (1986). Differences in neuropsychological test performance associated with age, education, and sex. In I. Grant & K.M. Adams (Eds.), *Neuropsychological assessment of neuropsychiatric disorders* (pp. 100–120). New York: Oxford University Press.

Heaton, R.K., Nelson, L.M., Thompson, D.S., Burkes, J.S., & Franklin, G.M. (1985). Neuropsychological findings in relapsing-remitting and chronic-progressive multiple sclerosis. *Journal of Consulting and Clinical Psychology, 53*, 103–110.

Heilman, K.M., Safran, A., & Geschwind, N. (1971). Closed head trauma and aphasia. *Journal of Neurology, Neurosurgery, and Psychiatry, 34*, 265–269.

Hooper, H.E. (1958). *The Hooper visual organization test manual.* Los Angeles: Western Psychological Services.

Jarvis, P.E., & Barth, J.T. (1985). *Halstead-Reitan battery: An interpretive guide.* Odessa, FL: Psychological Assessment Resources.

Jastak, J.F., & Jastak, S.R. (1984). *The Wide range achievement test–Revised manual.* Wilmington, DE: Guidance Associates.

Jennett, B. (1986). Head trauma. In A.K. Asbury, G.M. McKhann, & W.I. McDonald (Eds.), *Disease of the nervous system* (pp. 1282–1291). Philadelphia: W.B. Saunders.

Jennett, B., & Bond, M.R. (1975). Assessment of outcome after severe brain injury: A practical scale. *Lancet, 1*, 480–484.

Jennett, B., & Teasdale, G. (1981). *Management of head injuries.* Philadelphia: F.A. Davis.

Karzmark, P., Heaton, R.K., Grant, I., & Matthews, C.G. (1985). Use of demographic variables to predict full scale IQ: A replication and extension. *Journal of Clinical and Experimental Neuropsychology, 7*, 412–420.

Katz, M.M., & Lyerly, S.B. (1963). Methods for measuring adjustment and social behavior in the community: I. Rationale, description, discriminative validity and scale development. *Psychological Reports, 13*, 503–535.

Klonoff, P.S., Costa, L.D., & Snow, W.G. (1986). Predictors and indicators of quality of life in patients with closed-head injury. *Journal of Clinical and Experimental Neuropsychology, 8*, 469–485.

Klove, H. (1963). Clinical Neuropsychology. In F.M. Forster (Ed.), *The medical clinics of North America.* New York: W.B. Saunders.

Kwentus, J.A., Hart, R.P., Peck, E.T., & Kornstein, S. (1985). Psychiatric complications of closed head trauma. *Psychosomatics, 26*, 8–14.

Levin, H.S., Benton, A.L., & Grossman, R.G. (Eds.). (1982). *Neurobehavioral consequences of closed head injury.* New York: Oxford University Press.

Levin, H.S., Grafman, J., & Eisenberg, H.M. (Eds.). (1987). *Neurobehavioral recovery from head injury.* New York: Oxford University Press.

Levin, H.S., Grossman, R.G., & Kelly, P.J. (1976). Aphasic disorder in patients with closed head injury. *Journal of Neurology, Neurosurgery, and Psychiatry, 39,* 1062–1070.

Levin, H.S., Grossman, R.G., & Kelly, P.J. (1977). Impairment of facial recognition after closed head injuries of varying severity. *Cortex, 13,* 119–130.

Levin, H.S., Grossman, R.G., Rose, J.E., & Teasdale, G. (1979). Long-term neuropsychological outcome of closed head injury. *Journal of Neurosurgery, 50,* 412–422.

Levin, H.S., Grossman, R.G., Sarwar, M., & Meyers, C.A. (1981). Linguistic recovery after closed head injury. *Brain and Language, 12,* 360–374.

Levin, H.S., High, W.M., Goethe, K.E., Sisson, R.A., Overall, J.E., Rhoades, H.M., Eisenberg, H.M., Kalisky, Z., & Gary, H.E. (1987). The Neurobehavioral Rating Scale: Assessment of the behavioral sequelae of head injury by the clinician. *Journal of Neurology, Neurosurgery, and Psychiatry, 50,* 183–193.

Levin, H.S., O'Donnell, V.M., & Grossman, R.G. (1979). The Galveston Orientation and Amnesia test: A practical scale to assess cognition after head injury. *Journal of Nervous and Mental Disease, 167,* 675–684.

Lewis, R., & Kupke, T. (1977, May). *The Lafayette Clinic repeatable neuropsychological test battery: Its development and research applications.* Paper presented at the annual meeting of the Southeastern Psychological Association, Hollywood, FL.

Lezak, M.D. (1978). Living with the characterologically altered brain injured patient. *Journal of Clinical Psychiatry, 39,* 592–598.

Lezak, M.D. (1983). *Neuropsychological assessment* (2nd ed.). New York: Oxford University Press.

Mandleberg, I.A., & Brooks, D.N. (1975). Cognitive recovery after severe head injury: 1. Serial testing on the Wechsler Adult Intelligence Scale. *Journal of Neurology, Neurosurgery, and Psychiatry, 38,* 1121–1126.

Mattis, S. (1976). Mental status examination for organic mental syndrome in the elderly patient. In R. Bellack & B. Karasu (Eds.), *Geriatric psychiatry* (pp. 77–121). New York: Grune & Stratton.

McMillan, T.M., & Glucksman, E.E. (1987). The neuropsychology of moderate head injury. *Journal of Neurology, Neurosurgery, and Psychiatry, 50,* 393–397.

Milner, B. (1964). Some effects of frontal lobectomy in man. In J.M. Warren & K. Akert (Eds.), *The frontal granular cortex and behavior.* New York: McGraw-Hill.

Milner, B. (1971). Interhemispheric differences in the localization of psychological processes in man. *British Medical Bulletin, 27,* 272–277.

Newcombe, F. (1987). Psychometric and behavioral evidence: Scope, limitations, and ecological validity. In H.S. Levin, J. Grafman, & H.M. Eisenberg (Eds.), *Neurobehavioral recovery from head injury* (pp. 129–145). New York: Oxford University Press.

Newcombe, F., & Fortuny, L.A.I. (1979). Problems and perspectives in the evaluation of psychological deficits after cerebral lesions. *International Rehabilitation Medicine, 1,* 182–192.

Overall, J.E., & Gorham, D.R. (1962). The brief psychiatric rating scale. *Psychological Reports, 10,* 799–812.

Parsons, O.A., & Prigatano, G.P. (1978). Methodological considerations in clinical neuropsychological research. *Journal of Consulting and Clinical Psychology, 46*, 608–619.

Posner, M.I. (1987). Selective attention in head injury. In H.S. Levin, J. Grafman, & H.M. Eisenberg (Eds.), *Neurobehavioral recovery from head injury* (pp. 390–397). New York: Oxford University Press.

Raven, J.C. (1960). *Guide to the Standard Progressive Matrices*. New York: Psychological Corp.

Reitan, R.M. (1984). *Aphasia and sensory-perceptual deficits in adults*. Tucson, AZ: Reitan Neuropsychology Laboratories.

Reitan, R.M. (1986). Theoretical and methodological bases of the Halstead-Reitan Neuropsychological Test Battery. In I. Grant & K.M. Adams (Eds.), *Neuropsychological assessment of neuropsychiatric disorders* (pp. 3–30). New York: Oxford University Press.

Reitan, R.M., & Davison, L.A. (1974). *Clinical neuropsychology: Current status and applications*. New York: Winston/Wiley.

Rimel, R.W., & Jane, J.A. (1983). Characteristics of the head-injured patient. In M. Rosenthal, E.R. Griffith, M.R. Bond, & J.D. Miller (Eds.), *Rehabilitation of the head-injured adult* (pp. 9–21). Philadelphia: F.A. Davis.

Robinson, A.L., Heaton, R.K., Lehman, R.A.W., & Stilson, D.W. (1980). The utility of the Wisconsin Card Sorting Test in detecting and localizing frontal lobe lesions. *Journal of Consulting and Clinical Psychology, 48*, 605–614.

Ruff, R.M., & Light R. (1984). *Ruff-Light trail learning test*. Unpublished neuropsychological test.

Ruff, R.M., Evans, R., & Light, R.H. (1986). Automatic detection vs. controlled search: A paper approach. *Perceptual and Motor Skills, 62*, 407–416.

Ruff, R.M., Evans, R., & Marshall, L.F. (1986). Impairment of verbal and figural fluency following traumatic head injury. *Archives of Clinical Neuropsychology, 1*, 87–101.

Russell, E.W. (1979). Three patterns of brain damage on the WAIS. *Journal of Clinical Psychology, 35*, 611–620.

Ryan, T.V., & Ruff, R.M. (1988). The efficacy of structured memory retraining in a group comparison of head injured patients. *Archives of Clinical Neuropsychology, 3*, 165–179.

Sarno, M.T. (1984). Verbal impairment after closed head injury. *The Journal of Nervous and Mental Disease, 172*, 475–479.

Schacter, D.L., & Crovitz, H.F. (1977). Memory function after closed head injury: A review of the quantitative research. *Cortex, 13*, 150–176.

Squire, L.R., & Butters, N. (Eds.). (1984). *Neuropsychology of memory*. New York: Guilford.

Stroop, J.R. (1935). Studies of interference in serial verbal reactions. *Journal of Experimental Psychology, 18*, 643–662.

Teasdale, G., & Jennett, B. (1974). Assessment of coma and impaired consciousness: A practical scale. *Lancet, 2*, 81–84.

Thomsen, I.V. (1984). Late outcome of very severe blunt head trauma: A 10–15 year second follow-up. *Journal of Neurology, Neurosurgery, and Psychiatry, 47*, 260–268.

Van Zomeren, A.H. (1981). *Reaction time and attention after closed head injury*. Lisse, The Netherlands: Swets & Zeitlinger.

Wechsler, D. (1945). A standardized memory scale for clinical use. *Journal of Psychology, 19*, 87–95.

Wechsler, D. (1981). *Webster adult intelligence scale–Revised manual*. New York: Psychological Corp.

Wechsler, D. (1987). *Wechsler memory scale–Revised manual.* New York: Psychological Corp.

Wilson, R.S., Rosenbaum, G., Brown, G., & Grisell, J. (1979). An index of premorbid intelligence. *Journal of Consulting and Clinical Psychology, 46*, 1554–1555.

7

Cognitive Dysfunction and Psychoeducational Assessment in Traumatic Brain Injury

JOHN E. OBRZUT

GEORGE W. HYND

The last two decades have witnessed many advances in the development of neuropsychological theory and practice. Much of this work has led to more reliable assessment and intervention procedures that can be used not only with adults but also with children who experience head injuries and subsequent learning disorders. As Gaddes (1981) stated, although this new knowledge shows promise, in particular, for special education populations, some educators have distrusted its efficacy. These educators argue that attempts to relate behavior to the central nervous system (CNS) is speculative and not useful. However, Rourke and Gates (1981) contend that sophisticated neuropsychological study of central processing deficiencies in children have yielded incontrovertible evidence that brain dysfunction can play a major role in the etiology of such deficiencies.

Support for such a generalization comes from the work on subtypes of children with learning disabilities (see McKinney, 1984, for a review). In general, the most important data to emerge from subtype analyses are the findings that these subtypes tend to coincide with the intuitive feelings of teachers regarding the relative strengths and weaknesses of children (Doehring & Hoshko, 1977), and with the functional deficiencies thought to be associated with disturbances in specific brain regions (Fisk & Rourke, 1979; Petrauskas & Rourke, 1979; Satz & Morris, 1980). The evidence argues against a unitary syndrome theory of learning disabilities and demonstrates the feasibility of employing a neuropsychological approach to the study of homogeneous diagnostic groups within this category of exceptional children. Thus, the improved knowledge and techniques of neurology and neuropsychology show great promise in advancing our understanding of the head injured individual.

BASIC ASSUMPTIONS OF NEUROPSYCHOLOGY

The neuropsychological approach implies the study of brain-behavior relationships and accepts a causal association between these two variables. Specifically, as Gaddes (1985) summarizes, neuropsychology can provide valuable information about the development and functions of the normal brain. This information can help clinicians and educators better understand the perception, cognition, motor response, language development, and learning modes of a particular individual. Neuropsychology addresses deficits in learning that are related to impaired cerebral states. Also recognized is the direct relationship of brain deficits and their etiological significance to an individual's learning problem. In essence, the neuropsychological approach may be less useful in the case of an underachieving individual with a structurally normal brain. Neuropsychology acknowledges that the locus of a brain lesion may have greater causal significance than the extent or degree of dysfunction for a learning disability and recognizes that even documented localized brain damage must be viewed in a total social context.

PREVALENCE OF LEARNING DISORDERS

The prevalence of learning disorders varies in different settings, but in countries such as the United States, Canada, and parts of Europe the incidence of underachievers is about 15% (Gaddes, 1976), and approximately 7% of these have demonstrable neurological deficits (Myklebust & Boshes, 1969). These children have conclusive evidence of cerebral dysfunctions and display perceptual, cognitive, and/or motor impairments. It has even been estimated that 3% of all 3-year-olds have some type of language disorder and over 2% are severely impaired in linguistic expression. Thus, the best evidence is 2%

of school populations have hard signs that interfere with learning while another 5% have soft signs (Gaddes, 1985).

In light of this evidence it is difficult to argue against the neuropsychological model. The model contends that all behavior is mediated by the central nervous system (CNS) and its integrated and supporting physiological systems (Gaddes, 1985). When the physiological systems do not function properly, disruption of normal perception, cognition, or motor response can occur. Given this outcome, consideration of behavior only at the psychological level is inadequate. Further, the neuropsychological model stresses that learning disorders are problems in the acquisition of developmental skills, academic achievement, social adjustment, and *secondarily,* emotional growth and development, all of which may be the direct result of perceptual and linguistic processing deficits. Since recent evidence suggests that learning disabled children are not a homogeneous group (see McKinney, 1984, for a review), these children must be understood diagnostically in terms of the nature of their learning problems. A learning disability has been recently defined by federal legislation (P.L. 94–142) as

> a disorder in one or more of the basic psychological processes involved in understanding or in using language, spoken or written, which may manifest itself in an imperfect ability to listen, think, speak, read, write, spell or do mathematical calculations. The term includes such conditions as perceptual handicaps, brain damage, minimal brain dysfunction, dyslexia, and developmental aphasia. (*Federal Register*, 1976, p. 56977)

Therefore, it seems apparent that some knowledge of neuropsychology is required if one is to properly diagnose and treat the above condition.

While some argue that the neuropsychological approach stresses disease and chronicity and that brain damage is an irreversible disorder, there is evidence of substantial recovery of function when adequate retraining is provided (Luria, 1972; Rosner, 1974). Although neural fibers in the CNS do not regenerate once damage occurs, recovery of function in which these cells were involved prior to destruction may occur to some degree. Such recovery depends on the extent of retraining that is given to an individual who had brain damage. Thus, the two major tasks of neuropsychologists are to (a) assess the area of deficit and (b) address retraining (Golden, 1978). While retraining may be futile in cases of progressive brain disease (e.g., multiple sclerosis and Huntington's chorea), at least some recovery of function is expected in the case of nonprogressive types of brain damage. One needs to discriminate between these two types of brain damage in order to provide effective treatment. The classic error in psychology and medicine is that of providing exclusively behavioral treatment to an individual with an unidentified progressive neurological condition (Goldstein, 1979).

In most cases, complete recovery from severe head injury does not occur. Brain damage usually causes permanent reduction in capacity to function at the premorbid level. Therefore, the need is to evaluate the degree of discrepancy between a patient's objective (actual) capacity to perform and his or her subjective (perceived) level of performance. Another task for neuropsychologists is to specify the behaviors that may serve as appropriate targets for treatment (Goldstein, 1979).

THE ROLE OF PSYCHOEDUCATIONAL ASSESSMENT

Within the neuropsychological framework, the goal of psychoeducational assessment is to describe an individual's current level of cognitive, perceptual, motor, and linguistic abilities (Christensen, 1975; Obrzut, 1981; Reitan & Davison, 1974; Smith, 1975). Consistent with recent data showing a direct relationship between cognitive, behavioral, and central nervous system functioning, neuropsychological data have been viewed as offering potential insights into constructs measured by traditional tests employed in psychoeducational assessment (see, for example, Rattan, Rattan, Gray, & Dean, 1987). Since most of the consequences of head injury influence functioning in these areas, most diagnostic tests for brain damage have incorporated such tasks. Neuropsychologists use traditional psychometric tests that have validity, reliability, and adequate standardization as well as the interview or observation (rating scale) approach. The complexities of brain-behavior relationships in concert with time limitations often associated with progressive brain disease in patients seem to indicate that systematic assessment procedures are the most productive approach. Empirical research has supported the validity of predictions made on the basis of neuropsychological tests in such areas as diagnosis and prediction of outcome (Klove, 1974; Meier, 1974; Russell, Neuringer, & Goldstein, 1970) as well as in the work on subtypes of learning disorders (Satz & Morris, 1980).

The professional with a neuropsychological perspective working within an educational environment can provide better integration of behavioral and educational data and develop a more appropriate and relevant individual educational plan (IEP). This can be accomplished by developing recommendations that accurately reflect the differential assessment of cognitive abilities, identifying subtypes of learning disabilities, conducting developmental research, and identifying children with previously unsuspected neurologically based learning disorders. In addition, the neuropsychological perspective is beginning to have a significant impact on the provision of services to preschool children. The roles include early identification of high risk children, and provision of consultation services to parents of children who need special services upon entering school (see Obrzut & Hynd, 1983, for a review).

In summary, a neuropsychological perspective can be beneficial in asssessing and diagnosing the child's strengths and weaknesses. This perspective provides a broader knowledge base from which to interpret psychoeducational data. The information yielded from neurological and neuropsychological assessments can be used to form the basis of an ongoing process of evaluation in order that more effective treatment can be implemented. It is suggested that effective treatment should be based on knowledge concerning the complexity of relationships that exist between brain functions and behavior. Neuropsychological and psychoeducational tests can best elucidate these relationships, which are not readily achieved by interview or the more global types of observational techniques used by behavioral psychologists.

RELATIONSHIP OF MOTOR AND COGNITIVE DEFICITS IN CHILDREN WITH ACQUIRED BRAIN INJURY

Human behavior, according to Luria (1973), occurs with the participation of all parts of the brain, each part making its own special contribution to the work of the functional system as a whole. Neuropsychological assessment is therefore not used for localizing psychological processes to particular cortical areas but rather is used to determine (a) which groups of concertedly working brain zones are responsible for mediating behavior and (b) the unique contribution made by each zone. Luria asserts that in diagnosing children it is important for professionals who have obtained data from sensory screening and central processing assessment to understand three neuropsychological zones. Luria argues that (1) the primary projection zones receive sensory input via the peripheral nervous system and transmit sensations to the cerebral cortex; (2) the secondary association zones (bordering the primary zones) are responsible for analyzing, interpreting, and storing information; and (3) the tertiary zones, located between the various sensory association areas, are responsible for intersensory integration (Obrzut & Obrzut, 1982).

The Luria-Nebraska Neuropsychological Battery–Children's Revision (Golden, Hammeke, & Purisch, 1980) is an outgrowth of Luria's theories and is currently being used and modified for use in detecting brain damage in children from 8 to 12 years of age (Golden, 1981). The need for neuropsychological assessment, which depends upon the assumption of considerable localization of behavioral function within the brain, has also been the impetus for the development of the Halstead Neuropsychological Test Battery for Children (ages 9 to 14) (Reitan & Davison, 1974) and the Reitan-Indiana Neuropsychological Test Battery for Children (ages 5 to 8 years) (Reitan, 1969). These are the most widely used batteries currently available for the assessment of brain dysfunction. Nevertheless, a critical review of the associated research suggests caution in making diagnostic decisions based on the results of these batteries. Hynd, Snow, and Becker (1986) provide such a critical review.

While it is now becoming generally acknowledged that neuropsychological assessment provides a more thorough picture of cortical integrity than does normative IQ or achievement testing alone (Hynd & Willis, 1987), the interconnection between neurological and cognitive function is still not sufficiently understood to provide definitive assessment of learning deficits or to prescribe educational measures for remediation (Ellison, 1983). The ongoing search for an organic component for learning disabilities in children has nonetheless provided us with much insight and given us more of a basis for remediation than ever before.

EFFECTS OF BRAIN INJURY ON MOTOR AND COGNITIVE SKILLS

The effects of brain damage on a child's cognitive or motor function are various, depending on the etiology and extent of the lesion, the anatomical location, the child's age at onset, and the static or progressive nature of the damage.

In general, head injuries in childhood may result in significant intellectual impairment. Transient and minor abnormalities have been connected with lower intellectual function at preschool or school age in comparison to children who had normal neurologic exams in infancy. Some researchers have suggested that a child's age at the time of brain injury is important if the injury results from encephalitis, meningitis, or the therapeutic irradiation of the brain, and all tend to be more damaging when they occur during the infancy period. This is due to the greater susceptibility to injury of immature organs during their phase of most rapid development (Chadwick, Rutter, Thompson, & Shaffer, 1981). Neurologically abnormal infants account for most of the abnormal cognitive function found at 4 years of age. For example, significant correlations have been found between the Milani-Comparetti and Gidoni neurologic method of assessment (Milani-Comparetti & Gidoni, 1967) given in infancy and the motor subtests from the McCarthy Scales of Children's Abilities (McCarthy, 1972) for leg coordination, draw-a-design, and draw-a-child given at 4 years of age (Ellison, 1983).

In infants with hypotonia (lack of muscle tone) and spasticity/dyskinesia, it is likely that the motor abnormality will be resolved by preschool or early school years. Thus, *some* severe motor impairments are outgrown (Ellison, 1983). While it has been suggested that the hard signs of neurologic abnormality (such as hypotonia, spasticity) would be later found in soft signs such as inadequate coordination of hands, it must also be remembered that many of the lesser neurologic signs and symptoms tend to improve over time, many disappearing between 4 and 10 years of age (Ellison, 1983).

Severe generalized brain trauma has also been connected with consistently lower intellectual function. For example, Chadwick et al. (1981) found that mean WISC Full Scale IQ (Wechsler, 1949) scores were found to generally be 8½ points lower when the duration of unconsciousness was 72 hours or more than when unconsciousness occurred for a shorter period of time; and it was some 7½ points lower than those of noninjured children when there had been definite evidence of treatment for cerebral edema. The effects of brain trauma also tended to be somewhat more marked with respect to visuo-motor skills than verbal skills (Chadwick et al, 1981). In the case of open head injuries, general damage is less frequent and contra-coup effects are minimal or absent. Apparently the fracture of the skull absorbs much of the energy of the impact and acts as a kind of buffer. Therefore, unlike closed head injury, there is frequently no loss of consciousness. The main problem with open injuries is the depth of the lesion and how far it goes into the subcortical structures.

In contrast to substantial associations found between the extent of both general and localized brain injury and the severity of cognitive impairment, neither the child's age at injury nor the hemisphere damaged had much effect on the pattern of cognitive deficit (Chadwick et al., 1981). In analyzing the entire WISC battery, very few statistically significant differences were found. The mean score on the Similarities subtest of the WISC was significantly lower in children who were less than 5 years old at the time of injury, but this tendency was apparently on only some of the other subtests and there was *no* substantial difference in overall IQ according to age of child at time of injury. There was, however, a fairly consistent tendency in general for cognitive scores to be lower in the younger children within the subgroup of those with left-sided injuries. This difference reached statistical significance only in the case of the Similarities (verbal abstract reasoning) and Block Designs (nonverbal abstract reasoning) subtests, but the difference in Full Scale IQ was also substantial (7½ points), even though the difference failed to reach the .05 level of significance.

It is generally accepted that the pattern of cognitive deficits after unilateral lesions in adults differs according to which hemisphere is damaged, with verbal skill impairment resulting from left hemisphere damage and visuo-spatial impairment resulting from right hemisphere damage. The results of recent research, however, suggest that the two hemispheres of the brain are less rigidly specialized in their functions during early and middle childhood than is the case in adult life or after 15 years of age. Cognitive deficits associated with lateralized brain injuries tend to be less specific in childhood than in adult life (Gott, 1973; Nolan, Hammeke, & Barkley, 1983;

Selz & Wilson, in press). In studies by Chadwick et al. (1981), for example, there was some tendency for verbal skills to be more impaired with left hemisphere damage and visuo-spatial skills with right-sided lesions, but most of the differences were quite small and not statistically significant. On some tests from the Reitan battery, the findings went in the reverse direction. There was, however, a tendency for all tests of scholastic achievement to show greater impairment with *left* hemisphere lesions. Thus, the localization of children's functions and their connection to hemisphere of damage are far more complex than once thought.

A second major difference in effects of brain injury with respect to age at time of injury has to do with the type of cognitive tasks that are to be accomplished at that stage of development. For example, brain damage in young children impairs their ability to acquire knowledge in the manner that this knowledge is usually presented in the schools, and thus they fail at skills emphasized in the school years. Some of the greatest deficits are shown in language and symbolic skill attainment. In contrast, when brain damage occurs in adulthood after a normal childhood, language and acquired knowledge are spared (unless damage is to the language areas) and deficits exhibit themselves mainly in adaptive and problem solving ability (Selz & Wilson, 1987).

EFFECTS OF NEUROPSYCHOLOGICAL DEFICITS IN LEARNING DISABLED CHILDREN

Regarding the impact that impaired neurological function has on later school learning, it should be noted that the research is contradictory. Some of the controversy stems from different philosophies, creating two brain-behavior camps (localization theorists vs. functional theorists), and some stems from confounded research due to the fact that learning disabled children were at one time treated as a monolithic group.

Learning disabled children are now thought to suffer from a dysfunction of the central nervous system, but these children usually manifest more subtle neurological deficits than brain injured children. The kinds of deficits from which learning disabled children suffer are those of the higher cognitive functions, such as memory, with normal functioning on lower level abilities, such as motor tasks, when they are compared with normal children (Golden, 1981).

Learning disabled students have been found to perform in a relatively normal manner on measures with a strong motor component. However, the performance of learning disabled students tends to resemble that of brain damaged subjects on tests with strong cognitive or attentional demands (Selz & Wilson, in press). It has also been found that among the subscales of the McCarthy Scale of Children's Abilities, the greatest discrepancy between children with learning disabilities and normal children was performance on the memory scale, with the verbal scale showing the second greatest difference (the McCarthy Scale does entail a large number of motor tasks) (Prasse, Ellison, & Siewart, 1982). However, the research becomes somewhat contradictory unless one signifies the type of learning disability being examined and the age of the child.

In this regard Satz and his colleagues (Satz & Babbler, 1970; Satz, Friel, & Rudegair, 1976) have found that reading disabilities among 7- to 8-year-olds were related to sensory-motor-perceptual-mnemonic abnormalities, while among older children, reading disabilities appeared to be caused by language delay (Ellison, 1983). The best predictors of later reading disability found by Ellison (1983) were a finger-localization test, a recognition-discrimination test, name of day testing, and an alphabet recitation test. Overall performance on these tests was highly predictive of good and poor readers through follow-up at grade 4.

NEUROPSYCHOLOGICAL PROFILES OF CHILDREN WITH COMMON LEARNING AND BEHAVIOR PROBLEMS

In examining the relation of neurological deficits to learning disability, it is essential at this point to examine the various deficits that can constitute the label "learning disabled" (LD), and to note the various profiles on psychoeducational measures that identify these children.

It is not sufficient to categorize LD children based on their area of academic deficiency (reading vs. handwriting, for example). Recent research suggests that even reading disordered children can be further subdivided into three or more groups based on the neuropsychological function that is impaired (Nolan et al., 1983). Some children may be deficient in reading due to delays in language development while others may have delays in visual-spatial ability. Still others may experience delays in the sequential analysis of information. Rourke and Strang (1983) attempted to find a unique neuropsychological profile for specific categories of learning disabled children. They classified children with learning disabilities into three categories based on results from the Wide Range Achievement Test (Jastak & Jastak, 1965). Group 1 consisted of children who performed normally in reading, spelling, and math on the WRAT; Group 2 consisted of those children with impaired performance on reading/spelling but normal performance in math; and Group 3 consisted of students impaired in math performance but normal in reading/

spelling. The studies reported by Rourke and Strang (1983) indicated that children with learning disabilities who were better in the Arithmetic subtests of the WRAT compared to the Reading and Spelling subtests performed poorly on tests thought to tap abilities subserved by the left cerebral hemisphere. Children whose only deficit appeared on the Arithmetic subtest of the WRAT, with Reading and Spelling within normal limits, did poorly on measures of abilities thought to be subserved by the right hemisphere. Rourke and Strang (1983) later analyzed the math subtest errors of Group 3 and found that these youngsters performed differently than other major subtypes of math disabled children in that they tended to (a) make a larger number of errors, (b) make a wider variety of errors, and (c) exhibit some difficulty with the appreciation of mathematical concepts. The authors also offered two strategies to alleviate difficulties of children who exhibit neuropsychological math problems similar to Group 3 children: (1) Mechanical arithmetic should be made as verbal as possible, and (2) the teaching of such children must be highly systematic and concrete. These Group 3 children typically exhibited other educational difficulties, including reading comprehension, handwriting, general organizational abilities (e.g., organizing a notebook), and virtually any complex subject area.

The general findings by Rourke and Strang (1983) substantiate the theories of hemispheric localization. Learning disabled students who were reading/spelling impaired tended to have lower WISC-R Verbal IQ scores and poorer performance on the Halstead-Reitan measures of language skills as compared to learning disabled children, who were deficient only in math. The math group also showed a lower Performance IQ than Verbal IQ and more impaired visual-spatial skills on a neuropsychological battery.

Nolan et al. (1983), on the other hand, found no such discrepancy between Verbal and Performance IQ among learning disabled children according to whether they were reading or math disabled. They did find, however, that learning disabled children in general obtained a lower Verbal IQ than did normally functioning children. They did not find this discrepancy in Performance IQ between the two groups. Nolan et al. (1983) also subdivided their learning disabled group according to the same categories Rourke and Strang used—(1) Normals, (2) Reading/Spelling Impaired, and (3) Math Impaired. In comparing these groups on the Luria-Nebraska, Nolan et al. (1983) found no significant differences between the normal group and the math impaired group. In explaining why their research so directly contradicts that reported by Rourke and Strang, Nolan et al. (1983) indicated that Rourke and Strang's group of math students was larger and more severely impaired than Nolan et al.'s math impaired group, thus partially explaining why Nolan et al.'s group showed no deficiencies in Performance IQ or visual-spatial skills. Also, as Rourke and Strang (1978) and Barkley (1981) have suggested, at least two separate math impaired learning disabilities may exist: those due to visual-spatial deficits and those due to deficiencies in linguistic abilities.

This theory is important to remember in understanding the controversy that surrounds the psychoeducational instruments that categorize learning disabled students. The Arithmetic subtest of the WISC-R has a large verbal component and is regarded by many as measuring a verbal skill (it is also part of the Verbal IQ of the WISC-R). Furthermore, the Reasoning Cluster of the Woodcock-Johnson Psycho-Educational Battery–Test of Cognitive Abilities (WJPB-TCA) (Woodcock & Johnson, 1977) has been found to have greater sensitivity to verbal ability than the nonverbal reasoning skills of the sort tapped by the WISC-R Performance scale. Thus, the correlation between the Woodcock-Johnson Reasoning Cluster and the WISC-R Performance IQ is less than the correlation between the Reasoning Cluster and both the WISC-R Verbal and Full Scale IQ scores. Perhaps the Woodcock-Johnson Reasoning Cluster is not a valid measure of nonverbal cognitive ability for children with school problems and should not be used interchangeably with the WISC-R Performance IQ or with subtests such as the Category Test of the Halstead-Reitan Neuropsychological Battery (HRNB) to assess such skills.

NEUROPSYCHOLOGICAL DEFICITS IN READING PROFILES

The two basic theories in the research on reading are the developmental lag model and the deficit model. According to the developmental lag model there is an underlying lag mechanism in brain maturation that is thought to forecast the later onset of dyslexia. Thus, dyslexia is framed in a developmental model rather than a deficit model and is seen as a delay in the rate of acquisition of developmental skills rather than impairment in these skills.

According to the deficit model (subscribed to by Reitan & Davison, 1974), affected children probably will not catch up to their normal age-mates. This model also predicts a less than age-appropriate level of reading performance throughout the school years (Selz & Wilson, in press). Bakker (1983) suggests that reading disorders may stem from an imbalance in neurologic status, reflected by a lack of synchronism among abilities. Thus it may be that psychoeducational assessment should focus on the interrelationship among abilities rather than on the impairment of certain abilities. For example, some evidence shows that high IQ reading underachievers demonstrate impaired auditory sequence skills, minor receptive language difficulties, significantly low scores in Arithmetic, Digit Span, and Coding subtests of the WISC-R, and a Verbal/Performance IQ discrepancy within normal limits. The fact that there was no finger agnosia and that there were problems with orientational and relational concepts indicates in general that the main problem with this group of children may be selective attention. All weaknesses found with this group were highly loaded on an attention/concentration component, and this may be the primary factor underlying poor performance.

It has been suggested by Milich and Loney (1979), in their studies of hyperkinetic/minimal brain dysfunction (MBD) children, that a three-factor profile of the WISC-R is a more useful way to assess whether attentional deficits account for academic difficulties in children. The three factors suggested were (1) Verbal Comprehension: Similarities, Vocabulary, and Picture Arrangement; (2) Spatial Organization: Picture Completion, Block Design, and Object Assembly; and (3) Inattention-Memory: Information, Arithmetic, Digit Span, and Coding. The fact that this group of impulsive children also exhibited high scores on the Similarities and Object Assembly subtests has been said to suggest that these children may have a global rather than analytic strategy of information processing (Milich & Loney, 1979). Thus, not only with hyperkinetic/MBD children but also with high IQ reading underachievers, a three-factor profile including an Inattention-Memory factor may provide the most useful information.

The trend, then, is away from the sensory-motor, tactile kinesthetic techniques for screening children at risk for later reading problems toward tests of higher cognitive functioning. The most useful tests in classifying below average and above average readers may be the Vocabulary and Block Design subtests of the WISC-R and the Peabody Picture Vocabulary Test (PPVT-R) (Dunn & Dunn, 1981).

As a final note, it is useful to provide a typical example of research on reading impairment in order to examine some of the problems and sources of confusion in this area. Fox and Routh (1983) examined first graders with severe reading disabilities (average IQ) and found they were markedly deficient in phonemic segmenting compared to average readers and those with less severe reading problems. A follow-up 3 years later included the dysphonemic group, the members of which had all been retained 1 year. Though phonemic segmenting abilities had risen significantly, dysphonetic spelling patterns had emerged in this group by third grade. Fourth grade average readers spelled better phonetically (even though they had had no phonemic instruction) (Fox & Routh, 1983). Since the dysphonemic group of children could be classified as dysphonetic as opposed to dyseidetic, this study may indicate the problems that arise when trying to teach children through their weak modalities. It may also indicate that a retained group of below average readers should not be compared to a promoted group of average readers (who have had a wider exposure to vocabulary and who have not been taught through their weakest modality).

In summary, children and adolescents with learning and behavioral problems resulting from head injuries share some problems with individuals who experience learning disabilities. The evidence suggests that motor and cognitive deficits in children with learning disabilities parallel those found in children with acquired brain injury. In addition, there are also many similarities in the neuropsychological profiles, in general, and in reading profiles, in particular, between the two groups of children. It is important to acknowledge developmental considerations both in terms of outcome and treatment when assessing children with acquired brain injury.

REFERENCES

Bakker, D.J. (1983). Hemispheric specialization and specific reading retardation. In M. Rutter (Ed.), *Developmental neuropsychiatry* (pp. 498–506). New York: Guilford.

Barkley, R.A. (1981). Learning disabilities. In E. Mash & L. Terdal (Eds.), *Behavioral assessment of childhood disorders* (pp. 441–482). New York: Guilford.

Chadwick, O., Rutter, M., Thompson, J., & Shaffer, D. (1981). Intellectual performance and reading skills after localized head injury in childhood. *Journal of Child Psychology and Psychiatry, 22,* 117–139.

Christensen, A.L. (1975). *Luria's neuropsychological investigation.* New York: Spectrum.

Doehring, D.G., & Hoshko, I.M. (1977). Classification of reading problems by the Q-technique of factor analysis. *Cortex, 13,* 281–294.

Dunn, L.M., & Dunn, L.M. (1981). *Manual: Peabody picture vocabulary test–Revised.* Circle Pines, MN: American Guidance Service.

Ellison, P.H. (1983). The relationship of motor and cognitive function in infancy, pre-school and early school years. *Journal of Clinical Child Psychology, 12,* 81–90.

Federal Register. (1976). Education of handicapped children and incentive grants program, *41,* 56977.

Fisk, J.L. & Rourke, B.P. (1979). Identification of subtypes of learning disabled children at three age levels: A neuropsychological multivariate approach. *Journal of Clinical Neuropsychology, 1,* 289–310.

Fox, B., & Routh, D.K. (1983). Reading disability, phonemic analysis, and dysphonetic spelling: A follow-up study. *Journal of Clinical Child Psychology, 12,* 28–32.

Gaddes, W.H. (1976). Prevalence estimates and the need for definition of learning disabilities. In R.M. Knights & D.J. Bakker (Eds.), *The neuropsychology of learning disorders: Theoretical approaches* (pp. 3–24). Baltimore: University Park Press.

Gaddes, W.H. (1981). An examination of the validity of neuropsychological knowledge in educational diagnosis and remediation. In G.W. Hynd & J.E. Obrzut (Eds.), *Neuropsychological assessment and the school-age child: Issues and procedures* (pp. 27–84). New York: Grune & Stratton.

Gaddes, W.H. (1985). *Learning disabilities and brain function: A neuropsychological approach* (2nd ed.). New York: Springer-Verlag.

Golden, C.J. (1978). *Diagnosis and rehabilitation in clinical neuropsychology.* Springfield, IL: Thomas.

Golden, C.J. (1981). The Luria-Nebraska Children's Battery: Theory and formulation. In G.W. Hynd & J.E. Obrzut (Eds.), *Neuropsychological assessment and the school-age child: Issues and procedures* (pp. 277–302). New York: Grune & Stratton.

Golden, C.J., Hammeke, T.A., & Purisch, A.D. (1980). *The Luria-Nebraska neuropsychological battery: Manual.* Los Angeles: Western Psychological Services.

Goldstein, G. (1979). Methodological and theoretical issues in neuropsychological assessment. *Journal of Behavioral Assessment, 1,* 23–41.

Gott, P.S. (1973). Cognitive abilities following right and left hemispherectomy. *Cortex, 9,* 266–274.

Hynd, G.W., Snow, J., & Becker, M.G. (1986). Neuropsychological assessment in clinical child psychology. In B.B. Lahey & A.E. Kazdin (Eds.), *Advances in clinical child psychology* (pp. 35–86). New York: Plenum Press.

Hynd, G.W., & Willis, W.Q. (1987). *Pediatric neuropsychology.* Orlando, FL: Grune & Stratton.

Jastak, J.F., & Jastak, S.R. (1965). *The wide range achievement test.* Wilmington, DE: Guidance Associates.

Klove, H. (1974). Validation studies in adult clinical neuropsychology, In R.M. Reitan & L.A. Davison (Eds.), *Clinical neuropsychology: Current status and applications* (pp. 211–235). New York: Winston-Wiley.

Luria, A.R. (1972). *The man with a shattered world.* New York: Basic Books.

Luria, A.R. (1973). *The working brain.* Harmonds-Worth: Penguin Books.

McCarthy, D. (1972) *McCarthy scales of children's abilities.* New York: Psychological Corp.

McKinney, J.D. (1984). The search for subtypes of specific learning disability. *Journal of Learning Disabilities, 17,* 43–50.

Meier, M.J. (1974). Some challenges for clinical neuropsychology. In R.M. Reitan & L.A. Davison (Eds.), *Clinical neuropsychology: Current status and applications* (pp. 289–323). New York: Winston-Wiley.

Milani-Comparetti, A., & Gidoni, E.A. (1967). Routine developmental examination in normal and retarded children. *Developmental Medicine and Child Neurology, 9,* 631–638.

Milich, R.S., & Loney, J. (1979). The factor composition of the WISC for hyperkinetic/MBD males. *Journal of Learning Disabilities, 12,* 491–495.

Myklebust, H.R., & Boshes, B. (1969). *Final report, minimal brain damage in children.* Washington, DC: U.S. Department of Health, Education, and Welfare.

Nolan, D.R., Hammeke, T.A., & Barkley, R.A. (1983). A comparison of the patterns of the neuropsychological performance in two groups of learning disabled children. *Journal of Clinical Child Psychology, 12,* 22–27.

Obrzut, J.E. (1981). Neuropsychological procedures with school-age children. In G.W. Hynd & J.E. Obrzut (Eds.), *Neuropsychological assessment and the school-age child: Issues and procedures* (pp. 237–275). New York: Grune & Stratton.

Obrzut, J.E., & Hynd, G.W. (1983). Implications of neuropsychology for learning disabilities. *Journal of Learning Disabilities, 16,* 532–533.

Obrzut, J.E., & Obrzut, A. (1982). Neuropsychological perspectives in pupil services: Practical application of Luria's model. *Journal of Research and Development in Education, 15,* 38–47.

Petrauskas, R., & Rourke, B.P. (1979). Identification of subgroups of retarded readers: A neuropsychological multivariate approach. *Journal of Clinical Neuropsychology, 1*, 17–37.

Prasse, D., Ellison, P., & Siewart, J. (1982, March). *Neurological integrity and the McCarthy scales: Research-based qualifiers and applications.* Paper presented at the National Association of School Psychologists, Toronto.

Rattan, A.I., Rattan, G., Gray, J.W., & Dean, R.S. (1987). *Defining neuropsychological constructs of the WISC-R with learning disabled children.* Paper presented at the 19th Annual National Association of School Psychologists Convention, New Orleans.

Reitan, R.M. (1969). *Manual for administration of neuropsychological test batteries for adults and children.* Indianapolis, IN: Author.

Reitan, R.M., & Davison, L.A. (Eds.). (1974). *Clinical neuropsychology: Current status and applications.* New York: Winston-Wiley.

Rosner, B.B. (1974). Recovery of function and localization of function in historical perspective. In D.G. Stein, J.J. Rosen, & N. Butters (Eds.), *Plasticity and recovery of function in the central nervous system* (pp. 1–29). New York: Academic Press.

Rourke, B.P., & Gates, R.D. (1981). Neuropsychological research and school psychology. In G.W. Hynd & J.E. Obrzut (Eds.), *Neuropsychological assessment and the school-age child: Issues and procedures* (pp. 3–25). New York: Grune & Stratton.

Rourke, B.P., & Strang, J.D. (1978). Neuropsychological significance of variations in patterns of academic performance: Motor, psychomotor, and tactile-perceptual abilities. *Journal of Pediatric Psychology, 2*, 62–66.

Rourke, B.P., & Strang, J.D. (1983). Subtypes of reading and arithmetical disabilities: A neuropsychological analysis. In M. Rutter (Ed.), *Developmental neuropsychiatry* (pp. 473–488). New York: Guilford.

Russell, A., Neuringer, C., & Goldstein, G. (1970). *Assessment of brain damage: A neuro-psychological key approach.* New York: Wiley-Interscience.

Satz, P., & Babbler, D. (1970). *Reading retardation, neuropsychological, perceptual and psycholinguistic factors.* Rotterdam: University of Rotterdam Press.

Satz, P., Friel, J., & Rudegair, F. (1976). Some predictive antecedents of specific reading disability: A two, three, and four year follow-up. In J. Guthrie (Ed.), *Aspects of reading acquisition* (pp. 46–62). Baltimore: Johns Hopkins University Press.

Satz, P., & Morris, R. (1980). Learning disability subtypes: A review. In F.J. Pirozzolo & M.C. Wittrock (Eds.), *Neuropsychological and cognitive processes in reading* (pp. 109–141). New York: Academic Press.

Selz, M., & Wilson, S.L. (1989). Neuropsychological bases of common learning and behavior problems in children. In C.R. Reynolds (Ed.), *Handbook of child clinical neuropsychology: Issues and techniques of diagnosis, treatment, and training.* New York: Plenum Press.

Smith, A. (1975). Neuropsychological testing in neurological disorders. In W.J. Friedlander (Ed.), *Advances in neurology* (pp. 49–110). New York: Raven Press.

Wechsler, D. (1949). *Wechsler intelligence scale for children manual.* New York: Psychological Corp.

Woodcock, R.W., & Johnson, M.B. (1977). *Woodcock-Johnson psycho-educational battery.* Allen, TX: DLM Teaching Resources.

8

Disorders of Communication in Traumatic Brain Injury

THOMAS P. MARQUARDT

JULIE STOLL

HARVEY SUSSMAN

Brain-trauma-based communication deficits in adults occur at all levels of the communication process—from conceptualization of the idea to the biomechanics of speech production. The last two decades have witnessed the marriage of important conceptual frameworks for cognition, language, and speech, which subsequently have been yoked to provide at least an initial understanding of these communication deficits due to brain trauma. Efforts to clearly establish the important parameters of the disorder, however, have been impeded by a number of philosophical and methodological problems (Groher, 1984a). First, head trauma patients are heterogeneous in terms of type, site, and extent of brain damage that produces communication deficits. Open head injury, in which the skull has been penetrated, typically produces focal damage; closed head injury is more often characterized by diffuse bihemispheric damage. It would not be expected that major differences in lesions would produce similar communication deficits. Specific language deficits such as agrammatism and phonological disorders are long-term residuals of focal lesions of the language dominant hemisphere. Problems with the pragmatics of communication are frequent features of diffuse bi-hemispheric lesions. Second, the stage of recovery is an important determiner of the deficits observed. The semi-comatose patient observed immediately after blunt head injury bears little resemblance to the fully recovered patient with speech and language abilities near normal limits. Attempts to compare patients at different stages of recovery have produced terminological confusion because of the rapid changes in appearance of the communicative impairment. Third, because standardized assessment instruments sensitive to the unique communication deficits associated with brain trauma have not been available and subject groups have differed widely in severity of brain damage and stage of recovery, there has been an inability to directly compare performance on test instruments between experimental groups from different studies. Finally, studies of brain trauma have focused on medical management rather than communication deficits, and only recently has there been a concerted effort to characterize the features, recovery, and treatment of communicative function.

Our purpose is to delineate the unique features of communicative functioning after traumatic brain injury in adults and to provide a reasoned view of issues related to evaluation and treatment. The focus of this chapter is not with childhood language disorders following head injury, because of the great diversity that accompanies such injuries as well as a variety of developmental issues that have to be taken into consideration (Ewing-Cobbs, Levin, Eisenberg, & Fletcher, 1987). Terminology is discussed. Specific characteristics of speech and language following focal and diffuse traumatic brain injury are presented. Also discussed are assessment and treatment strategies using both cognitive and language frameworks.

PERSPECTIVES ON NOMENCLATURE

Early research on the communication problems of brain trauma patients focused on penetrating head injuries, mostly from missile wounds (Goldstein, 1948; Luria, 1970; Schiller, 1947). The language of these subjects resembled, symptomatically, patients with focal lesions due to vascular infarct and was appropriately termed *aphasic*. Specific deficits were found in auditory comprehension, oral expression, reading, and writing, which allowed these patients to be assigned to different types of taxonomically derived classifications of aphasia (e.g., Broca's, Wernicke's). Major studies of war-related head trauma and subsequent communication problems continue to provide new information. Mohr et al. (1980) studied the effects of head wounds in 1,030 Vietnam veterans and found aphasia occurred in 244 of the patients. Aphasia resolved in 84 cases within 10 years. In a follow-up study, Ludlow et al. (1986)

divided the patients with nonfluent aphasia occurring within 6 months following injury into two groups: 13 with persistent nonfluent aphasia, and 26 without symptoms of aphasia. The recovered group demonstrated problems only in written expressive syntax, while the group with persistent aphasia showed syntactic processing deficits in all language modalities, with only minor problems in other language faculties. The point to be made is that focal damage subsequent to missile wounds to the dominant hemisphere produces clusters of speech and language deficits that historically have been viewed as similar in important respects to communication deficits associated with vascular lesions. Diffuse lesions would not be expected to produce the same result.

During the past two decades there has been a parallel consideration of the communication problems due to nonpenetrating head wounds or closed head injury (CHI). In general, two views have been developed regarding how these disorders, which result from widespread frequently nonfocal lesions, might best be conceptualized. One view holds that the CHI-based communication deficits are effectively considered as forms of aphasia and/or related disorders. For example, Levin (1981) cited anomic aphasia and Wernicke's aphasia as the two most frequently occurring types of syndromes secondary to acute diffuse brain damage. In a series of studies, Sarno and her colleagues (Sarno, 1980, 1984; Sarno, Buonaguro, & Levita, 1986) reported that all closed head injured postcoma patients evidenced linguistic impairment on formal testing, although these deficits may not have been observable in conversation. Based on the results of subtests from the Neurosensory Center Comprehensive Examination for Aphasia (Spreen & Benton, 1977), Sarno divided the population of head injured patients into three groups of relatively similar size. The first group included aphasic patients with pervasive verbal impairment that affected performance. Patients with dysarthria and "subclinical" aphasia were included in the second group. These patients had higher verbal performance on the language measures than the aphasic subjects of Group 1 and demonstrated dysarthria which ranged from mild articulatory imprecision to completely unintelligible speech. Performance of the patients of Group 3 was characterized by deficits in visual naming, word fluency, and the Token Test with the degree of impairment less than for the patients of the dysarthric group. The Token Test (DeRenzi & Vignolo, 1962) is composed of a series of tasks in which the subject is asked to manipulate large and small circles and squares of differing colors in response to instructions that increase in length and complexity; this test is considered to be highly sensitive to auditory comprehension deficits. Sarno concluded that the findings could be viewed as indicating a severity continuum from most severely impaired (aphasia) to least impaired (subclinical aphasia) and that fully two-thirds of all postcomatose head injured patients are less linguistically intact than they might appear from conversational interaction. Similarly, Kertesz and McCabe (1977) described the communication deficits of posttrauma patients as aphasia. They noted that the communication deficits rapidly resolved in approximately half the cases but that some of these patients demonstrated aphasia more than a year after onset.

It is not unexpected that patients early in recovery are "aphasic" due to the severity of the initial confused language and jargon. Such language deficits ameliorate quickly, however, leaving only about 2% frank aphasia following blunt head injury (Heilman, Safran & Geschwind, 1971). Levin, Grossman, Sarwar, and Meyers (1981) found that approximately 42% of their sample of 21 CHI patients regained cognitive, language, and social skills. Half of the remaining group demonstrated a generalized language deficit. The remaining six patients presented with a linguistic disturbance, most commonly anomia, that was associated with mild acute injury and normal comprehension. Groher (1977) tested 14 patients within approximately 10 days of brain damage and then at monthly intervals for 5 months. The patients initially demonstrated a marked depression in speech and language performance in all language modalities when compared to other aphasic subjects. At the end of 6 months, however, their performance had significantly improved, but they continued to show deficits in auditory processing and difficulty in spelling and sentence construction.

It is expected that in most cases of CHI, speech and language functioning rapidly recover to a point where the primary residuals are not major obstacles to oral communication. This does not imply that speech and language functioning is "normal" if premorbid functioning is used as the referent; only that on tests used to assess aphasic symptomatology, these patients perform at nearly normal levels within the limits of the assessment instrument. Continued subtle deficits in auditory processing, sentence construction, and anomia often remain. More importantly, however, significant deficits in the use of language as a tool of cognition and socialization, not captured by assessment instruments for aphasia, serve as the primary obstacles to effective communication.

A second view of communicative functioning secondary to CHI focuses on the impact of cognitive disorganization. Problems in reasoning, judgment, attention, sequencing, and memory are used to account for observed problems in communication. Darley (1964) was perhaps the earliest researcher to apply the label "language of confusion" to the deficits associated with diffuse brain damage. He described the syndrome as one in which patients had difficulty recognizing, understanding, and responding to the environment. They also have short-term memory deficits and disorganized reasoning, are disoriented in time and space, and present with behavior that is less adaptive and appropriate than normal. Halpern, Darley, and Brown (1973) compared groups of patients with the language of confusion, aphasia, apraxia of speech, and the language of generalized intellectual impairment on a series of language tasks. The label of language of confusion was not reserved for patients with traumatic lesions, since 5 of the 10 subjects in this group had other etiologies such as hemorrhage or tumor. The diagnosis of language of generalized intellectual impairment appeared to be a label for patients with dementia, since 8 of the 10 subjects of this group demonstrated "degeneration" without identification of the type or etiology of degeneration. Although results must be interpreted with caution because the etiology of brain damage was trauma in only half the cases, Halpern, Darley, and Brown found that the confused patients were moderately impaired in arithmetic, reading comprehension, writing to dictation, and relevance based on a rating scale for aphasia (Sklar, 1966). They were mildly impaired in communicative adequacy, auditory comprehension, syntax, naming, auditory retention, and fluency. The deficits observed on the language tasks were ascribed to impaired cognitive processes. For example, they noted that these patients "gave bizarre responses to various stimuli, indicating that clearness of thinking and accuracy of remembering were impaired. They seemed unaware of the irrelevance of their responses and made no attempt at correction" (p. 170). The language of confusion subjects were best differentiated from the other groups on the basis of relevance, reading comprehension, and writing of words to dictation.

In general, language from this vantage point is described anecdotally as fragmented, irrelevant, or bizarre (Wertz, 1978). Hagen (1984) described confused language as "receptive/expressive language that may be intact phonologically, semantically, and syntactically, yet is lacking in meaning because the behaviorial responses are irrelevant, confabulatory, circumlocutory, or tangential in relation to a given topic, and lacking a logicosequential relationship between thoughts" (p. 246). Ylvisaker and Szekeres (1986) and Szekeres, Ylvisaker, and Holland (1985) described cognitive-language deficits that were viewed as impairments of language learning or use that are indicative of more generalized cognitive deficits including disorganized discourse, inefficient integration of language, poor verbal learning, and inadequate use of language. Hagen (1984) argued that the language dysfunction in closed head injury is a secondary consequence of the underlying impairment/disorganization of nonlinguistic processes that support language. He concluded that CHI patients demonstrated language disorders that were a product of both linguistic and cognitive factors.

These two views of communication deficits in closed head injury are not imcompatible. During the early stages of recovery, specific language deficits as well as communication impairments arising from cognitive disorganization characterize the disorder. Groher (1977) observed, "I believe that closed head trauma patients initially manifest both aphasic (a reduced capacity to interpret and formulate language symbols) and confused (faulty short-term memory, mistaken reasoning, inappropriate behavior, poor understanding of the environment and disorientation) language skills" (p. 220). With recovery, residual deficits in receptive and expressive language remain, but the primary problems are in language use where thought content is confused and seldom relevant to the discussion. Hagen (1981), based on experience with 2,500 head injured patients, divided them into three groups after the early recovery phase characterized by diffuse symptomatology. These groups included (a) patients with disorganized language secondary to cognitive disorganization who may have a coexisting specific language disorder, (b) those with a specific language disorder and coexisting minimal cognitive disorganization, and (c) those with attention, retention, and recent memory impairment but without language dysfunction.

At this point, it would be helpful if some of the specific linguistic/communicative deficits of the patients were dealt with in more specific terms. The purpose of this short discussion is to highlight the most prominent features of the communicative impairment in closed head injury.

LANGUAGE DEFICITS IN TRAUMATIC BRAIN INJURY

The most commonly documented residual linguistic deficit in closed head injury is a persistent word retrieval impairment with associated circumlocution and verbal paraphasias (Heilman et al., 1971; Levin, Grossman, & Kelly, 1976; Najenson, Sazbon, Fiselzon, Becker, & Schechter, 1978; Thomsen, 1975). Qualitative measures of word fluency and visual confrontation naming reveal marked decreases in number of words able to be retrieved in timed tests such as the Boston Diagnostic Aphasia Examination (Goodglass & Kaplan, 1972) and the Neurosensory Center Comprehensive Examination for Aphasia (Spreen & Benton, 1977). This finding is not surprising due to the memory and attentional problems of this population. Few responses in a 1-minute time period would also be anticipated because of the slowness of processing and motoric performance. There is, however, large variability in the qualitative performance in the CHI population. Adamovich and Henderson (1983, 1985) observed the strategies used to retrieve words in left cerebrovascular accident, right cerebrovascular accident, closed head injured, old normals, and young normals. They found that the CHI group changed strategies more often during the task than either of the normal groups. Exploration of the qualitative performance on word fluency tests is seldom reported, yet would appear to be helpful in determining compensatory intervention.

Intuitively, the anomic language disturbance seen in CHI is not "aphasia." Prigatano, Roueche, and Fordyce (1985) argued that communication inadequacies seen in CHI are "nonaphasic" in contrast to the classic Broca's or Wernicke's aphasia subsequent to cerebrovascular accident. Excessive talkativeness and tangential speech are two nonaphasic language disturbances identified by Prigatano et al. that are integrally tied to the anomic deficit and lack of connected thought or cohesion.

Expressing the aphasia/nonaphasia dilemma, Holland (1982) observed that "if the language problems seen in closed head injury patients don't look like aphasia, sound like aphasia, act like aphasia, feel, smell or taste like aphasia, then they aren't aphasia" (p. 345). Aphasia denotes a disorder encompassing far more than just anomia. Aphasia entails significant difficulty across language modalities, usually sparing social/pragmatic skills. It is precisely this use of language in a social context that appears to be the common deficiency in the majority of patients with closed head injury. Holland noted that patients with aphasia communicate better than they talk, but the opposite appears to be the case for the head injured. What she meant is that aphasic patients effectively utilize compensatory strategies and residual speech and language skills to communicate efficiently in many social contexts. In contrast, patients with closed head injury are ineffective communicators, even though speech and language skills are relatively unimpaired. Formal language tests have been unable to capture the rambling ineffective communication of the brain trauma patient in social interaction.

Recently pragmatics (how languge is used in a social context) has emerged as a focus of language assessment in head injured individuals. Milton, Prutting, and Binder (1984) defined pragmatics as "behaviors which have the potential, if used inappropriately, to disrupt or penalize conversational interchanges" (p. 114). They examined language behaviors during unstructured conversation using the Pragmatic Protocol (Prutting & Kirchner, 1983). Mean percentage use of appropriate behaviors for the normal group of five subjects was 99.4%; for the closed head injured group it was 76%. The behaviors most frequently judged inappropriate were those of prosody, affect, topic selection, topic maintenance, turn taking, and conciseness. In a later study, Mentis and Prutting (1987) analyzed the cohesion of three head injured and three normal adults. Although the sample was small, several interesting findings emerged. The Halliday and Hasan (1976) cohesion analysis was used to judge whether semantic relations, or cohesive ties, appeared within conversational and/or narrative samples of head injured adults. In the development of a topic, the identification of referents and of semantic relations among referents must be established. By viewing grammar and vocabulary, the extent of interdependence of linguistic elements can be determined. For example, in the sentence *Mary gave it to John*, the obligatory referent for *it* must have been previously mentioned. In the normal speaker, interpretation of some linguistic elements is made only by referring to established referents. In the head injured patient, these cohesive ties frequently are missing and ambiguity results. The study revealed that although sentence level syntactic abilities were adequate, the head injured subjects used fewer cohesive ties and a different distribution than the normal subjects. The CHI subjects also used incomplete ties or referred to something not evident from the text. Abnormal cohesive patterns could be related to linguistic processing deficits, compensatory strategies, or pragmatic breakdown. The researchers concluded that difficulties with semantic relational concepts could underlie cohesion errors in discourse. Irvine and Behrmann (1986) investigated language form and use and cognitive ability in three CHI patients. Based on aphasia battery performance, tests of receptive and expressive language, and a profile of communicative appropriateness that took into consideration responses to the interlocutor, control of semantic content, cohesion, fluency, sociolinguistic sensitivity, and nonverbal communication, they concluded that there is no one language disorder characteristic of closed head injury and that the interactions between language use and form are subject specific and may be attributed to cognitive impairment or other factors.

In summary, the majority of CHI patients demonstrate no language structure problems with only mild to moderate impairment in content due to word retrieval difficulties. Social interaction skills are markedly deficient, reflecting a disturbance in the use of language (pragmatics). Lack of cohesion in discourse may violate social context demands, reflecting a direct language disturbance or a cognitive and concomitant language problem. The relationship between cognition and language for more abstract communicative tasks, however, remains inseparable. Further investigation of linguistic competence in CHI in discourse contexts is needed. In addition, pre- and post-onset factors such as motivation and personality need to be explored in greater detail given the social interaction problems of these patients.

SPEECH DEFICITS AFTER TRAUMATIC BRAIN INJURY

Severe closed head injury produces heterogeneous deficits in neuromuscular control of the speech mechanism. To a large extent neuromuscular speech disorders have been cited as chronic residuals in patients after the early stages of primary language recovery have been completed (Levin, 1981). Thomsen (1984), in a follow-up of 40 severely impaired patients with blunt head injury, found that all 15 patients who demonstrated dysarthria on initial examination at approximately 4 months postonset of brain damage continued to demonstrate dysarthria 10 to 15 years later. Groher (1977), in a study of 14 patients, reported that all demonstrated dysarthria after regaining consciousness. Nine demonstrated spastic dysarthria and five a mixed type of spastic-ataxic involvement. Two of the patients with spastic dysarthria and all five with mixed dysarthria evidenced mild intelligibility problems 6 months after onset of brain damage. Groher (1984a) also noted that Kaplan, Phillip, and Halper

(1979) reported mild residual dysarthria in several patients 2 to 6 months after brain damage.

Given the incidence of dysarthria following brain damage, there is strikingly little information that details the type or severity of neuromuscular speech involvement. The most frequently occurring deficits appear to result from bilateral damage to pyramidal and extrapyramidal tracts producing spastic dysarthria. Spastic dysarthria is characterized by imprecise articulation, harsh voice quality, reduced stress, monopitch, and monoloudness and is usually found in conjunction with spastic quadriplegia. The shearing acceleration/deceleration forces caused by blunt brain damage as well as direct insult also may produce brainstem and cerebellar damage producing flaccid and ataxic types of dysarthria. Nasal emission, hypernasality, breathiness, and consonant imprecision are features of flaccid dysarthria; excess and equal stress, irregular articulatory breakdown, distorted vowels, and harsh voice quality are features of ataxic dysarthria (Darley, Aronson, & Brown, 1975). More commonly it would be expected that head injury will cause an admixture of these different types of dysarthria with the specific speech production deficits dependent on the site and extent of brain damage. Less commonly damage to the basal ganglia may produce hypokinetic or hyperkinetic forms of dysarthria. Kent, Netsell, and Bauer (1975), in a cinefluorographic study, and Lehiste (1965), in an acoustic analysis, provided case studies of dysarthria following brain trauma which detailed deficits in lingual movement and slowed rate and incoordination in articulatory activity. However, with minor exceptions, detailed examination of dysarthria in an extensive sample of brain trauma patients has yet to be completed.

Levin et al. (1983) reported that 9 of 350 patients (3%) were mute for varying periods even though communication was recovered through a nonspeech modality. Subcortical lesions, primarily of the putamen and internal capsule, were found in four patients, and left hemisphere lesions without subcortical damage were found in four of five patients. The left hemisphere damaged subjects showed a longer period of impaired consciousness indicative of severe diffuse brain injury and long-term linguistic deficits. Von Cramon (1981) reviewed 11 patients with acute traumatic mutism due to brainstem damage. The patients demonstrated breathy voicing and a strained type of phonation. Intensity gradually increased with a corresponding decrease in breathiness. All of the patients showed some dysphonia and restricted intonational pitch ranges within a year of the head trauma. Articulation was characterized by reduced rate, reduced ability to maintain occlusions, and stable constrictions of the upper airway and particular problems in control of the front part of the tongue that continued for as long as the patients were studied. Four of the patients also demonstrated hypernasality. In a follow-up study, Vogel and von Cramon (1983) investigated phonetic errors in five patients with dysarthria following traumatic mutism.

Initially, the subjects could not spread or round the lips or protrude the tongue to the lips on nonspeech tasks. During recovery, the subjects were requested to produce a series of two-syllable words containing all standard German consonants, vowels, diphthongs (two vowels produced within the same syllable), and selected consonant clusters. The words also were investigated by spectrographic analysis. Two of the patients were able to produce identifiable speech sounds in less than 2 weeks, while the other three patients required between 3 and 7 weeks. With the exception of one patient who demonstrated Parkinsonian-like speech production, articulation was near normal limits by approximately 3 months. In general, key features of the dysarthria included difficulty in gaining articulatory closure, particularly for the back of the tongue, and problems in developing turbulent airflow and in tongue placement for some vowels.

Several additional studies have focused on the dysphonic component of posttraumatic dysarthria. Hartmann and von Cramon (1984), in an acoustic analysis of 14 patients, found two subgroups: one showing breathy and tense voice quality that gradually normalized and a second group that initially was normal or lax with a breathy quality which subsequently became more tense. Finitzo et al. (1987) found voice disorders subsequent to brain trauma in seven patients from a larger pool of 70 patients with spasmodic dysphonia. In contrast, Sapir and Aronson (1985) reported two cases of aphonia subsequent to head trauma, one with spastic dysarthria and one with ataxic dysarthria, who regained phonation after a single session of symptomatic voice therapy. They argued that the most likely explanation was that the aphonia was due to an affective disorder due to frontal lobe damage rather than laryngeal paralysis or apraxia of phonation.

Other deficits in speech motor control also have been identified subsequent to head trauma. Zazula (1984) found impaired ability to produce intonational contours in patients with moderate to severe brain trauma. Lazurus and Logemann (1987), in a radiographic investigation, studied 53 closed head injury patients referred for swallowing problems. They found that 81% of the patients had a delayed or absent swallowing reflex, 50% demonstrated reduced tongue control, and 33% had reduced peristalsis. To demonstrate the diversity of speech disorders associated with head trauma, Cooper (1983) and Helm-Estabrooks, Yeo, Geschwind, Freedman, and Weinstein (1986) report the onset and/or relapse of stuttering following brain damage.

In summary, dysarthria and associated deficits in phonation and swallowing are common residuals in CHI. They frequently are camouflaged by disorganization and fragmentation of oral expression, which have been the focus of more recent research. The presence of dysarthria in its most severe form may necessitate the use of alternative and/or augmentative communication systems to bypass the impaired speech production apparatus.

RECOVERY OF COMMUNICATIVE FUNCTION AFTER TRAUMATIC BRAIN INJURY

Determining the recovery of function following brain damage is important for several reasons. First, treatment effects cannot be factored from the total recovery of function unless spontaneous (nontreatment) recovery is known; spontaneous recovery is the yardstick against which treatment effects are measured. Second, communicative functioning can serve as an important indicator of improved neurological functioning during the acute stage. The dense relationship between cognitive and linguistic functions allows measures of communication to serve as a mirror of the neurological functioning of the patient. Finally, a pattern of recovery based on known variables allows prognostic decisions to be made relative to the patient's eventual level of functioning.

Most studies of missile-wound-based head trauma are retrospective investigations of wartime injuries. Wepman (1951), for example, studied 68 aphasic patients at least 6 months postonset of brain damage. Based on a treatment program that included speech therapy, reading, writing, spelling, and mathematics educational training, he found that 51% were much improved, 35% were improved, and 14% were unchanged. Mohr et al. (1980) and Ludlow et al. (1986) studied head injured patients from the Vietnam War era and found specific residual aphasic deficits 10 to 15 years or more following brain damage. To a large extent, these studies revealed primary recovery as well as residual aphasias during the first 6 months following brain damage.

Given the relative recency of major interest in closed head injury, the number of studies that have tracked recovery or evaluated performance during two or more fixed time frames is striking. In a number of cases, these studies have not dealt specifically with communicative functioning. Overgaard et al. (1973), for example, investigated factors that might be beneficial in predicting final outcome in 201 patients with head trauma due to motor vehicle accidents. Initial neurological examinations and a detailed neurological examination 24 to 36 months later revealed that abnormal motor activity was the most important unfavorable sign in younger patients; history and length of unconsciousness were the most unfavorable signs for older patients. Basic clinical signs, age, and posttraumatic blood pressure were significantly related to functional recovery 2 to 3 years postinjury.

A group of patients were examined at 4.5 months, 2.5 months, and 10 to 15 years after blunt head injury by Thomsen (1984). Based on questionnaires completed by the patient, relatives, or staff, she found that although physical functioning, speech, and memory remained severely impaired in many cases, the psychosocial problems associated with the neurological insult were the most serious concern, with permanent deficits in personality and emotion reported in two-thirds of the cases. Scherzer (1986) investigated the effects of a cognitive retraining program in 32 adults with severe head injury and with an average postcoma recovery period of 59 months. The patients were provided with a 30-week treatment program that included cognitive and perceptual remediation, problem-solving learning, counseling, exercise and relaxation, social skills, and prevocational training, The greatest improvement occurred in psychomotor tests of attention, visual information processing, memory, and complex reasoning. The treatment effects were robust as measured 3 to 12 months after completion of the program.

Levin et al. (1987) evaluated 57 patients with minor head injury 1 week and 1 month after head trauma on a battery of memory, attention, and information processing tasks and compared their performance with 56 control subjects. A subset of 32 patients also was evaluated 3 months later. Based on statistical comparisons of performance, they concluded that a single uncomplicated minor head injury does not produce permanent disabling neurobehavioral impairment in most patients without history of substance abuse or pre-existing neuropsychiatric problems.

These three exemplars of studies of minor versus severe head injury in treated and untreated conditions at chronic and acute stages point out that major recovery is to be expected from spontaneous recovery and as a function of cognitively based treatment. Studies of communicative recovery have been sparse, but provide a scaffolding for consideration of expected residual deficits following brain damage.

Najenson et al. (1978) observed 15 patients with prolonged coma after brain damage for a year or more. Estimates of communicative performance were based on ratings of auditory comprehension, visual comprehension, speech, oral expression, reading, and writing, because the subjects were too severely impaired to complete standardized tests. No treatment of communicative deficits was reported. Nine of the subjects demonstrated significant recovery, while six remained in a vegetative state. Six of the nine who recovered demonstrated "complete" recovery of semantic functions, and three showed residual aphasic deficits. Eight of the subjects who recovered demonstrated a residual dysarthria. In an earlier study, Najenson et al. (1975) evaluated 40 patients with closed and open head trauma who had regained consciousness within 3 months. Twenty of the patients were characterized as aphasic based on results from the Functional Communication Profile (Taylor, 1963). Substantial variability characterized the recovery patterns of the patients. Expressive skills preceded the recovery of receptive skills, and after 6 months most difficulty was noted on reading and narrative writing tasks.

Thomsen (1975) examined 12 patients after diffuse closed head injury and approximately 30 months later using nonstandardized speech and language tasks. She found that four of the patients had not improved and that, as a group, the patients demonstrated residual aphasia and dysarthria. In a case study, Thomsen (1981) described a 44-year-old man with severe head trauma and pronounced global aphasia. The patient received intensive treatment from 10 weeks to 2 years following the injury, and an evaluation of language, learning, and memory was completed and a questionnaire dealing with cognitive, behavioral, and emotional changes was completed by the patient's spouse. Treatment was geared to the functional level of the patient. Initially it took the form of afferent input for naming of body parts and activities for improving automatic speech. Later treatment tasks included work on antonyms and synonyms. Twelve years later the patient was reevaluated with the same group of tests. Between the two assessment periods, the patient demonstrated marked improvements in language and cognitive function that were reflected in daily living activities.

Groher (1977) completed a detailed study of language and memory recovery in 14 patients. The 14 closed head injured subjects were tested using the Porch Index of Communicative Ability (Porch, 1971) and the Wechsler Memory Scale (Wechsler, 1948) after regaining consciousness and then at 30-day intervals for 120 days. The patients initially showed depressed performance on gestural, verbal, and graphic tasks, with gestural ability most impaired. All language skills showed improvement during the first month and up to 4 months, but scores revealed decreased performance on expressive and receptive tasks 4 months after brain damage. Comprehension of reading material was poor up to 4 months after insult. The patients were able to converse readily and make their needs known, but 9 of the 14 carried on conversations that were inappropriate in length, and thought content was frequently confused and irrelevant. Graphic skills were characterized by spelling errors, poor syntax, and incomplete sentence construction. All memory tasks, with the exception of orientation, were within normal limits by the end of 4 months. Groher concluded that it is the "discrepancy between the seemingly 'normal' ability to communicate and a poor performance in organizational and retention skills which becomes such a devastating liability for the patient who suffers closed head trauma with resultant language or memory disorders" (p. 220).

In general, the studies of recovery of communicative functioning suggest that there is a marked resolution of linguistic deficits in the near term (30 to 60 days) followed by improvement that may continue for a year or more. At the end of the early recovery period, continued language deficits can be observed from standardized testing, particularly in naming but also in auditory comprehension, reading, and writing. The degree of specific language deficit, however, is related to the severity of the brain injury, with more severe brain trauma producing more severe residual effects and with minor closed head injury producing no significant lasting effects. The primary residuals following the early rapid improvement are semantic and pragmatic communication deficits characterized by problems related to relevance, topic maintenance, inhibition of verbal output, and logical organization of expression.

ASSESSMENT

Given the potential for focal and diffuse damage to multiple sites, it is not surprising that communicative deficits in head injury are extremely heterogeneous. In many ways, the assessment of these patients is more demanding than in aphasia or dysarthria alone, because there is no single battery of standardized measures that effectively captures the salient characteristics of the disorder. Moreover, the magnitude of associated cognitive deficits and rapid changes in neurological functioning following onset demand that the assessment of communicative skills dovetail with other measures of performance that are outside the province of many speech/language pathologists.

During the early stages of recovery when language and cognitive disorganization is greatest, formal testing frequently cannot be completed because the patient is confused, disoriented, and cannot participate fully in stimulus response tasks. During this period of time, as noted by Hagen (1984), a methodology should be employed that effectively allows for describing, categorizing, and scaling the type and severity of cognitive and language impairment. Standardized testing must await initial recovery.

Hagen (1981, 1984) described four areas of assessment in head trauma. The areas included categorizing spontaneous responses to random environmental stimuli; scaling responses to stimuli not controlled by the patient; administration of a language battery; and assessment of cognitive and verbal abilities. He suggested that the four assessment areas may mirror longitudinally the recovery of the patient or may be carried out in combination depending on the level of functioning. Categorizing spontaneous responses included observations, based on daily activities and language tests, to identify the level of disorientation, confusion, distractibility, and impulsivity; reduced initiation and inhibition; concreteness; reduced cognitive flexiblility; disorganization; and reductions in judgment. It is clear that although these behaviors may be reflected in communicative functioning, they are not direct estimates of speech and language abilities.

Hagen (Hagen & Malkmus, 1979) used the Levels of Cognitive Functioning Scale to track changes in behavioral responses over time. The eight-level behavior scale varies from Level I (no response) to Level VIII (purposeful and appropriate) where the patient can recall and integrate events, is responsive to the environment, and shows carry-over for new learning but may continue to demonstrate decreased ability relative to premorbid levels in language, abstract reasoning, and judgment. Hagen suggested that, at a minimum, cognitive assessment should include evaluation of attentional abilities, discrimination, temporal ordering, memory, categorization, association/integration, analysis/synthesis, and maintenance of goal-directed behavior. Since phonology, syntax, and semantics may appear within normal limits, he recommended that assessment of language functioning should be guided by an effort to determine the level of language integrity using tests of intelligence and learning.

Ylvisaker and Szekeres (1986) presented a similar view of assessment. They noted that the formal test situation may mask the deficits of the brain injured patient. Formal testing provides a quiet environment without distractions, an interactive examiner who provides concise explanations for tasks, and tests that do not test learning over repeated sessions or generalization of newly learned strategies and skills to different environments. The test situation has the effect of attenuating observed problems in attention, memory, motivation, the efficiency of information processing, and fatigue. They suggested that formal assessment of the brain injured patient include observation of the patient in a variety of environments to evaluate the effects of setting on the efficiency of information processing, behavior appropriateness, and stress; a detailed interview of the family to identify the highest and lowest levels of functioning based on behavior in a familiar environment; and diagnostic therapy to determine the rate of new learning and the generalization of these skills to other settings. A series of diagnostic questions (e.g., What is the level of semantic knowledge? What are the effects of processing demands on language comprehension?) for receptive language, expressive language, integrating language and verbal reasoning, and verbal memory and new learning are provided as gateways for diagnostic decision making.

Hagen (1984) and Ylvisaker and Szekeres (1986) view communication as if it were hung on a scaffolding of cognition. In the absence of significant structural language problems, communication deficits are due to underlying problems in attention, memory, inhibition, and organization of information, and are assessed accordingly. Evaluation protocols are framed to include assessment of both language and cognition. However, since there are almost no formal measures of language in conversational settings, specific deficits and levels of functioning are estimated from informal detailed observations of behavior coupled to selected tests of cognition.

In patients with severe head trauma, a no less macroscopic view of evaluation is assumed, but there is a more detailed analysis of specific speech and language deficits. It is necessary to determine areas of relatively normal function and areas of specific deficit, a process that might best be carried out using an assessment battery for aphasia such as the Boston Diagnostic Aphasia Examination (Goodglass & Kaplan, 1972) or the Porch Index of Communicative Ability (Porch, 1971). Also of value in determining communicative functionality is Communicative Abilities in Daily Living (Holland, 1980). Additional tests may need to be selected to examine in more detail auditory comprehension, oral expression, naming, reading and writing skills, and pragmatics. Milton et al. (1984), for example, demonstrated the utility of a protocol to assess pragmatic function in head injury. The protocol was designed to be sensitive to interactional features of the communicative situation. It includes 32 behaviors that cross all levels of language functioning including phonology, syntax, semantics, and pragmatics. The instrument is divided into three speech act categories: (a) utterance act that includes ways the message is presented (verbal, nonverbal, and paralinguistic), (b) propositional act (behaviors that provide the linguistic meaning), and (c) illocutionary and perlocutionary acts (reciprocal acts that govern discourse). Based on a sample of unstructured conversation, behaviors are recorded but the frequency is not taken into consideration because even a single occurrence may be reason enough to target it for remediation. A severity index based on frequency of inappropriate behaviors is used, because some pragmatic deficits may be more penalizing than others and frequency does not address this qualitative aspect of performance.

A major consideration in assessment is speech performance. Although many head injured patients late in recovery demonstrate relatively normal structural language coupled with problems with pragmatics and higher level verbal functioning, there also is a relatively high incidence of significant dysarthria, particularly in severe head trauma. Perhaps the overriding feature of dysarthria in head injury is weakness due to damage to the pyramidal tract and lower motor neurons. When communicative functioning is addressed through a cognitive filter, these oftentimes severe problems are viewed as relatively less important. The assessment of dysarthria requires a detailed analysis of the anatomic and functional integrity of the speech production apparatus as well as more global measures of intelligibility. The motor speech examination (Darley et al., 1975) is composed of a series of observations relative to the anatomic integrity of the speech production apparatus and a group of nonverbal and verbal tasks that assess facial, lingual, velopharyngeal (mechanism for closing the passageway between oral and nasal cavities), mandibular, and laryngeal functioning that should be a pro forma part of the examination of the patient. The Assessment of Intelligibility of Dysarthric Speech (Yorkston & Beukelman, 1981) provides six types of information: single word intelligibility, sentence intelligibility, speaking rate in words per minute, rate of intelligibile speech based on number of intelligible words per minute, and communication efficiency (defined as the rate of intelligible speech compared to normal speakers). In cases of severe head injury, assessment of the anatomic and functional integrity of the speech production apparatus and determination of intelligibility are minimum prerequisites of the examination.

Severe neuromuscular deficits may be sufficient to preclude oral expression as a primary means of communication. In these cases, a detailed examination must consider cognititve, linguistic, motor, and sensory functioning to determine which augmentative or alternative systems provide the most efficient means of communication. This assessment typically requires the aid of occupational and physical therapists because of the need to determine residual motor functioning of the extremities and the critical need for positioning of the patient in using the system. Finally, dysphagia is not an uncommon consequence of neuromuscular impairment in severe head injury. Detailed assessment of the speech production apparatus for vegetative functioning coupled to radiographic assessment of mastication and deglutition typically are completed to determine the effects of weakness and incoordination and to plan a course of remediation (Groher, 1984b).

In summary, assessment of the head injured patient requires consideration of cognitive deficits that impact on higher order language functioning, impaired language form that may be observed at early stages of recovery or as a more permanent residual of severe injury, and neuromuscular-based speech and swallowing disorders that may coexist with cognitive and language impairment. Quite obviously, the assessment battery will be chosen to assess the most important domains of cognition, language, and speech to determine the patient's residual skills and major areas of deficit.

TREATMENT

There appears to be an implicit assumption that cognition should serve as the vehicle for dealing with communication disorders subsequent to brain trauma. Although it is intuitively logical that improved attention, memory, verbal reasoning, and organization of information should have the effect of increasing the efficiency of communication in these patients, there are no experimental studies of treatment efficacy using this approach. Until generalization of improved cognitive abilities to communication skills can be shown experimentally, it would seem more appropriate to deal with the communication deficits directly. With only a few exceptions, most descriptions of treatment of communication deficits are based on cognitive retraining.

Adamovich and Henderson (1985) suggested that deficits in speech, voice, and swallowing are subject to traditional treatment methods. For the more incapacitating communication problems arising from cognitive processing deficits, they propose a four-stage treatment hierarchy geared toward changing and modifying behavior and then generalizing these behaviors to other environments. The first stage includes alerting and stimulation tasks to improve attention and perception. Specific tasks include auditory stimulation and tracking from gross nonspeech to finely discriminated speech sounds; identification of environmental sounds; and verbal stimulation to elicit vocalizations. The second stage, orientation, entails repetitive review with the patient of time, place, and person activities. The third stage, operative training, includes tasks to improve discrimination, organization, memory, and high-level "thought processing" (convergent thinking, deductive reasoning, inductive reasoning, divergent thinking, and multiprocess reasoning). The final stage, self-reliant functioning, focuses on carry-over of new skills to functional situations through home visits and group therapy that requires organization of ideas and conversational skills (turn taking, self-monitoring, etc.).

Hagen (1984) gears treatment to the cognitive level of the patient. If the patient is not responsive or exhibits generalized or localized responding, the purpose of treatment is to increase awareness of the environment by talking with the patient and managing external stimuli. For confused and/or agitated patients, treatment is focused on increasing awareness and reducing agitation by environmental management. When the patient continues to be confused but is no longer agitated, the purpose of treatment is to provide a setting conducive to purposeful and appropriate responses to stimuli. Particularly important at this point is the maintenance of a structured environment in terms of physical setting and daily scheduling, the use of verbal descriptions to describe tasks as they are performed and to review the daily routine, and slowed repetitive presentation of questions and instructions. Daily routine completed with minimal supervision is the goal for patients who have reached a cognitive level where behavior is appropriate and purposeful. At this point the patient appears "normal" because of the structured nature of the environment.

A primary feature of Hagen's approach to treatment is that cognition-based tasks serve as the framework for treatment of "cognitive-linguistic disorganization." He suggests that the critical factor in language rehabilitation is to match the cognitive functioning level of the patient with the stimulus input so that the patient can process stimuli in an organized manner that in turn allows language to be used in an organized manner. Treatment is designed to facilitate the development of 13 abilities ranging from attention to suppression of irrelevant stimuli to modification of a response. What is particularly noteworthy about this approach is the lack of reciprocity in task selection. Apparently cognition facilitates language, but language may not be critical to cognitive rehabilitation.

A similar framework of treatment is provided by Ylvisaker and Szekeres (1986). Here again the organizing framework is one of cognitive abilities without a direct addressing of communication deficits. For example, cognitive-language activities proposed for the middle stage of recovery (restricted attention, shallow perception, weak memory/learning, poor access to stored contents, weak organizing skills, severely impaired executive and metacognitive functions) include tasks for selective attention and comprehension, access to past experiences, semantic knowledge and organizational principles, organizing processes, reasoning and problem solving, metacognitive functioning, and orientation. Although verbal skills are intrinsic to the tasks, the focus is on improved cognitive functioning rather than improved communication abilities.

In contrast, several investigators (e.g., Davenport, 1981; Smith, 1984) have dealt directly with specific speech and language disorders that may result from head trauma including treatment methods for aphasia, dysarthria, apraxia, and dysphagia. The treatment methodology for these disorders would not be expected to differ significantly from treatment provided for patients with aphasia due to cerebrovascular accidents (Chapey, 1981; Marquardt, 1982).

Recently, treatment techniques have evolved that deal directly with the impaired communication system of CHI patients. These techniques differ from the approaches of Hagen (1984) and Ylvisaker and Szekeres (1986) in that communication rather than cognition becomes the focus of treatment. Yorkston, Stanton, and Beukelman (1981) described a language-based compensatory training program for a CHI patient. The purpose of the program, encompassed within a broader program of rehabilitation, was to use relatively intact language functioning to compensate for impaired sequencing ability. The program contained three parts. In the first phase, the patient rehearsed a story as she sequenced a series of 10 pictures. She checked the accuracy of the sequencing, with feedback from the clinician, by retelling the story. During the second phase, the patient read written descriptions of the pictures as they were sequenced. In the third phase, the sequencing task was repeated with written cues. Results showed improved sequencing ability that was maintained without treatment. Performance on similar tasks also was improved but to a lesser extent than the trained task. The researchers concluded that one important role of the speech/language pathologist may be to determine whether language ability is sufficient to serve as a compensatory system for overriding cognitively based deficits in organization and sequencing.

Gajar, Schloss, Schloss, and Thompson (1984) investigated the effectiveness of a self-monitoring and feedback paradigm on the development of group conversational behaviors in two head injured patients. The two patients demonstrated perseverative responding, failures in topic maintenance, interruptions, and inappropriate laughter. The subjects were included in a group of four and were provided with a light signal corresponding to positive or negative interactions. The signal was initially controlled by the experimenter (feedback) and then by the group (self-monitoring). Feedback and self-monitoring had a positive effect on the conversational behaviors of the two patients tested, and positive communication interactions were higher in frequency during the treatment phases than during associated baseline periods.

Ehrlich and Sipes (1985) carried out a group treatment program for improving communication skills in six patients with CHI. The patients demonstrated problems in message repair and revision, reduced cohesion and coherence in narratives, poor topic maintenance, and intermittent inattention to messages from other speakers. Two therapists functioned as role models, providing examples of appropriate communicative behaviors, and utilizing verbal and gestural cues to facilitate improved communication skills. Within the group discussions, the therapists introduced models relative to nonverbal communication, communication in context, message repair, and cohesiveness of narrative and demonstrated appropriate and inappropriate behaviors. Two patients also completed similar role-playing activities. The role-playing activities were videotaped and then were played back for group analysis and discussion. Treatment effects compared to goals were evaluated clinically by observing the functioning of each patient during the role playing, during the videotape playback of the role playing, and within the spontaneous communication of the group discussion. A rating scale based on the pragmatic protocol of Prutting and Kirchner (1983) was used to provide an empirical evaluation of change. Results showed that all six patients improved when pre- and posttreatment performances were compared. Most improvement was noted in topic maintenance, initiation of conversation, syntax, cohesion, and communication repair. Gains were less in intelligibility, listening, and lexical selection. Little to no change was found in body posture, interruption, prosody, facial expression, and the variety of language use. Ehrlich and Sipes concluded that the patients were more effective communicators at the end of treatment. Specifically, they demonstrated greater awareness of the speaker's goal in communication, greater sensitivity to the listener's needs, and improved use of turn-taking behaviors such as topic maintenance and repairs of communication breakdowns.

These later studies are important because they demonstrate the utility of treatment programs that directly deal with the communication problems after the course of spontaneous recovery. These language-based programs reflect a shift from a passive cognitive framework to a more direct targeting of residual language abilities to enhance communication effectiveness. There is no clear-cut reliance on generalization from improved cognitive functioning to improved ability to utilize communication in social interaction. It is important to note that language-based treatment of communication disorders in CHI emphasizes the compensatory nature of treatment by maximizing residual skills, not by retraining lost functions. This basic premise also underlies cognitive retraining activities (Prigatano, 1987).

CONCLUSIONS

Traumatic brain injury produces communication residuals typically associated with focal and diffuse lesions. The assessment protocols and treatment methodology for the two types of lesions vary as a function of the communication residuals demonstrated. In missile wounds, the symptomatology is similar to patients with focal lesions due to cerebrovascular accidents who demonstrate aphasia with retention of pragmatic communication abilities. Accordingly, traumatic brain injury patients with focal damage respond to many of the similar treatment modalities traditionally offered to those with aphasia due to cerebrovascular accident. Tests of language form are the primary assessment instruments for patients with aphasia due to missile wounds to the head. In contrast, in CHI with nonfocal damage, there is a rapid improvement in language form but with a significant deficit in the ability to utilize communication for the purposes of social interaction. Sentential tests of language form do not capture the nonaphasic language of this population. Current research is directed toward investigation of linguistic competence in narrative and conversational discourse. For patients with CHI, both the tools of evaluation and the methodology of treatment are presently based on a cognitive processing model that has yet to be demonstrated as sufficient for capturing important aspects of the communication impairment. Only additional data will allow a decision to be made regarding its long-range utility in rehabilitation of the communication deficits of brain injured patients.

REFERENCES

Adamovich, B., & Henderson, J. (1983). Treatment of communication deficits resulting from traumatic head injury. In W. Perkins (Ed.), *Current therapy of communication disorders: Language handicaps in adults* (pp. 105–117). New York: Thieme & Stratton.

Adamovich, B., & Henderson, J. (1985). Can we learn more from word fluency measures with aphasic, right brain injured and closed head trauma patients? In R. Brookshire (Ed.), *Clinical Aphasiology Conference proceedings* (pp. 124–130). Minneapolis: BRK.

Chapey, R. (1981). *Language intervention strategies in adult aphasia.* Baltimore: Williams & Wilkins.

Cooper, E. (1983). A brain-stem contusion and fluency: Vicki's story. *Journal of Fluency Disorders, 8*, 269–274.

Darley, F.L. (1964). *Diagnosis and appraisal of communication disorders.* Englewood Cliffs, NJ: Prentice-Hall.

Darley, F., Aronson, A., & Brown, J. (1975). *Motor speech disorders.* Philadelphia: F.A. Davis.

Davenport, M. (1981). Speech therapy. In C.D. Evans (Ed.), *Rehabilitation after severe head injury* (pp. 51–75). New York: Churchill Livingstone.

DeRenzi, E., & Vignolo, L. (1962). The token test: A sensitive test to detect receptive disturbances in aphasics. *Brain, 85*, 665–678.

Ehrlich, J., & Sipes, A. (1985). Group treatment of communication skills for head trauma patients. *Cognitive Rehabilitation*, 32–37.

Ewing-Cobbs, L., Levin, H.S., Eisenberg, H.M., & Fletcher, J.M. (1987). Language functions following closed-head injury in children and adolescents. *Journal of Clinical and Experimental Neuropsychology, 9*, 575–592.

Finitzo, T., Pool, K., Freeman, F., Cannito, M., Schaefer, S., Ross, E., & Devous, M. (1987). Spasmodic dysphonia subsequent to head trauma. *Archives of Otolaryngology—Head and Neck Surgery, 13*, 1107–1110.

Gajar, A., Schloss, P., Schloss, C., & Thompson, C. (1984). Effects of feedback and self-monitoring on head trauma youths' conversation skills. *Journal of Applied Behavior Analysis, 17*, 353–358.

Goldstein, K. (1948). *Language and language disturbances*. New York: Grune & Stratton.

Goodglass, H., & Kaplan, E. (1972). *The assessment of aphasia and related disorders*. Philadelphia: Lea & Febiger.

Groher, M. (1977). Language and memory disorders following closed head trauma. *Journal of Speech and Hearing Research, 20*, 212–223.

Groher, M. (1984a). Communication disorders. In M. Rosenthal, E. Griffith, M. Bond, & J. Miller (Eds.), *Rehabilitation of the head injured adult* (pp. 155–165). Philadelphia: F.A. Davis.

Groher, M. (1984b). *Dysphagia: Diagnosis and management*. Stoneham, MA: Butterworths.

Hagen, C. (1981). Language disorders secondary to closed head injury: Diagnosis and treatment. *Topics in Language Disorders, 1*, 73–87.

Hagen, C. (1984). Language disorders in head trauma. In A. Holland (Ed.), *Language disorders in adults* (pp. 245–281). San Diego: College-Hill Press.

Hagen, C., & Malkmus, D. (1979, November). *Intervention strategies for language disorders secondary to head trauma*. American Speech-Language-Hearing Association Convention Short Course, Atlanta, GA.

Halliday, M.A., & Hasan, R. (1976). *Cohesion in English*. London: Longman.

Halpern, H., Darley, F., & Brown, J. (1973). Differential language and neurologic characteristics in cerebral involvement. *Journal of Speech and Hearing Disorders, 38*, 162–173.

Hartmann, E., & von Cramon, D. (1984). Acoustic measurement of voice quality in dysphonia after severe closed head trauma: A follow-up study. *British Journal of Disorders of Communication, 19*, 153–261.

Heilman, K., Safran, A., & Geschwind, N. (1971). Closed head trauma and aphasia. *Journal of Neurology, Neurosurgery, and Psychiatry, 34*, 265–269.

Helm-Estabrooks, N., Yeo, R., Geschwind, N., Freedman, M., & Weinstein, C. (1986). Stuttering: Disappearance and reappearance with acquired brain lesions. *Neurology, 36*, 1109–1112.

Holland, A. (1980). *Communicative abilities in daily living*. Baltimore: University Park Press.

Holland, A. (1982). When is aphasia aphasia? The problem of closed head injury. In R. Brookshire (Ed.), *Clinical Aphasiology Proceedings* (pp. 345–349). Minneapolis: BRK.

Irvine, L., & Behrmann, M. (1986). The communicative and cognitive deficits following closed head injury. *The South African Journal of Communication Disorders, 33*, 49–54.

Kaplan, P., Phillip, P., & Halper, A. (1979). *Recovery of self-care activities in patients with traumatic brain damage*. Paper presented at the Third Annual Post-Graduate Course on the Rehabilitation of the Traumatic Brain-Injured Adult, Williamsburg, VA.

Kent, R., Netsell, R., & Bauer, L. (1975). Cineradiographic assessment of articulatory mobility in the dysarthrias. *Journal of Speech and Hearing Disorders, 40*, 467–480.

Kertesz, A., & McCabe, P. (1977). Recovery patterns and prognosis in aphasia. *Brain, 100*, 1- 18.

Lazarus, C., & Logemann, J. (1987). Swallowing disorders in closed head trauma patients. *Archives of Physical Medicine and Rehabilitation, 68*, 79–84.

Lehiste, I. (1965). Some acoustic characteristics of dysarthric speech. *Bibliloteca Phonetica, 2*, 1–124.

Levin, H. (1981). Aphasia in closed head injury. In M.T. Sarno (Ed.), *Acquired aphasia* (pp. 427–463). New York: Academic Press.

Levin, H., Grossman, R., & Kelly, P. (1976). Aphasic disorder in patients with closed head injury. *Journal of Neurology, Neurosurgery, and Psychiatry, 39*, 1062–1070.

Levin, H., Grossman, R., Sarwar, M., & Meyers, C. (1981). Linguistic recovery after closed head injury. *Brain and Language, 12*, 360–374.

Levin, H., Madison, C., Bailey, C., Meyers, C., Eisenberg, H., & Guinto, F. (1983). Mutism after closed head injury. *Archives of Neurology, 40*, 601–606.

Levin, H., Mattis, S., Ruff, R., Eisenberg, H., Marshall, L., Tabaddor, K., High, W., & Frankowski, R. (1987). Neurobehavioral outcome following minor head injury: A three-center study. *Journal of Neurosurgery, 66*, 234–243.

Ludlow, C., Rosenberg, J., Fair, C., Buck, D., Schesselman, S., & Salazar, A. (1986). Brain lesions associated with nonfluent aphasia fifteen years following penetrating head injury. *Brain, 109*, 55–80.

Luria, A. (1970). *Traumatic aphasia: Its syndrome, psychology and treatment.* The Hague: Mouton.

Marquardt, T.P. (1982). *Acquired neurogenic disorders.* Englewood Cliffs, NJ: Prentice-Hall.

Mentis, M., & Prutting, C. (1987). Cohesion in the discourse of normal and head-injured adults. *Journal of Speech and Hearing Research, 30*, 88–98.

Milton, S., Prutting, C., & Binder, G. (1984). Appraisal of communicative competence in head injured adults. In R.H. Brookshire (Ed.), *Clinical Aphasiology Conference proceedings* (pp. 114–123). Minneapolis: BRK.

Mohr, J., Weiss, G., Caveness, W., Dillon, J., Kistler, J., Meirowsky, A., & Rish, B. (1980). Language and motor disorders after penetrating head injury in Viet Nam. *Neurology, 30*, 1273–1279.

Najenson, T., Groswasser, Z., Stern, M., Schechter, I., Daviv, C., Berghaus, N., & Mendelson, L. (1975). Prognostic factors in rehabilitation after severe head injury: Assessment six months after trauma. *Scandinavian Journal of Rehabilitation Medicine, 7*, 101–110.

Najenson, T., Sazbon, I., Fiselzon, J., Becker, E., & Schechter, I. (1978). Recovery of communicative functions after prolonged traumatic coma. *Scandinavian Journal of Rehabilitation Medicine, 10*, 15–21.

Overgaard, J., Hvid-Hansen, O., Land, A., Pedersen, K., Christensen, S., Haase, J., Hein, O., & Tweed, W. (1973). Prognosis after head injury based on early clinical examination. *Lancet*, 631–635.

Porch, B. (1971). *Porch index of communicative ability* (rev. ed.). Pala Alto, CA: Consulting Psychologists Press.

Prigatano, G.P. (1987). Recovery and cognitive retraining after craniocerebral trauma. *Journal of Learning Disabilities, 20*, 10, 603–613.

Prigatano, G., Roueche, J., & Fordyce, D. (1985). Nonaphasic language disturbances after closed head injury. *Language Sciences, 7*, 217–229.

Prutting, C., & Kirchner, D. (1983). Applied pragmatics. In T.M. Gallagher & C.A. Prutting (Eds.), *Pragmatic assessment and intervention issues in language* (pp. 29–64). San Diego: College-Hill Press.

Sapir, S., & Aronson, A. (1985). Aphonia after closed head injury: Aetiologic considerations. *British Journal of Disorders of Communication, 20*, 289–296.

Sarno, M.T. (1980). The nature of verbal impairment after closed head injury. *Journal of Nervous and Mental Disease, 168*, 685–692.

Sarno, M.T. (1984). Verbal impairment after closed head injury: Report of a replication study. *Journal of Nervous and Mental Disease, 172*, 475–479.

Sarno, M., Buonaguro, A., & Levita, E. (1986). Characteristics of verbal impairment in closed head injured patients. *Archives of Physical Medicine and Rehabilitation, 67*, 450–455.

Scherzer, B. (1986). Rehabilitation following severe head trauma: Results of a three year program. *Archives of Physical Medicine and Rehabilitation, 67*, 366–373.

Schiller, F. (1947). Aphasia studied in patients with missile wounds. *Journal of Neurology, Neurosurgery, and Psychiatry, 10*, 183–197.

Sklar, M. (1966). *Sklar aphasia scale: Protocol booklet.* Los Angeles: Western Psychological Services.

Smith, R. (1984). Treatment of communication disorders. In M. Rosenthal, E. Griffith, M. Bond, & J. Miller (Eds.), *Rehabilitation of the head injured adult* (pp. 355–366). Philadelphia: F.A. Davis.

Spreen, O., & Benton, A.L. (1977). *Neurosensory center comprehensive examination for aphasia* (rev. ed.). Victoria, BC: University of Victoria, Neuropsychology Laboratory.

Szekeres, S.F., Ylvisaker, M., & Holland, A.L. (1985). Cognitive rehabilitation therapy: A framework for intervention. In M. Ylvisaker (Ed.), *Head injury rehabilitation: Children and adolescents* (pp. 219–246). San Diego: College-Hill Press.

Taylor, M. (1963). A measurement of functional communication in aphasia. *Archives of Physical Medicine and Rehabilitation, 46*, 101–107.

Thomsen, I. (1975). Evaluation and outcome of aphasia in patients with severe closed head trauma. *Journal of Neurology, Neurosurgery, and Psychiatry, 38*, 713–718.

Thomsen, I. (1981). Neuropsychological treatment and longtime follow-up in an aphasic patient with very severe head trauma. *Journal of Clinical Neuropsychology, 3*, 43–51.

Thomsen, I. (1984). Late outcome of very severe blunt head trauma: A 10–15 year second follow-up. *Journal of Neurology, Neurosurgery, and Psychiatry, 47*, 260–268.

Vogel, M., & von Cramon, D. (1983). Articulatory recovery after traumatic mutism. *Folia Phoniatrica, 35*, 294–309.

von Cramon, D. (1981). Traumatic mutism and the subsequent reorganization of speech functions. *Neuropsychologia, 19*, 801–805.

Wechsler, D. (1948). *Wechsler memory scale.* New York: Psychological Corp.

Wepman, J. (1951). *Recovery from aphasia.* New York: Ronald Press.

Wertz, R. (1978). Neuropathologies of speech and language: An introduction to patient management. In D.F. Johns (Ed.), *Clinical management of neurogenic communicative disorders* (pp. 1–101). Boston: Little, Brown.

Ylvisaker, M., & Szekeres, S. (1986). Management of the patient with closed head injury. In R. Chapey (Ed.), *Lan-*

guage intervention strategies in adult aphasia (pp. 474–490). Baltimore: Williams & Wilkins.

Yorkston, K., & Beukelman, D. (1981). *Assessment in intelligibility of dysarthric speech.* Austin, TX: PRO-ED.

Yorkston, K., Stanton, K., & Beukelman, D. (1981). Language-based compensatory training for closed head injured patients. In R. Brookshire (Ed.), *Proceedings of the Clinical Aphasiology Conference* (pp. 293–299). Minneapolis: BRK.

Zazula, T. (1984). Perception and production of intonation in moderate and severe head injuries. *Dissertation Abstracts International, 45,* 36–48.

PART III

INTERVENTION ISSUES

9

Neuropsychiatric Evaluation and Treatment of Traumatic Brain Injury

TONA L. McGUIRE

CARRIE E. SYLVESTER

Neuropsychiatric problems following severe head injuries are among the most disabling sequelae. In the acute phase of recovery, considerable attention is given to recovery of basic functions such as walking and talking. Failure to adequately emphasize behavioral and social factors may be compatible with an apparently good recovery, but can leave the patient with major psychosocial dysfunction.

As survival of persons who have experienced head injuries has improved, attention has turned to the cognitive, social, and psychiatric problems that mar the outcome of those individuals. This chapter focuses on the evaluation and management of neuropsychiatric sequelae of severe head injuries. Psychopharmacologic and psychotherapeutic interventions are discussed in the contexts of hospitalization and long-term follow-up at home and in the community.

NEUROPSYCHIATRIC SEQUELAE

Confusion in describing neuropsychiatric sequelae can result from lack of distinction between reports of minor versus severe head injury. A minor head injury consists of brief loss of consciousness (usually less than 20 minutes) with some disorientation and confusion, but no specific neurological findings or subsequent deterioration (Levin et al., 1987). Behavioral difficulties have been described following even minor head injuries (Casey, Ludwig, & McCormick, 1986) as well as mild cognitive deficits early in recovery from such minor injuries (Levin et al., 1987). Behavioral morbidity reported in the minor head injury group, such as affective lability, anxiety, and discipline problems in children, resembles that seen in the severely injured group. The behaviors seen following minor head injury are, however, thought to be directly related to the experience of an anxiety producing event, rather than reflecting presumed extensive organic pathology. Although some controversy remains, data from a multicenter study suggest that behavioral and cognitive morbidity in mild head injuries resolves, in most cases, within a few months (Levin et al., 1987).

Organic cognitive and affective changes may have variable courses and have symptoms presenting episodically, becoming static, or resolving gradually or rapidly (Chadwick, Rutter, Brown, Shaffer, & Traub, 1981; Chadwick, Rutter, Shaffer, & Shrout, 1981). They may be considered in the context of stages of recovery as described by Divack, Herrle, and Scott (1985). Early stage behaviors such as agitation are often related to decreased ability to process information in general. In the middle stage, the ability to understand the environment improves, but there is often decreased motivation and compliance. The head injured patient in the late stages of recovery may appear normal, but unrecognized cognitive deficits may impair social, academic, or occupational performance.

Another standard system for categorizing behaviors of the head injured patient is the organic mental disorders as defined in DSM III-R (American Psychiatric Association, 1987). *Delirium* following head injury is typically observed in early recovery, presenting primarily as fluctuating levels of consciousness. There is often difficulty with maintaining attention, and frequently there are perceptual disturbances such as hallucinations or illusions. The sleep-wake cycle is disrupted, with variations ranging from near stupor to significant insomnia. Psychomotor disturbances may include restlessness and tremors. The time frame for delirium is usually less than a month following resolution of coma. It may present alone or may be superimposed on an individual with evidence of trauma induced dementia.

Loss of intellectual function is the primary feature of *dementia* and can involve memory, judgment, or higher reasoning. Changes may also occur in affect and personality. When the individual becomes aware of the deterioration of cognitive abilities, anxiety and depression may be precipitated. These changes are often observed in the middle stages of recovery. As the more severe cognitive deficits in head injured individuals resolve, changes may remain leading to diagnoses of *organic personality syndrome, intermittent explosive disorder* (organic aggressive syndrome), *organic delusional syndrome, organic hallucinosis, organic mood syndrome, organic anxiety syndrome,* or *atypical/mixed organic mental syndrome.* Clinical features within these diagnostic categories may vary depending on location of the brain injury. These personality changes, which can be both quite subtle and unfortunately permanent, are seen in late stages of recovery.

Psychiatric dysfunction following head injury is commonly seen, and is related to the extent of injury, length of coma, premorbid personality, and environmental factors (Lishman, 1968). It is important to recognize that brain injury can exacerbate pre-existing psychopathology or cause premorbid personality traits to reach pathological proportions (Yudofsky & Silver, 1985). Damage to the frontal lobes is especially common and can lead to a distinctive cluster of symptoms (Silver, Yudofsky, & Hales, 1987). These may include decreased motivation and problems with maintaining concentration and attention. Poor social judgment accompanied by difficulty in planning or an apparent lack of concern for the future is often seen.

A most disturbing symptom is emotional "incontinence," or rapidly alternating and uncontrollable emotional states (Pincus & Tucker, 1985; Schiffer, Cash, & Hearndon, 1983). For example, there may be sudden onset of crying or laughing precipitated by minimal stimulation and often unrelated to any true feelings of humor or sadness. Temporal lobe injuries, especially left-sided injuries with seizures, are substantially associated with later psychiatric disability (Hillbom, 1960; Lishman, 1968). Significant personality disturbances and atypical psychoses have been observed in patients with penetrating injuries to the temporal lobes. Substantial discord exists among investigators as to the symptoms that may be most specifically associated with temporal lobe epilepsy or damage, but those most commonly agreed upon include aggression and anger; altered sexuality; hypergraphia; enhanced contemplative, religious, and philosophical ideation; humorless sobriety, circumstantiality, and viscosity; and schizophreniform psychosis (Fedio, 1986).

Another perspective has been provided by studies in animal populations and with adult stroke patients which suggest that some affective disorders are specifically related to both extent and site of the injuries with special reference to frontal lobe damage and disruption of noradrenergic pathways (Kwentus, Hart, Peck, & Korstein, 1985; Robinson, 1983). In addition, research characterizing the psychological symptoms of subcortical dementia and postmortem examinations revealing damage to subcortical structures in brain injured patients indicate that many of the behaviors commonly seen in these patients are due to diffuse subcortical damage rather than to localized injuries (Cummings, 1986a, 1986b; Lishman, 1978). This is especially noteworthy in the case of patients with late onset intermittent explosive disorder in whom diffuse cortical and subcortical lesions may cause aggression without other apparent and localizing cognitive or personality symptoms (Silver et al., 1987).

Psychoses with schizophrenic features have been said to have an increased incidence following head injury (Kwentus et al., 1985; Lishman, 1978). Although premorbid personality has been implicated as a predisposing factor, it should be noted that in epileptic patients who develop psychosis there is less probability of premorbid personality disorder or family history of psychosis than in patients with idiopathic schizophrenia (Cummings, 1986a, 1986b). Paranoid psychoses have also been noted in early stages of recovery as well as in long-term follow-up of head injured patients. This is at least in part due to suspiciousness caused by limitations in cognitive function leading to misinterpretation of the behavior and social cues of others. The subsequent paranoia may be further aggravated by others' response to the patient's displays of anger due to disinhibition of emotions. Another psychotic disorder that has been described as a sequela of head injury is mania with or without depression, but this is apparently a rare occurrence (Bracken, 1987; Clark & Davison, 1987). The presence of mania with associated grandiosity and intrusiveness sufficient to require strict setting of limits is another mechanism for paranoia and other interpersonal difficulties in the head injured patient.

Depression and anxiety are very common following brain trauma (Levin, Grossman, Rose, & Teasdale, 1979; Lipsey, Robinson, Pearlson, Rao, & Price, 1983; Lishman, 1978; Robinson, 1983). In some individuals, this is obviously a response to the recognition of cognitive limitations and personality changes. The affective symptoms may also resemble symptoms known to occur with brain injury, thus rendering identification of etiology nearly impossible. Irritability, difficulty with transitions, and apathy or anhedonia are some such frequently troublesome symptoms. Death by suicide increases with the length of time since injury, and seems to be related to personality changes causing disruptions in relationships and occupational functioning (Hillbom, 1960).

Consequences of severe head injury have been described in more detail in adults than in children. The neuropsychiatric features of child and adolescent patients have usually been described in terms of specific behaviors exhibited, rather than by diagnostic categories. Difficulties with conduct or attention, including aggression, destructiveness, and impulsivity, have received the most attention (Blau, 1936; Brown, Chadwick, Shaffer, Rutter, & Traub, 1981; Filley, Cranberg, Alexander, & Hart, 1987; Richardson, 1963). Depressive symptoms have, nevertheless, been particularly noted in adolescents (Chadwick, 1985; Jacobson et al., 1986; Rutter, 1981).

Evaluation and treatment of the head injured child or adolescent are complicated by a variety of issues. These include any psychological or cognitive dysfunction that preceded the injury, developmental factors, family and social issues, and complications directly related to the brain injury itself (Klonoff, 1971). For example, children and adolescents who were impulsive and engaged in hazardous activities were, not surprisingly, also those more likely to suffer head injury (Craft, Shaw, & Cartlidge, 1972; Mannheimer & Mellinger, 1967). Further, anhedonia, or inability to experience pleasure, is a prominent feature of depression in childhood and adolescents (Poznanski, 1982). Attempts to relieve that bored, anhedonic feeling may also lead to increased exposure to risk. It, therefore, becomes difficult to ascertain whether the restlessness and impulsivity sometimes seen in these patients are new behaviors. Similar concerns regarding premorbid risk-taking behavior have also been raised in discussions of adult brain injury (Malec, 1985; Yudofsky & Silver, 1985).

Psychological disturbance late in recovery has been found to occur more frequently in the patient with family discord or parental psychiatric disorder (Brown et al., 1981). The presence of parental major depression, bipolar affective disorder, anxiety disorder, or sociopathy is also an indication of possible preinjury psychopathology in the child (Cadoret, 1978; Weissman, Leckman, Merikangas, Gammon, & Prusoff, 1984). Controlled studies have, however, documented an increase in psychiatric problems associated with severe brain injury in patients who would not otherwise be considered at risk (Brown et al., 1981; Rutter, 1981).

PSYCHOPHARMACOLOGIC INTERVENTIONS

There have been few controlled studies of the medical treatment of posttraumatic organic psychiatric symptoms. There are fewer studies of psychopharmacologic interventions for pediatric patients. Therefore, we have reviewed what is generally understood about the psychopharmacology of posttraumatic psychiatric symptoms with reference to special information about children and adolescents when possible.

Beta-adrenergic Agents

Aggressive, violent, or agitated behaviors present significant management difficulties in the patient with delirium, dementia, or intermittent explosive disorder. Propranolol (Inderal), a beta-adrenergic blocking agent, has been the most evaluated psychoactive medication used in head injured patients with temper or rage outbursts (Jenkins & Mauruta, 1987; Mattes, 1986). Beta-adrenergic blockade reduces physical symptoms of sympathetic nervous system arousal associated with fear and anger such as sweating, trembling, and rapid heart rate. Beta-adrenergic blocking agents should not be used in patients with asthma, diabetes mellitus, and a number of cardiac conditions. There is a risk of adverse reaction in patients who are concurrently on neuroleptic (formerly antipsychotic or major tranquilizer) medications such as haloperidol (Haldol) or a monoamine oxidase inhibitor antidepressant such as phenelzine (Nardil). The dosage regimen for propranolol recommended for adults by Silver and Yudofsky (1985) begins at 20 mg. three times/day with gradual increase to 640 mg./day if no response or adverse effects are observed before reaching that dose. If no response occurs after 4 weeks at maximum dosage, the trial is considered adequate. If the patient's behavior or cognition deteriorates, the possibility of central nervous system toxicity due to propranolol must be entertained (Remick, O'Kane, & Sparling, 1981). It is also important to note that this medication should be gradually tapered over 10 to 14 days to avoid rebound hypertension when it is discontinued.

Greendyke and Kanter (1986) recently demonstrated the efficacy of pindolol (Visken), a beta-blocking agent with partial intrinsic sympathomimetic activity, in doses of 40 to 60 mg./day. They reported pindolol to have faster onset of action than propranolol without the side effects of low blood pressure and excessive slowing of the heart.

Anticonvulsants

Anticonvulsants have been used for treating rage outbursts for nearly 20 years (Monroe, 1975). They have been used primarily in patients with both seizures and uncontrolled rage, a situation that occurs in head injured patients. Carbamazepine (Tegretol) has become the drug of first choice for patients with seizures and rage outbursts, especially when the epileptic focus is in the temporal lobe (Reynolds, 1982). That is in part because, despite the risk of bone marrow suppression, carbamazepine is reported to have a different, but no more hazardous, side effect profile than phenytoin (Dilantin) (Hart & Easton, 1982). It is important, however, to be aware of a variety of adverse effects of carbamazepine which include behavioral and psychological changes such as irritability, agitation, and psychosis (Evans, Clay, & Gualtieri, 1987). Further, it is necessary to consult the current annual edition of *The Physicians' Desk Reference* published by Medical Economics for recommendations for hematological and other biological monitoring for this or any pharmacological agent. This requirement should be especially observed when the medication is to be chronically used. The usual dosage of carbamazepine is 20 to 30 mg./kg./day in three divided doses. Treatment is started in adults at 200 mg. daily with a maximum daily dose of 600 to 1,200 mg. The usual therapeutic plasma concentration is between 6 to 12 micrograms/ml. with central nervous system side effects beginning to appear at about 9 micrograms/ml. (Rall & Schleifer, 1985).

Benzodiazepines

Although benzodiazepines such as diazepam (Valium) have been reported to be useful in treating aggressive behavior (Barin, Hanchett, Jacob, & Scott, 1985), they have also been implicated in disinhibition of aggressive impulses (Bach-y-Rita, Lion, Climent, & Ervin, 1971). Further, few data exist regarding their use in children except as anticonvulsants. Psychoactive effectiveness of the anticonvulsant benzodiazepines may, therefore, be observed when severe behavioral dyscontrol is suspected to be due to posttraumatic seizure activity. Oxazepam (Serax) is a particularly potent anticonvulsant, and is also the most rapidly metabolized benzodiazepine, so that, in the event of disinhibition or excessive drowsiness, it would clear quickly (Baldessarini, 1985). Another short-acting benzodiazepine that has been recommended for *severe* anxiety in the head injured population is lorazepam (Ativan). For the adult who has not suffered head trauma, the usual daily dose of oxazepam is 30 to 60 mg./day and for lorazepam is 2 to 6 mg./day (Baldessarini, 1985). These dosages are, however, probably excessive for many head injured individuals. Therefore, it is prudent to avoid the use of these medications, but when a trial seems indicated, to begin with a fraction of the usual dose and to advance the dose slowly.

Neuroleptic (Antipsychotic) Medications

Aggressive behavior may be due to psychotic thinking such as hallucinations or paranoid delusions, but the use of neuroleptic medications has been discouraged in the head injured patient due to the potential for those medications to block recovery of cognitive function (Feeny, Gonzalez, & Law, 1982). The animal study upon which that recommendation was based also demonstrated that physical restraints retard recovery of cognitive function. Management of individual patients must, therefore, take into consideration that the use of physical restraints in human beings may prevent access to rehabilitative therapy sessions including school or occupational therapy. Other factors to be considered include degree of psychic pain and cognitive disorganization beyond that explained by the traumatic lesion.

Brain injury causes patients to be more sensitive to the sedative and anticholinergic side effects of neuroleptic medications (Silver et al., 1987). Dystonias, akathisias, and Parkinsonian side effects are also a significant concern because movement disorders that could be elicited or exacerbated by neuroleptic medications are a common, if perhaps subtle, feature of subcortical dementia (Cummings & Benson, 1983). The usual daily dose of chlorpromazine (Thorazine) in psychotic adults without head injury is 300 to 800 mg. (Baldessarini, 1985). The starting dose of chlorpromazine is 5 mg. three times/day for the agitated brain damaged adult in whom some sedation is a desired effect (Yudofsky & Silver, 1985). In the more common situation when sedation is undesirable, less sedating neuroleptic medications such as fluphenazine (Prolixin) or haloperidol (Haldol) have been recommended. Further, the higher potency neuroleptic thiothixene (Navane) has been reported to be associated with fewer side effects than the more sedating thioridazine (Mellaril) in schizophrenic adolescents (Realmuto, Erickson, Yellin, Hopwood, & Greenberg, 1984). In psychotic, but not head injured, adults, the usual daily dose of fluphenazine hydrochloride is 1 to 20 mg., of haloperidol is 6 to 20 mg., and of thiothixene is 6 to 30 mg. (Baldessarini, 1985). The recommended beginning dosages for brain injured adults are fluphenezine 0.5 mg. twice/day, and haloperidol 0.5 mg. twice/day (Yudofsky & Silver, 1985). It is also noted that significant side effects have been seen in brain injured adults at maximum haloperidol doses exceeding 5 mg. daily and that movement disorders caused by neuroleptics clear very slowly.

Antihistamines and Hypnotics

The psychopharmacologic interventions described above are for significant rage, aggression, or other behavioral dyscontrol that is persistent or frequently recurrent. It is important to remember that there is little or no information about the use of these agents in children except for the use of anticonvulsant agents. Because of that, diphenhydramine (Benadryl), an antihistamine that produces sedation, is commonly used in young children for both sedation and relief of anxiety (Jaffe & Magnuson, 1985). Barin and colleagues (1985) have reported successful use of the antihistamine hydroxyzine pamoate (Vistaril) to manage isolated episodes of aggression, but without reference to controlled studies. The use of antihistamines in head injured individuals, as with the previously discussed medications, bears special risks. The antihistamines lower the seizure threshold and may cause incoordination, blurred vision, or a variety of undesirable anticholinergic side effects such as dry mouth, nausea, and abdominal cramping (Jaffe & Magnuson, 1985).

Barbiturate medications and long-acting benzodiazepine hypnotics such as flurazepam (Dalmane) are contraindicated in the head injured population, because they can further disrupt the frequent traumatic disturbances in sleep patterns (Yudofsky & Silver, 1985). Chloral hydrate, which is usually employed as a sleep inducing agent, is still occasionally used when a calming or hypnotic effect is desired in children who are displaying acute excitement (Baldessarini, 1985). There is no information, however, about the use of chloral hydrate in a head injured population.

Antidepressants

Tricyclic antidepressants in very low doses, such as amitriptyline (Elavil) 25 mg. twice/day, have been used for management of agitation or emotional lability in patients with a variety of central nervous system disorders (Schiffer et al., 1983). Antidepressants are also considered, of course, in the patient in whom a diagnosis of major depression is entertained, especially when psychomotor retardation or vegetative symptoms such as anorexia are interfering with general recovery. Preinjury symptoms and a family history of major depression responding to antidepressant medication may be very good clues to potential medication response as well as guiding specific choice of medication. Although amitriptyline was found not beneficial in treating depression following minor head trauma, none of those head injured patients had a variety of symptoms, such as worse symptoms in the morning or change in weight or activity, that are usually associated with a high probability of response to antidepressant medication (Baldessarini, 1985; Saran, 1985). Nortriptyline (Pamelor) has been demonstrated, in a careful, double-blind study, to successfully treat poststroke depression (Lipsey, Robinson, Pearlson, Rao, & Price, 1984). One recommendation is the use of nortriptyline or desipramine (Norpramin) because of their favorable side effect profiles (Silver et al., 1987). Silver and coauthors further note that antidepressant effects in depressed head injured patients may be expected with one-third to one-half the usual dose. The usual adult dose of nortriptyline is 75 to 150 mg./day, with a usual starting dose of 10 mg./day recommended for the head injured patient (Baldessarini, 1985; Silver et al., 1987). Desipramine is an active metabolite of imipramine (Tofranil) with fewer side effects, but is somewhat more arousing such that it may be of limited use in an agitated, depressed patient (Blackwell, Stefopoulos, Enders, Kuzuma, & Adolphe, 1978; Rancurello, 1985). The usual adult dose of desipramine is 100 to 200 mg./day, with a recommended starting dose in the head injured patient of 10 mg. three times/day (Baldessarini, 1985; Silver et al., 1987).

There are no controlled studies of the use of antidepressants in head injured children and adolescents. Further, there are limited data on the efficacy of antidepressants in children and adolescents (Campbell & Spencer, 1988). Imipramine has been the most commonly, longest used pediatric antidepressant medication. There is evidence that imipramine is effective in depressed prepubertal children (Puig-Antich et al., 1987). The starting dose in depressed children without head injury is 1.0 to 1.5 mg./kg./day, with gradual advancement over 10 to 20 days (Campbell & Spencer, 1988). Although doses up to 5 mg./kg./day are mentioned, these have only been approved for investigational purposes and are probably high for a head injured population. It is important to consult the current annual *Physicians' Desk Reference* published by Medical Economics for the maximum clinical dose, which was conservatively set at 2.5 mg./kg./day, but is subject to change as more data are compiled. Major depression in adolescents apparently responds poorly to tricyclic antidepressants (Ryan et al., 1986). This low response rate is similar to that in young adults in the reproductive age range and thought to be related to high sex hormone secretion (Puig-Antich, Ryan, & Rabinovich, 1985). There are, therefore, no data specifically addressing the medical management of major depression in the head injured adolescent population, which is a significant knowledge gap considering that age group's affinity for vehicles, skateboards, and risky exploration.

Lithium

Because mania secondary to head trauma alone is rare and mania in childhood and adolescence is uncommon, other secondary causes of mania such as tricyclic antidepressants should be considered prior to initiating treatment (Bracken, 1987; Clark & Davison, 1987; Strober & Carlson, 1982; Sylvester, Burke, McCauley, & Clark, 1984). The treatment of choice for mania is lithium with or without an antipsychotic medication. Treatment or prevention of manic-depressive symptoms are the only approved uses for lithium. Even in therapeutic dosage of 300 mg. to 2,400 mg./day with blood levels of 0.75 to 1.0 mEq/L., lithium is a toxic medication that can cause confusion, lethargy, and a fine resting tremor which interferes with handwriting (Baldessarini, 1985). These neurological effects are clearly especially undesirable in a head injured population. There is, however, some anecdotal information that lithium may benefit some brain damaged individuals (Oyewumi & LaPierre, 1981; Rosenbaum & Barry, 1975). Carbamazepine is another option that is receiving increasing attention (Baldessarini, 1985; Evans et al., 1987). It may have obvious, though as yet untested, benefits in the seizure-prone head injured individual with symptoms of mania. The decision to use lithium depends upon the patient's prior history and family history as well as consideration of other options such as response to antipsychotic medication or carbamazepine and the side effects of those medications.

Stimulants

Central nervous system stimulants may be indicated for apathy, psychomotor slowing, inattentiveness, and poor concentration in head injured individuals. Caffeine, dextroamphetamine (Dexedrine), and methylphenidate (Ritalin) are commonly used stimulants that may be effective in controlling those symptoms. Their use must be carefully monitored in head injured children because they may increase stereotypic (repetitive) and aggressive behaviors (Glenn, 1986). In the situation where accident proneness was a consequence of attention deficit disorder/hyperactivity, the use of a stimulant to manage impulsivity or inattentiveness is possibly indicated. The dosages and the need for close monitoring with the school have been a focus of intensive study (Rapport et al., 1988; Kupietz, Winsberg, Richardson, Maitinsky, & Mendell, 1988; Richardson, Kupietz, Winsberg, Maitinsky, & Mendell, 1988). The starting dose for dextroamphetamine (Dexedrine) is 5 mg. daily to twice daily for children 6 years or older. The maximum dose is 40 mg., with a daily dose range of 0.15 to 0.5 mg./kg. The starting dose for methylphenidate (Ritalin) is 5 mg. twice daily, with a maximum dose of 60 mg. and daily dose range of 0.3 to 1.0 mg./kg. (Donnelly & Rapoport, 1985).

PSYCHOTHERAPEUTIC INTERVENTIONS

Some adult and adolescent patients may benefit from primarily supportive psychotherapy with some additional focus on achieving recognition of the effects of their behavior on others. Traditional individual psychotherapy for the head injured patient is frequently impeded by posttraumatic cognitive limitations and by a premorbid, externally oriented personality lacking in introspective tendencies (Malec, 1985). Individual therapy is also sometimes rendered less effective by environmental factors. These environmental factors include inconsistent expectations of the patient, which may be due to inadequate communication or to conflicts between the patient's family and personnel who have frequent contact with the patient (McGuire & Rothenberg, 1986). A comprehensive, eclectic approach, with attention to bereavement, medical management, social skills training, and family issues (especially with regard to discharge planning), is, therefore, crucial to facilitate adequate psychosocial adaptation in these patients.

It is important to recognize that the response to the loss of usual cognition and interpersonal relationships will produce symptoms of bereavement in family members and, to a degree depending upon remaining self-awareness, in the patient. Families and individuals vary in their progression through the stages of shock, denial, anger, depression, and adjustment (Clayton,

Desmarais, & Winokur, 1968). Erroneous assumptions that the patient or family members are suffering from prolonged psychopathology can be prevented by recognizing that new challenges, such as arranging school or job placement, may precipitate another wave of grief (Jacobson et al., 1986). Faced with those challenges, the family or patient may display considerable exacerbation of anger or guilt. Issues relating to premorbid psychopathology may also surface at that time so that differentiating bereavement from depression or anger exhibited by family members can be difficult. Friends and relatives may have cut off verbal communication or may avoid the patient and family due to their own discomfort. Thus, the family and patient might become increasingly isolated at a time when the need to ventilate feelings is urgently felt. The goal of therapy is, therefore, to allow the family and individual patient to express their sad, angry, guilty, and ambivalent emotions in an appropriate, accepting setting.

Certainly, as Gloag (1985) emphasizes, an attempt needs to be made to treat the "head injured family" by offering methods of structuring areas of life in which the injured patient is likely to need support. In the late stages of recovery, the family of head injured adults should participate in their cognitive retraining and be taught specific strategies to help them become as functional as possible. Family members may discover difficulties in treating the head injured patient consistently when there is considerable variability in behavioral symptoms resulting from the cognitive deficits associated with dementia. If the recovery reaches a plateau and family members realize that the changes may be permanent, apparently unpredictable behaviors, especially in the area of social judgment, may severely tax the family's coping skills and adaptability (Jacobson et al., 1986). Family members should be encouraged to participate in psychotherapy for themselves. It is important because failure to do so makes adaptation to the "new" family member extremely difficult. Marital therapy may be warranted when there is a committed spouse who wishes to maintain the relationship.

Parents of head injured children need to be taught both specific intervention strategies and general behavioral management principles. As the child begins the transition from hospital to home, the techniques can be practiced, revised, and adapted before discharge (Divack et al., 1985). Staff and parents can model and practice prosocial behavior with the child. As an adjunct to standard recreational therapy activities, videotaped practice with an emphasis on social skills retraining may be enormously helpful, if the social skills retraining is specifically tailored for the head injured child. These activities can be done individually or with small groups of children. The issue of guilt tends to be important to parents of a head injured child. There is sometimes an attitude that the child has endured so much that he or she should not have any limits placed on behavior. Parents need much support and education on the importance of consistent discipline and structure for any child, and especially for the head injured child.

DISCHARGE PLANNING

As previously mentioned, new challenges can precipitate relapse of the patient's and family's grieving processes. It is important to initiate discharge planning early and to expect some ambivalence and resistance as discharge approaches. Although discharge is generally a long-awaited milestone, many families are frightened by the prospect of managing the care of the head injured patient by themselves. They acutely feel the loss of support, might panic, and can refuse to allow discharge. A calm, accepting, but firm stance by the staff will help most families through this time. Discharge should be approached from a transitional framework. While the patient is hospitalized, the head injured patient's family can gradually assume a larger share of the care-giving responsibilities. Discharge can then be preceded by progressively longer passes to the home environment until the family feels confident of its ability to manage.

With some families, however, denial may be so strong that the family pushes for premature discharge. Cognitive deficits, behavior problems, or organic psychiatric symptoms may be completely ignored as the family insists that everything will be fine if only the patient could be home. Sometimes the only helpful approach is to allow the family to assume care, providing this does not place the patient at risk for harm. Generally, once full-time responsibility for the inadequately rehabilitated head injured patient is experienced by the family, they quickly reconsider. They should be allowed to request help with dignity, as "I told you so" is neither helpful nor humane.

Issues are similar for the head injured child or adolescent, although in planning for discharge the psychological status of the parents is as crucial as that of the child. Unfortunately, because psychopathology, such as depression, that causes some children to be at risk for these injuries also may occur in one or both parents, some families are unable to accommodate to the stress of returning their cognitively or behaviorally impaired child to their home. If the family is unable to recognize that their home is an inappropriate environment, child protection services may need to be enlisted.

It is helpful, with the patient's and family's permission, to communicate directly with those persons in the patient's community who have any special need to understand the cognitive and behavioral limitations imposed by the injury. The most obvious persons are the patient's individual classroom teachers and athletic coaches. Others who might be considered are scout leaders, employers, and other major preinjury support figures in the child's or adolescent's life with whom some continued contact and understanding would be beneficial.

There is a subgroup of head injured individuals whose aggressive and impulsive behavior causes them to be dangerous to themselves or others; this precludes most home settings following the acute recovery phase. For these patients, admission to an inpatient psychiatric setting may be necessary to provide intensive behavioral treatment and medication management. Following this treatment, some individuals will be ready to return to the community. Others, however, may require the structure of a group residential setting, or may need to be enrolled in a day treatment program with return home for evenings and weekends.

Families making the decision to have the patient go to a secondary treatment facility or group residential setting require much support. Such a decision may seem entirely appropriate to professionals working with the patient, but may still be perceived as failure or rejection by the parents, spouse, extended family, friends, or by the patient himself. Other families may reject such treatment options vigorously, only to change their minds once the daily care of the patient becomes overwhelming and disruptive. They may then experience a profound sense of failure, which is sometimes expressed as anger directed at the patient. Again, therapy at such a point is useful in clarifying issues for the family and offering acceptance and support.

LONG-TERM FOLLOW-UP OF THE HEAD INJURED PATIENT

Psychological functioning following discharge from the hospital may vary with time, the initial euphoria of returning home dissolving in the reality of daily activities. Studies of adult patients have demonstrated that cognitive and personality changes following head injury have a significant impact on social and vocational functioning (Oddy & Humphrey, 1980). For example, some individuals may be able to return to work following rehabilitation, but are unable to form adequate interpersonal relationships (Prigatano et al., 1984). Communication and behavioral deficits can significantly interfere with the development and maintenance of normal social relationships. Communication problems can be manifest as dysarthrias such as monotone or nasal speech, or unusual rate of speech production. In addition, cognitive processing difficulties can produce language that is tangential and socially inappropriate (Ylvisaker, 1986). Such inappropriate and odd speech may cause others to withdraw. This further isolates the affected individual and decreases opportunity to practice social skills.

For children, a critical arena of functioning is the school setting. The child's workplace is school, where he or she is less able to depend on old learning than is an adult in many work situations. Thus resistance to attending school or completing work, as well as behavior problems, may develop as academic work becomes progressively more difficult. However, because in many head injured children well-learned skills such as reading may be intact, it may be years before more subtle decreased abilities relative to their peers become apparent (Shaffer, Bijur, Chadwick, & Rutter, 1980). In addition, neuropsychological assessment done early in recovery may not reveal such major problems. As more is expected from the child over time, however, a pattern of repeated failure may cause depression, anxiety, and poor self-concept.

Often the only available classroom placement for the head injured child or adolescent is with children identified as learning disabled. Although similarities have been reported in learning disabled and head injured children, school difficulties appear to be greater for the head injured child (Cohen, Joyce, Rhoades, & Welks, 1985). These difficulties are related not only to academic problems (Ewing-Cobbs, Fletcher, & Levin, 1985), but are also secondary to communication, behavior, and socialization problems. School is, for most children and adolescents, where the majority of social interaction with peers and unrelated adults takes place.

Some children with communication and behavior problems may be unaware of their own behavior and lack the internal feedback to self-correct. They are, however, usually aware of the consequences of their lack of ability, the sense that other people don't like them. For the child with significant cognitive and language problems, standard social skills training, which relies on an adequate memory and good attentional abilities, may be inappropriate. The child might not be able to appreciate nuances of social behavior. He or she may also be unable to practice situations in advance with "What should you do if ..." games, but may be able to learn more appropriate interactions with directions such as "Don't stand too close" or "Remember to ask before you join a game." Work with young adults has suggested that cognitive and social retraining following head injury, with a focus on acceptance of deficits and learning compensatory strategies, can positively influence social and family relationships as well (Prigatano et al., 1984).

For families of both the child with marked residual deficits and the child with less overt problems, adjustment is likely to wax and wane. Grief over the loss of the "healthy child" may tend to resurface as major milestones in the child's life either are reached or would have been reached. For example, classmates returning to school in September may painfully remind parents that their child must attend a special school or class. Impulsive and aggressive behavior from the child who exhibited few premorbid behavior problems quickly refutes the pretense that all is as it was before. It may be necessary to repeatedly offer therapy focused on bereavement to both family and patient when new stages of life are reached.

For the adolescent other developmental issues also play an important role in psychological functioning (Jacobson et al., 1986). Parents who are unsure of their child's judgment or abilities may not encourage appropriate individuation and separation. The wish to avoid any further physical or emotional injury may also produce overprotectiveness. In that situation, normal adolescent exuberance, assertion of independence, or introspection may be mislabeled as evidence of the sequelae of brain injury. Family therapy may allow parents to voice their fears, assess their perceptions, and develop appropriate strategies for helping their adolescent become as independent as possible.

Siblings are frequently the invisible victims of chronically disabling disorders, and sibling relationships may deteriorate over time (Oddy & Humphrey, 1980). Having suffered through the family trauma of the injury and hospitalization, siblings may next be required to readjust their home life to accommodate their recovering brother or sister. Resentment is common as the parents' time, energy, and financial resources are poured into helping the injured child. Guilt following the angry feelings may leave siblings feeling confused and alone. Family therapy and individual supportive psychotherapy may help by allowing them to openly discuss their feelings and to be reassured that such reactions are expected and accepted.

SUMMARY

Severe head injury carries with it the potential for significant neuropsychiatric sequelae. Difficulties related to brain damage are further complicated by family, school, occupational, interpersonal, and social factors. School and career planning, social skills remediation, individual psychotherapy for selected patients, family therapy interventions for most families, and medical management must be carefully integrated. It should be anticipated that interventions with head injured patients and their families need to occur over an extended period and must adapt to the individual's changing needs. Attention must be paid to maintaining adequate communication among physician, teacher, psychologist, family, and patient, all of whom must truly work together as a team to facilitate an optimal outcome.

REFERENCES

American Psychiatric Association. (1987). *Diagnostic and statistical manual of mental disorders* (3rd ed., rev.). Washington, DC: American Psychiatric Association.

Bach-y-Rita, G., Lion, J.R., Climent, C.E., & Ervin, F.R. (1971). Episodic dyscontrol: A study of 130 violent patients. *American Journal of Psychiatry, 127*, 1472–1478.

Baldessarini, R.J. (1985). *Chemotherapy in psychiatry: Principles and practice.* Cambridge, MA: Harvard University Press.

Barin, J.J., Hanchett, J.M., Jacob, W.L., & Scott, M.B. (1985). Counseling the head injured patient. In M. Ylvisaker (Ed.), *Head injury rehabilitation: Children and adolescents* (pp. 361–379). San Diego: College-Hill.

Blackwell, B., Stefopoulos, A., Enders, P., Kuzuma, R., & Adolphe, A. (1978). Anticholinergic activity of two tricyclic antidepressants. *American Journal of Psychiatry, 135,* 722–724.

Blau, A. (1936). Mental changes following head trauma in children. *Archives of Neurology, 35,* 733–769.

Bracken, P. (1987). Mania following head injury. *British Journal of Psychiatry, 150,* 690–692.

Brown, G., Chadwick, O., Shaffer, D., Rutter, M., & Traub, M. (1981). A prospective study of children with head injuries: III. Psychiatric sequelae. *Psychological Medicine, 11,* 63–78.

Cadoret, R.J. (1978). Psychopathology in adopted-away offspring of biologic parents with antisocial behavior. *Archives of General Psychiatry, 35,* 176–184.

Campbell, M., & Spencer, E.K. (1988). Psychopharmacology in child and adolescent psychiatry: A review of the past five years. *Journal of the American Academy of Child and Adolescent Psychiatry, 27,* 269–279.

Casey, R., Ludwig, S., & McCormick, M.C. (1986). Morbidity following minor head trauma in children. *Pediatrics, 78,* 497–502.

Chadwick, O. (1985). Psychological sequelae of head injury in children. *Developmental Medicine and Child Neurology, 27,* 69–79.

Chadwick, O., Rutter, M., Brown, G., Shaffer, D., & Traub, M. (1981). A prospective study of children and head injuries: II. Cognitive sequelae. *Psychological Medicine, 11,* 49–61.

Chadwick, O., Rutter, M., Shaffer, D., & Shrout, P. (1981). A prospective study of children with head injuries. *Journal of Clinical Neuropsychology, 3,* 101–120.

Clark, A.F., & Davison, K. (1987). Mania following head injury: A report of two cases and a review of the literature. *British Journal of Psychiatry, 150,* 841–844.

Clayton, P., Desmarais, L., & Winokur, G. (1968). A study of normal bereavement. *American Journal of Psychiatry, 125,* 168–178.

Cohen, S.B., Joyce, C.M., Rhoades, K.W., & Welks, D.M. (1985). Educational programming for head injured students. In M. Ylvisaker (Ed.), *Head injury rehabilitation: Children and adolescents* (pp. 383–410). San Diego: College-Hill.

Craft, A.W., Shaw, D.A., & Cartlidge, N.E.F. (1972). Head injuries in children. *British Medical Journal, 4,* 200–203.

Cummings, J. (1986a). Organic psychoses: Delusional disorders and secondary mania. *Psychiatric Clinics of North America, 9,* 293–311.

Cummings, J. (1986b). Subcortical dementia. *British Journal of Psychiatry, 149,* 682–697.

Cummings, J.L., & Benson, D.F. (1983). *Dementia: A clinical approach.* Boston: Butterworth.

Divack, J.A., Herrle, J., & Scott, M.B. (1985). Behavior management. In M. Ylvisaker (Ed.), *Head injury rehabilitation: Children and adolescents* (pp. 349–360). San Diego: College-Hill.

Donnelly, M., & Rapoport, J.L. (1985). Attention deficit disorders. In J.M. Wiener (Ed.), *Diagnosis and psychopharmacology of childhood and adolescent disorders* (pp. 180–197). New

York: Wiley.

Evans, R.W., Clay, T.H., & Gualtieri, C.T. (1987). Carbamazepine in pediatric psychiatry. *Journal of the American Academy of Child and Adolescent Psychiatry, 26*, 2–8.

Ewing-Cobbs, L., Fletcher, J.M., & Levin, H.S. (1985). Neuropsychological sequelae following pediatric head injury. In M. Ylvisaker (Ed.), *Head injury rehabilitation: Children and adolescents* (pp. 71–90). San Diego: College-Hill.

Fedio, P. (1986). Behavioral characteristics of patients with temporal lobe epilepsy. *Psychiatric Clinics of North America, 9*, 267–281.

Feeny, D.M., Gonzalez, A., & Law, W.A. (1982). Amphetamine, haloperidol, and experience interact to affect rate of recovery after motor cortex injury. *Science, 217*, 855–857.

Filley, C., Cranberg, L., Alexander, M., & Hart, E. (1987). Neurobehavioral outcome after closed head injury in childhood and adolescence. *Archives of Neurology, 44*, 194–198.

Glenn, M.B. (1986). CNS stimulants: Applications for traumatic brain injury. *Journal of Head Trauma Rehabilitation, 1*, 74–76.

Gloag, D. (1985). Rehabilitation after head injury: 2. Behavioral and emotional problems, long term needs, and the requirement for services. *British Medical Journal, 290*, 913–915.

Greendyke, R.M., & Kanter, D.R. (1986). Therapeutic effects of pindolol on behavioral disturbances associated with organic brain disease: A double-blind study. *Journal Clinical Psychiatry, 47*, 423–426.

Hart, R.G., & Easton, J.D. (1982). Carbamazepine and hematological monitoring. *Annals of Neurology, 11*, 309–312.

Hillbom, E. (1960). After-effects of brain injuries. *Acta Psychiatrica et Neurologica Scandinavica Supplement, 142*, 1–195.

Jacobson, M., Rubinstein, E., Bohannon, W., Soundheimer, D., Cieci, R., Toner, J., Gong, E., & Heald, F. (1986). Follow-up of adolescent trauma victims: A new model of care. *Pediatrics, 77*, 236–241.

Jaffe, S.L., & Magnuson, J.V. (1985). Anxiety disorders. In J.M. Wiener (Ed.), *Diagnosis and psychopharmacology of childhood and adolescent disorders* (pp. 199–214). New York: Wiley.

Jenkins, S.C., & Mauruta, T. (1987). Therapeutic use of propranolol for intermittent explosive disorder. *Mayo Clinical Proceedings, 62*, 204–214.

Klonoff, H. (1971). Head injuries in children: Predisposing factors, accident conditions, and sequelae. *American Journal Public Health, 61*, 2405–2417.

Kupietz, S.S., Winsberg, B.G., Richardson, E., Maitinsky, S., & Mendell, N. (1988). Effects of methylphenidate dosage in hyperactive reading-disabled children: I. Behavior and cognitive performance effects. *Journal of the American Academy of Child and Adolescent Psychiatry, 27*, 70–77.

Kwentus, J., Hart, R., Peck, E., & Korstein, S. (1985). Psychiatric complications of closed head trauma. *Psychosomatics, 26*, 8–17.

Levin, H.S., Grossman, R.G., Rose, J.E., & Teasdale, G. (1979). Long-term neuropsychological outcome of closed head injury. *Journal of Neurosurgery, 50*, 412–422.

Levin, H.S., Mattes, S., Ruff, R.M., Eisenberg, H.M., Marshall, L.F., Tabaddor, K., High, W.M., & Frankowski, R.F. (1987). Neurobehavioral outcome following minor head injury: A three center study. *Journal of Neurosurgery, 66*, 234–243.

Lipsey, J.R., Robinson, R.R., Pearlson, G.D., Rao, K., & Price, T.R. (1983). Mood change following bilateral hemisphere brain injury. *British Journal of Psychiatry, 143,* 266–273.

Lipsey, J.R., Robinson, R.R., Pearlson, G.D., Rao, K., & Price, T.R. (1984). Nortriptyline treatment of post-stroke depression: A double-blind study. *The Lancet, 1,* 297–300.

Lishman, W.A. (1968). Brain damage in relation to psychiatric disability after head injury. *British Journal of Psychiatry, 114,* 373–410.

Lishman, W. (1978). *Organic psychiatry.* Oxford: Blackwell Scientific Publications.

Malec, J. (1985). Personality factors associated with severe traumatic disability. *Rehabilitation Psychology, 30,* 165–172.

Mannheimer, D., & Mellinger, G. (1967). Personality characteristics of child accident repeaters. *Child Development, 38,* 491–502.

Mattes, J.A. (1986). Psychopharmacology of temper outbursts: A review. *Journal of Nervous and Mental Disease, 174,* 464–470.

McGuire, T.L., & Rothenberg, M.B. (1986). Behavioral and psychosocial sequelae of pediatric head injury. *Journal of Head Trauma Rehabilitation, 1,* 1–6.

Monroe, R.R. (1975). Anticonvulsants in the treatment of aggression. *Journal of Nervous and Mental Disease, 160,* 119–126.

Oddy, M., & Humphrey, M. (1980). Social recovery during the year following severe head injury. *Journal of Neurology, Neurosurgery, and Psychiatry, 34,* 798–802.

Oyewumi, L.K., & LaPierre, Y.D. (1981). Efficacy of lithium in treating mood disorder occurring after brain stem injury. *American Journal of Psychiatry, 138,* 110–112.

Pincus, J.H., & Tucker, G.J. (1985). Disorders of intellectual functioning. In *Behavioral neurology* (3rd ed., pp. 151–216). New York: Oxford University Press.

Poznanski, E.O. (1982). The clinical characteristics of childhood depression. In L. Grinspoon (Ed.), *Psychiatry, 1982: Annual review* (pp. 296–307). Washington, DC: American Psychiatric Press.

Prigatano, G.P., Fordyce, D.J., Zeiner, H.K., Roueche, J.R., Pepping, M., & Wood, B.C. (1984). Neuropsychological rehabilitation after closed head injury in young adults. *Journal of Neurology, Neurosurgery, and Psychiatry, 47,* 505–513.

Puig-Antich, J., Perel, J.M., Lupatkin, W., Chambers, W.J., Tabrizi, M.A., King, J., Goetz, R., Davies, M., & Stiller, R.L. (1987). Imipramine in prepubertal major depressive disorders. *Archives of General Psychiatry, 44,* 81–89.

Puig-Antich, J., Ryan, N., & Rabinovich, H. (1985). Affective disorders in childhood and adolescence. In J.M. Wiener (Ed.), *Diagnosis and psychopharmacology of childhood and adolescent disorders* (pp. 151–178). New York: Wiley.

Rall, T.W., & Schleifer, L.S. (1985). Drugs effective in the therapy of the epilepsies. In A.G. Gilman, L.S. Goodman, T.W. Rall, & F. Murad (Eds.), *The pharmacological basis of therapeutics* (7th ed., pp. 446–472). New York: Macmillan.

Rancurello, M. (1985). Clinical applications of antidepressant drugs in childhood behavioral and emotional disorders. *Psychiatric Annals, 15,* 88–100.

Rapport, M.D., Stoner, G., DuPaul, G.J., Kelly, K.L., Tucker, S.B., & Schoeller, T. (1988). Attention deficit disorder and methylphenidate: A multilevel analysis of dose-response effects on children's impulsivity across settings. *Journal of the American Academy of Child and Adolescent Psychiatry, 27,* 60–69.

Realmuto, G.M., Erickson, W.D., Yellin, A.M., Hopwood, J.H., & Greenberg, L.M. (1984). Clinical comparison of thiothixene and thioridazine in schizophrenic adolescents. *American Journal of Psychiatry, 141,* 440–442.

Remick, R.A., O'Kane, J., & Sparling, T.G. (1981). A case report of toxic psychosis with low-dose propranolol therapy. *American Journal of Psychiatry, 138,* 850–851.

Reynolds, E.H. (1982). The pharmacological management of epilepsy associated with psychological disorders. *British Journal of Psychiatry, 141,* 549–557.

Richardson, E., Kupietz, S.S., Winsberg, B.G., Maitinsky, S., & Mendell, N. (1988). Effects of methylphenidate dosage in hyperactive reading-disabled children: II. Reading achievement. *Journal of the American Academy of Child and Adolescent Psychiatry, 27,* 78–87.

Richardson, F. (1963). Some effects of severe head injury: A follow-up study of children and adolescents after protracted coma. *Developmental Medicine and Child Neurology, 5,* 471–482.

Robinson, R. (1983). Investigating mood disorders following brain injury. An integrative approach using clinical and laboratory studies. *Integrative Psychiatry, July–August,* 35–45.

Rosenbaum, A.H., & Barry, M.J. (1975). Positive therapeutic response to lithium in hypomania secondary to organic brain syndrome. *American Journal of Psychiatry, 132,* 1072–1073.

Rutter, M. (1981). Psychological sequelae of brain damage in children. *American Journal of Psychiatry, 138,* 1533–1534.

Ryan, N.D., Puig-Antich, J., Cooper, T., Rabinovich, H., Ambrosini, P., Davies, M., King, J., Torres, D., & Fried, J. (1986). Imipramine in adolescent major depression: Plasma levels and clinical response. *Acta Psychiatrica Scandinavica, 73,* 275–288.

Saran, A.S. (1985). Depression after minor closed head injury: Role of dexamethasone suppression test and antidepressants. *Journal of Clinical Psychiatry, 46,* 335–338.

Schiffer, R.B., Cash, J., & Hearndon, R.M. (1983). Treatment of emotional lability with low-dosage tricyclic antidepressants. *Psychosomatics, 24,* 1094–1096.

Shaffer, D., Bijur, P., Chadwick, O., & Rutter, M. (1980). Head injury and later reading disability. *Journal of the American Academy of Child Psychiatry, 19,* 592–610.

Silver, J.M., & Yudofsky, S.C. (1985). Propranolol for aggression: Literature review and clinical guidelines. *International Drug Therapy News, 20,* 9–12.

Silver, J.M., Yudofsky, S.C., & Hales, R.E. (1987). Neuropsychiatric aspects of traumatic brain injury. In R.E. Hales & S.C. Yudofsky (Ed.), *Textbook of neuropsychiatry* (pp. 179–190). Washington, DC: American Psychiatric Association.

Strober, M., & Carlson, G. (1982). Bipolar illness in adolescents with major depression: Clinical, genetic, and psychopharmacologic predictors in a three- to four-year prospective follow-up investigation. *Archives of General Psychiatry, 39,* 549–555.

Sylvester, C.E., Burke, P.M., McCauley, E.A., & Clark, C.J. (1984). Manic psychosis in childhood: Report of two cases. *Journal of Nervous and Mental*

Disease, 172, 12–15.

Weissman, M.M., Leckman, J.F., Merikangas, K.R., Gammon, G.D., & Prusoff, B.A. (1984). Depression and anxiety disorders in parents and children: Results from the Yale family study. *Archives of General Psychiatry, 41*, 845–852.

Ylvisaker, M. (1986). Language and communication disorders following pediatric head injury. *The Journal of Head Trauma Rehabilitation, 1*, 48–56.

Yudofsky, S.C., & Silver, J.M. (1985). Psychiatric aspects of brain injury: Trauma, stroke, and tumor. In R.E. Hales & A.J. Frances (Ed.), *Psychiatry update–APA annual review* (pp. 142–158). Washington, DC: American Psychiatric Association.

10

Behavioral Change Strategies for Children and Adolescents with Traumatic Brain Injury

ANN V. DEATON

Persons with severe brain injuries are surviving in ever-increasing numbers. Because of the multiplicity of behavioral and cognitive changes that result from brain injury, outcome remains variable. Some patients demonstrate astounding "spontaneous" recovery while others continue to have significant impairments. It is this latter group that requires innovative treatment strategies if they are to re-enter society as productive members. The reason for this is that one of the most enduring, and potentially incapacitating, effects of brain injury is that of personality and behavioral change. The effects of a brain injury on behavior are complex, multiply determined, and unique to each individual (Heaton & Pendleton, 1981). While the potential sequelae have been well documented in adults (e.g., Brooks, 1984; Jennett & Teasdale, 1981), the study of children and adolescents with brain injuries has not been nearly so extensive. Developmental issues and time of injury also complicate the study of child and adolescent head injury. Moreover, the development of treatment methodologies has been slow and effortful as professionals and families have struggled to understand the sequelae of a condition that is estimated to affect over 3% of all children by 15 years of age (Rivara & Mueller, 1986).

The goal of this chapter is to provide an overview of the range of problem behaviors typically occurring in head injured children and adolescents and to describe potential approaches for behavioral intervention and change. The review will be limited, insofar as possible, to the *behavioral* effects of head injury and how to change or manage them. Obviously, behavior cannot be considered in isolation from the cognitive and psychosocial effects of head injury and, where necessary, these topic areas will be incorporated in the discussion.

While focusing on identifiable behaviors, however, this chapter is not limited to behaviors and interventions that occur only in the school setting. The school will not always be the sole or the optimal setting for effecting behavior change with the brain injured child or adolescent. Educators, as well as other professionals, may find that discussion of interventions in other environments is instructive in identifying what they can and cannot accomplish in the school setting. In particular, this discussion may enable the reader to decide when to expand programs into the home, to refer the child to another professional in the community, or to recommend an inpatient facility for treatment.

AN OVERVIEW OF COMMON MALADAPTIVE BEHAVIORS FOLLOWING BRAIN INJURY

Although no two brain injured persons have precisely the same pattern of abilities and deficits, some effects of brain injury occur frequently enough to mention. For the sake of simplicity, these may be categorized as self-care, cognitive, and interpersonal behaviors. Self-care skills include such behaviors as not eating, poor toileting skills, inability to dress oneself, and inability to remain safe without supervision. These skills deficits are likely to occur primarily following a severe head injury, and can have a devastating effect on the child's health, self-esteem, and capacity to participate in the school setting; further, these deficits are likely to affect the potential educational placements available to the child.

Second, some behaviors appear primarily cognitive in nature, such as distractibility, irritability, impulsivity, failure to initiate activities, poor decision making, and failure to shift from one activity or subject to another. In many environments, these deficits interfere with the head injured child's ability to adapt to the smallest changes in routine (e.g., a school assembly that causes a class to be canceled) or to plan appropriately how to deal with change.

Finally, behaviors that can be viewed as interpersonal skills deficits include poor anger control, extreme attention seeking behavior (e.g., self-injury), failure to respond appropriately to others' social cues, and failure to monitor one's own behavior for appropriateness. Lezak (1987) and Oddy (1984) have suggested that disinhibited behaviors (i.e., saying or doing things that one would ordinarily inhibit) are one of the most common sequelae of head injury in children. When these behaviors are displayed by the head injured child, they can lead to rejection by peers and helping professionals alike. In addition, Barin, Hanchett, Jacob, and Scott (1985) have suggested that these behaviors increase the risk of further injury in that risk taking occurs due to problems in judgment and the head injured child's difficulty accepting the injury-related changes.

As special educators will recognize, some of these behaviors (e.g., impulsivity) are common to individuals who have not sustained a specific brain injury. Certainly, some of those who suffer head injuries may have already been predisposed to behavioral difficulties (Rutter, 1981). There is little doubt, however, that severe head injury results in an increase in behavioral problems and that the more severe the head injury, the more likely that subsequent behavioral difficulties will result (Divack, Herrie, & Scott, 1985; Goethe & Levin, 1984). In one study, the rate of behavioral problems (e.g., social inappropriateness, impulsivity) was three times as great in severely head injured persons as in matched controls (Brown, Chadwick, Shaffer, Rutter, & Traub, 1981). Other authors have noted a tendency for preinjury behaviors to become exaggerated and therefore problematic. McGuire and Rothenberg (1986), for example, cited a case of an adolescent whose clowning was viewed as cute and endearing before his injury but as inappropriate afterwards. Thus, the behaviors may not be entirely new, but may reflect exacerbations of preinjury tendencies.

MISCONCEPTIONS ABOUT THE BEHAVIORS OF BRAIN INJURED PERSONS

Behavioral problems that are the result of brain injury are often referred to as "organic." Unfortunately, this label is sometimes interpreted as meaning that these behaviors are not subject to change and that attempts to do so would be futile. The fact is that very few brain injured persons have fully lost the ability to learn some new behaviors or to relearn old ones, though the learning process may be different and more difficult for the brain injured individual. With sufficient structure, consistency, and repetition, brain injured persons can usually learn to adapt at some level to their environment.

A second frequent misconception about the behavioral changes that may accompany brain injury is that all are maladaptive problem behaviors that need to be eliminated or unlearned (e.g., physical aggression, impulsivity, overly affectionate behavior). In addition to attempting to decrease these maladaptive behaviors, programs of behavior change also seek to increase adaptive behaviors (e.g., eating, communicating, dressing). In fact, the main goal of a behavioral change program may be to help the brain injured individual to learn or relearn positive, adaptive skills in order to function in a less restrictive environment. Moreover, improving adaptive skills is often central to the brain injured individual's self-esteem and independence.

A third misconception is that the inappropriate behaviors of brain injured persons are deliberate or intentional. This explanation is sometimes given as a reason for punishing these behaviors so that the brain injured child will learn. Such is often the case when children with brain injuries are disruptive in the classroom and are therefore suspended from school. However, as Savage (1987) has suggested, the traditional disciplinary model is inappropriate for the student whose behavior is a result of brain injury. The underlying reason for the problem behavior must be identified in order to change it. Children may refuse school work, for example, because the time limits imposed for completion ensure that they will fail. Thus, refusal protects their tenuous sense of self-esteem and control.

BEHAVIOR CHANGE THEORY

Literature on behavior modification theories and strategies has proliferated since the 1950s. While it will not be reviewed in detail here, readers needing a general review or introduction will find *Child Behavior Analysis and Therapy* (Gelfand & Hartmann, 1984) an excellent book. In brief, the basic premise of behavioral approaches is that behavior has antecedents (events that elicit or precede behaviors) and consequences (events that follow behaviors). By manipulating these, the behavior can be changed. Procedures have been developed to increase desired behaviors, to decrease maladaptive behaviors, and to shape existing behaviors into more complex or appropriate ones. Though these principles and methods have been applied to the behavioral difficulties of a number of different populations, little of the work has been carried out with traumatically brain injured individuals, who are unique with respect to the suddenness of their injuries and the catastrophic changes and discontinuity brought about in their lives. Moreover, they differ from the populations of previously studied individuals (e.g., mentally retarded individuals, conduct disordered children and adolescents) with regard to their learning histories (pre- and postinjury), their cognitive abilities, and their dramatically altered self-perceptions. These unique characteristics of this population require that the effectiveness of behavioral change strategies be evaluated anew and, if needed, modified.

The process of applying and evaluating the efficacy of behavioral change with brain injured individuals is a rather recent one. There are few published guidelines, though clinical experience and anecdotal evidence are accumulating quickly as the need and potential value of behavioral approaches with this population are recognized. For example, Malec (1984) outlined four basic assumptions that should be addressed in the brain injured individual when some form of behavioral intervention is being attempted. These are as follows:

1. Behavior disturbances after head injury represent inadequate personal and interpersonal self-regulation skills (e.g., an adolescent who makes frequent sexual advances to others without comprehending the impact on social interactions and relationships).

2. If a behavior is a change from preinjury style of behavior, it is most likely the result of a change in cognitive and learning abilities (e.g., a girl who was cooperative and docile before her injury may appear oppositional afterward because she does not understand or remember when others ask her to do something).

3. Normal responses to the stress of severe injury depend on normal cognitive functioning, and are affected by cognitive impairment (e.g., being able to grieve significant injury-related losses may not be possible if one has lost the cognitive ability to be aware of the losses).

4. Self-management skills may be learned or relearned if programs are implemented to help the brain injured person to compensate for cognitive or neuropsychological deficits. On the other hand, maladaptive behaviors that are inappropriately reinforced and thereby learned may persist even when the underlying cognitive deficits are no longer present. (For example, some children and adolescents become agitated and aggressive as they are coming out of coma. If they are rewarded for those behaviors with increased attention and primary reinforcers such as food, they may learn that agitation and aggression are good ways of getting their needs met.)

The above assumptions demonstrate that an essential component of adaptive behavior is the ability to monitor one's own behavior. This is, unfortunately, one of the areas commonly affected by brain injury. Thus, brain injured persons can be expected to require external feedback and structure to become aware of the inappropriateness or appropriateness of their actions. If inappropriate, they are likely to require environmental contingencies that will enable them to relearn adaptive behaviors.

BEHAVIOR CHANGE STRATEGIES

Behavioral intervention is sometimes thought of as something that is "done *to*" or "carried out *on*" the identified patient. The ethics of using these strategies, especially with a cognitively impaired population, thus need to be addressed. In general, the focus should be on cooperative, collaborative aspects, with all participants agreeing on the behaviors that need to be changed and how to change them (Gelfand & Hartmann, 1984). Tynan, Pearce, and Royall (1986) have addressed the issue of informed consent with the brain injured population where the injured person has relatively intact cognitive functioning. These authors describe a case where a nonverbal adolescent used self-abusive behavior to communicate frustration and fatigue. In such a case, it is necessary to provide an alternate behavior or strategy that can serve the same essential function (i.e., communication) for the child. In this case, contingent physical restraint was combined with teaching the use of an alternative communication device. These strategies eventually allowed near elimination of the self-abuse. Obviously, the ideal is to have a situation in which the planned changes are perceived as beneficial by both the head injured person and those others who have initiated the change. An approach that ignores the need for all participants to have a say is not likely to create a significant amount of investment in the problem solving process on the injured individual's part (Vredevoogd, 1986) and, as a consequence, is less likely to be successful.

A frequent error made in attempting to change a behavior is to proceed too quickly to the implementation of a strategy before adequately (a) defining the behavior; (b) evaluating its function, etiology, and frequency; (c) identifying all the potential resources available; and (d) listing all the possible strategies for intervention. Going through this sequential process carefully will facilitate the selection of a successful intervention. Each of these steps, essential to any plan to change behavior, is addressed below.

Defining the Problem Behavior

Setting the stage for effective behavior change with the brain injured child requires a measurable and precise definition of the target behavior. At the outset of the behavior change process, the specific behavior in need of change is not always available. A teacher may state, for example, that a head injured boy who has recently returned to school is "simply unmanageable and cannot be made to do anything in the classroom." One way of arriving at a more specific definition is to think of examples of this child's being unmanageable. If the teacher comes up with the example that the child punches anyone who asks him to do something, the problem becomes more clear: to eliminate the child's punching behavior. In addition, the situation preceding the behavior is clear: Demands are made of the head injured child just before he punches someone. One way of ensuring that the target behavior has been adequately defined is to check with all those working with the child to see if they agree about the behavior's occurrence and nonoccurrence. This is typically a simple matter with a behavior such as physical aggression, but it is more difficult when the problem is social inappropriateness or uncooperativeness.

Second, the appropriate dimension (i.e., duration, frequency, intensity) of the target behavior needs to be specified (Gelfand & Hartmann, 1984). The most important characteristic of attention, for example, may be its duration. The goal for a brain injured child who can attend to an activity for only 20 seconds may be to increase the attention span to 5 minutes. In contrast, the changes desired in an aggressive child may be decreased frequency of aggressive episodes, decreased intensity of the aggression, or the ability to quickly return to a task following an aggressive outburst.

Identifying the Function, Etiology, and Rate of the Target Behavior

Once the target behavior is known, an initial assessment, or baseline period, will be required to adequately evaluate the function of the behavior, its underlying cause or immediate precipitants, and its salient dimensions (i.e., frequency, intensity, duration, etc.). A hallmark of brain injury is that the injured person's behavior can be extremely variable from one day or time of day to another, making the initial assessment difficult and, at times, impossible. When possible, the baseline measure should include time of occurrence, a description of the behavior, and the exact events preceding and following the behavior. Though this may initially appear burdensome and unnecessary, the following case illustrates the value of a thorough baseline assessment.[1]

> *Case 1:* Jason, 16, remained in a residential rehabilitation center 3 years after sustaining a severe head injury. Unfortunately, he remained severely cognitively and behaviorally impaired, with a fluent aphasia characterized by his being able to articulate clearly but with vacant content. On a measure of receptive vocabulary (Peabody Picture Vocabulary Test, Dunn, 1965), Jason scored at chance level, perseverating on choosing the picture located on the upper left of each page. Jason was unable to return to his family and community because of apparently unprovoked physical aggression occurring several times per day. Since Jason was unable to explain why he was aggressive, a baseline evaluation was completed to identify the frequency and specifics of Jason's aggression as well as the circumstances immediately preceding and following it.

[1] Case examples are based upon actual patients. However, some of the details have been changed to preserve patients' anonymity.

During the baseline period, Jason punched or kicked someone an average of 3.5 times per day. Reviewing the events occurring just before this behavior showed that Jason never attacked people who did not approach him first. Just before he lashed out, Jason appeared startled. On closer examination, it was noted that he struck only those who approached him from the right side. Immediately after he attacked someone, staff typically backed away until Jason appeared calm, and then returned to complete the activity. Following this baseline period, neuropsychological and visual field exams were undertaken that showed Jason to have a complete right visual field loss consistent with damage to the posterior left hemisphere. It was presumed that Jason struck out because he was startled and frightened when approached from his blind side without warning. This baseline assessment clarified the cause and function of the target behavior and thereby dictated the selection of an appropriate intervention: in this case, approaching Jason from the left side or greeting him aloud before approaching from the right. This intervention decreased the episodes of physical aggression to approximately twice per week, a level that allowed Jason to be transferred to a facility close to his home.

Identifying Resources for Behavioral Intervention

As noted in the preceding example, implementing an effective intervention for changing Jason's aggression involved drawing on the resources of the staff who worked directly with the injured individual. The strategy chosen in this case required little training or effort on the part of these staff and was clearly preferable to getting hit by Jason. Some behavioral interventions, however, can require significant additional resources to carry out and are therefore much more costly, in terms of time, effort, and monetary expenditures. Identifying the available resources in advance of selecting an intervention strategy should facilitate choosing a feasible strategy because it is consistent with the available resources. These resources may include (a) the child himself, including memory, motivation, ability to learn, and so forth; (b) the professionals, including staff:student ratio, staff training, individual traits (e.g., patience, perseverance), and so forth; (c) the family, including ability to consistently carry out programs at home, provision of relevant information for selecting reinforcers, and so forth; and (d) the setting, including inherent reinforcements, peers, financial resources, and so forth.

Resources are constantly changing as the individual child and situation change. As time passes after an injury, the child and family often become increasingly valuable as resources since the child's overall abilities are improving and the family is becoming more knowledgeable about the effects of the brain injury. During an initial period of posttraumatic amnesia, for example, the head injured child's ability to learn and carry out any new behavior will be poor. Moreover, the child will probably be unmotivated to learn because of failing to recognize deficits or the need for compensation. As memory improves, more active self-monitoring on the part of the head injured child becomes possible. Families, professionals, and the child may also receive specific training that enables them to become resources. For example, a course in the management of aggressive behavior can be offered to teach those working with the brain injured child how to react to physical aggression. When able to handle aggression in a manner that minimizes reinforcement of aggression and the risk of physical injury, families and professionals can prevent the behavior from being inadvertently reinforced (e.g., by removal from a difficult, frustrating situation) and can maintain the child in the least restrictive setting. Training in behavioral management strategies such as the use of token economies and appropriate reinforcers may also provide additional resources. In the following example, the role of resources in arriving at an appropriate behavioral change strategy will become clear.

Case 2: Billy, 11, sustained an injury in a fall, after which a hematoma was evacuated from the right frontotemporal area of his brain. Five months later, he returned to school but continued to be confused and distractible. His verbal IQ of 87 suggested low average verbal abilities; Billy scored significantly below average on the two performance subtests he was able to complete. Motor speed was slow with either hand and Billy had difficulty learning and retrieving new information, especially following interference (Rey Auditory Verbal Learning Test: Trial VII = 5/15 words) (Rey, 1964). When uncertain of what was expected of him, Billy's reaction was to withdraw to a corner of the room. The baseline evaluation showed that nearly all episodes of withdrawal occurred when the environment was loud and crowded. Possible strategies for decreasing Billy's withdrawal included using his peers to provide him with support and feedback, providing Billy with one-to-one staff, rewarding Billy for participation, teaching Billy how to ask for help when he was confused, or providing home tutoring for a while before returning Billy to a classroom setting.

Unfortunately, in this case resources were limited. Billy's peers in the classroom were not viewed as a significant resource because many of them had emotional difficulties that made it difficult for them to focus on Billy's needs and to actively help him. The school system did not have adequate staff to provide Billy with one-to-one staff or to provide him with much in the way of home tutoring. On the other hand, Billy himself was motivated to do well in school and his parents and teacher all wanted to help him to become successful again. Billy, his parents, his teacher, and a neuropsychologist sat down together and decided on a private signal Billy could use to let his teacher know when he was overwhelmed. She, in turn, promised to come and help him within 2 minutes of seeing his signal. In addition, Billy's parents agreed to give Billy a favorite snack when he came home for each day he was able to stay in class without withdrawing more than one time. They also agreed to take him on a special outing once a week if he stayed in class for 4 of 5 days. This strategy enabled Billy to begin to be successful again and to get help when he needed it. Also, he was no longer teased by peers (who did not know his secret signal) about running to sit in the corner.

This case demonstrates that even with limited resources (e.g., little control over how peers behave, inadequate personnel), it is still possible to select a strategy that is effective in changing the brain injured child's behavior and enabling him or her to be successful. Relying on resources that do not exist or over which you have no control is likely to yield an ineffective strategy, and failure to change a behavior may further reduce available resources (e.g., the child's self-esteem, the parents' willingness to cooperate).

Strategies for Behavior Change

How can one identify potential strategies for changing the behavior? Obviously, the strategies will depend upon the nature of the behavior, its function, and the available resources. For the injured child who refused to respond to requests, for example, possible strategies include rewards for compliance, time out, removal to a less stressful situation, ignoring of noncompliance, loss of privileges or attention, more attention given to cooperative children in the immediate environment, and avoidance of frustrating situations, among many other possibilities. Depending upon the function of the behavior, its cause, and other characteristics of the brain injured child (e.g., ability to pick up on subtle social cues such as the teacher reinforcing more appropriate peers nearby), any of these strategies (and others) may be appropriate. Table 10.1 suggests some possible change strategies for noncompliant behavior. As noted in this table, noncompliance that is designed to avoid frustration or failure can be approached with a preventive strategy (e.g., alternate difficult tasks with easy, enjoyable ones to reduce the frustration level). Alternatively, if the noncompliance is designed to avoid having to do the task at all, the strategy may be a specific response to the noncompliance when it occurs (e.g., brief time out followed by a return to the activity through to completion). As Jacobs (1987) has noted, the best behavioral management strategy for the brain injured individual is that which uses "as few of your resources as possible, but as many as necessary, to achieve your goals."

One rule of thumb in the selection of a strategy is to choose the least intrusive procedure that will be effective. In general, this means that reinforcement is to be preferred to punishment. There are at least two reasons to follow this recommendation. First, reinforcement (and time out from reinforcement) is more likely than punishment alone to lead to lasting changes in the behavior of the brain injured person (Eames & Wood, 1985). Second, punishment may lead to depression, decreased initiative, and lower self-esteem in the injured individual, who may already be experiencing these problems and viewing himself or herself in a negative light (Malec, 1984). In the case of dangerous behaviors such as self-abuse, physical restraint may be necessary and may be the least intrusive intervention that is effective in

TABLE 10.1
Noncompliance with Task Demands in the Brain Injured Individual: Pairings of Antecedents and Consequences with Potential Interventions

Possible Antecedents	Possible Interventions
Does not understand task demands	— Provide clear, concrete instructions, in writing if needed — Model task completion
Does not begin task	— Give prompts — Reinforce each instance of initiative, however minor (e.g., picks up a pencil)
Unable to do task	— Simplify task — Provide training in underlying skills
Is not motivated	— Make task more interesting or relevant — Give desired rewards for task completion
Possible Consequences	
Avoids failure or frustration by not complying	— Alternate difficult tasks with easy, enjoyable ones — Provide tasks at which child will succeed
Gets out of doing task	— Must complete task before going on to other activities, regardless of time to completion
Receives attention for not doing task	— Is timed out or ignored while noncompliant — Is reinforced with attention for cooperation — Other children in environment are reinforced for their cooperation
Gets to assert independence/ control over situation	— May be offered choices when appropriate

preventing bodily damage. However, this intervention alone is unlikely to produce any lasting change unless coupled with rewards for positive, appropriate behavior. For example, Sand, Trieschmann, Fordyce, and Fowler (1970) have described the use of a two-faceted approach to decrease the tantrums of a 7-year-old boy who had been traumatically head injured more than 2 years earlier. In this case, time outs were given contingent on tantrum behavior, while appropriate behaviors were rewarded with tokens that could be exchanged for rewards. When receiving attention was made contingent on positive behaviors instead of negative ones, this brain injured child quickly became more compliant.

Implementation and Evaluation

Once a strategy or strategies have been selected, it is essential that they be implemented consistently and that their effectiveness be evaluated. Because many brain injured persons have impairments in the area of attention and memory (Auerbach, 1986), it is often useful to provide concrete feedback in the form of graphs or charts to remind them of gains. Particularly if progress is slow, videotaping at various intervals may also provide for concrete comparisons between previous and current levels of functioning.

Not all programs will be effective, regardless of how well planned they are, and there are a number of possible options to consider if a behavioral program is not effective. First, it may be useful to assess whether the program is being consistently implemented. Divack et al. (1985) have noted that less than 100% consistency in implementation can result in a program's failure. For example, in Case 2, Billy's program for reducing withdrawal from confusing situations might be ineffective if the teacher sometimes failed to provide him with help within the agreed upon time period of 2 minutes.

A second cause for failure is that additional resources may be required. In Case 1, Jason might continue to be aggressive toward those who don't know him because they may approach him from his blind side without warning. Since it is not feasible to educate everyone about Jason's unique needs, an additional resource in this case would be training for Jason in routine visual scanning in order to minimize surprises.

Third, a program may not work because the strategy selected was inappropriate or not powerful enough. Most commonly, this is a result of the chosen reinforcement not being truly reinforcing to that particular brain injured child. For example, free time may be anxiety provoking rather than rewarding to the injured child who functions best with a high degree of structure. Along these lines, Grimm and Bleiberg (1986) have noted particular difficulty finding effective reinforcers for the brain injured individual who lacks motivation and initiative as a result of frontal lobe damage. Difficulties can sometimes be remedied by choosing a different reinforcer, decreasing the time interval necessary for reinforcement (e.g., rewarding Billy for each class period during which he does not withdraw), and providing more structure.

Finally, an intervention may prove ineffective because the target behavior was not ideal. This can happen when the chosen behavior has been poorly defined and the criteria for adequate performance increase as the head injured child's skills increase (e.g., "uncooperativeness" may be defined initially as refusal to complete a task but later as grumbling about it). Another possibility is that the chosen behavior is difficult to change because it has been occurring for a long time with considerable reinforcement; this type of behavior would be likely to require a lengthy intervention period (e.g., when a head injured child's refusal to eat has resulted in the child receiving preferred foods such as ice cream). Finally, the target behavior may have been inappropriate because the child is unable to perform it. This can occur when the injury involves organically based limitations; for example, the child may be unable to establish a consistent swallow; or a child interrupts because he or she is too cognitively limited to focus on multiple social cues. If the target behavior is inappropriate, the most useful approach is to further define the target behavior or to select a new behavior that may be more readily changed.

Wood (1984) has suggested that psychopharmacologic interventions can sometimes be a useful adjunct to behavioral management. The reported success of such interventions as aids to behavioral control has been variable, and professional attitudes are mixed. Some authors have reported that medications can lead to a decrease in the injured child's ability to learn (e.g., Barin et al., 1985; Dean, 1986). However, these same authors have also noted instances in which medications can be helpful in increasing attention (Dean, 1986) and decreasing agitation (Barin et al., 1985), thereby facilitating learning and behavioral change.

Generalization

Once a behavior has been learned (in the case of deficits) or extinguished (in the case of excesses), it is usually desirable to have this change generalize to other situations. Moreover, it may be possible to shift the control for the behavior back to the brain injured individual and away from external sources. Once again, because of the cognitive impairments often accompanying a brain injury, generalization may need to be specifically taught and in some cases may be an impossible task. Divack and colleagues (1985) note that generalization will be facilitated by gradual rather than abrupt changes, and this is particularly true with the brain injured individual. The basic process is that of moving from primary (concrete) to secondary reinforcers, from immediate to delayed feedback, and from continuous to intermittent reinforcement. In short, the movement is toward a schedule and type of reinforcement more often found in natural environments (Divack et al., 1985). Plans for generalization therefore need to take into account the environments in which the injured person will be expected to function and the characteristics of those settings. Some relapses should be expected as attempts are made to decrease the levels of reinforcement. However, if the relapse is severe or prolonged, it may be necessary to re-establish control over the behavior before again attempting to phase out the external controls more gradually. Unfortunately, as previously mentioned, some brain injured individuals will not be able to generalize. In such cases, after exhausting various methods, the goal of generalization should be abandoned and functional skills should be taught in the settings in which they are expected to occur.

ADDITIONAL MODES OF INTERVENTION TO CHANGE BEHAVIORS

Although most of this chapter has dealt with strategies for changing specific behaviors of individuals, group interventions and environmental modifications can also be effective in addressing some of the more common behaviors occurring in brain injured individuals. These strategies may also be more viable in cases where available resources are limited.

Group Interventions

Group interventions have the advantages of providing peer support, feedback, and modeling, and may therefore be particularly appropriate for head injured children and adolescents seeking acceptance by their peer group. Group interventions allow the brain injured child to feel less isolated and provide an opportunity for demonstrating competencies and successfully helping peers, thereby increasing self-esteem. Barin and colleagues (1985) have also noted that group interventions with injured children may facilitate return to a more normative group of noninjured peers by providing some practice and some degree of inoculation against teasing. Some examples of focused groups include self-assessment, social skills, and problem solving. Model formats for these kinds of groups with adolescents and young adults have been developed (e.g., Ben-Yishay, 1980; Deaton, 1986; Helffenstein & Wechsler, 1982; Prigatano, 1986), though the individuals in the group, the setting, and the available resources will also help determine the format. Initial studies indicate their effectiveness in improving communication and social skills (Ben-Yishay, 1980; Helffenstein & Wechsler, 1982) and awareness of injury-related deficits and residual assets (Deaton, 1986). Unfortunately, there are no known studies on the effectiveness of group interventions with younger brain injured children.

For brain injured children and adolescents who may not have insight into their behaviors, some groups may teach a standard approach to problem situations that can be routinely applied to avoid inappropriate behaviors. Groups in inpatient or school settings may also provide for the feedback of peers outside of group settings in the natural environment. This is an important advantage since the ultimate goal of group interventions, as with any behavioral management strategy, is to promote generalization. Generalization can also be promoted by fading prompts and emphasizing self-initiation and self-monitoring as the group members progress.

> *Case 3:* Evan, a 17-year-old injured in an automobile accident while intoxicated, returned to treatment 2 years after his injury when his parents reported that his behavior could not be managed in their home. Still of average intelligence, Evan had difficulties in the areas of gross motor skills (remained nonambulatory), memory (could remember only two of four objects 5 minutes later), and frustration tolerance. Evan had frequent tantrums in the home when his needs or expectations were not being met. The tantrums consisted of screaming, hitting his fist against nearby objects, and hitting anyone who happened to be nearby. Evan's parents responded to all tantrums immediately with a solicitous attitude, asking him what they could do for him and quickly following his wishes. Evan's homebound teacher had refused to work with him following several such episodes.
>
> Soon after admission to a rehabilitation facility, Evan was found appropriate for inclusion in a high-level social skills group using videotaped feedback and for a self-assessment group designed to facilitate accurate self-awareness in head injured adolescents. Initially, Evan expressed his frustration in each of these groups in his usual manner; that is, he had a tantrum. In the social skills group, the response to his tantrum was a brief physical restraint by the therapist to maintain Evan's and others' safety. This was followed by reviewing the videotaped tantrum with Evan, after which he was never observed to have a tantrum in this group while being videotaped. In the self-assessment group, peers did not confront Evan about his tantrums immediately but, rather, reinforced tantrums by letting him have the floor to talk about himself. After several such attention-getting tantrums, however, Evan's peers began to ignore his tantrums or to confront him about interrupting. The incidence of tantrums in this group showed a marked decrease. Generalization of these improvements to the living unit required a separate, unit-based program that used peer feedback in addition to staff feedback and proved effective in decreasing but not eliminating Evan's tantrums. Generalization to home and school settings was expected to require additional training of the significant care providers in these environments.

Environmental Modifications

"For the severely impaired or those in the early stages of recovery, a carefully structured environment becomes perhaps the treatment of choice for maintaining attention and reducing behavior problems" (Grimm and Bleiberg, 1986, p. 512). As discussed in Prigatano's chapter (Chapter 12, this volume), some of the cognitive changes that can result from brain injury include distractibility, memory impairment, difficulty switching from one idea or activity to another (cognitive inflexibility or perseveration), and poor self-monitoring skills. These difficulties typically result in failure to complete tasks or in inadequate performance of tasks in a variety of settings. The modification of antecedent conditions to behaviors is often overlooked as a method of behavior change (Divack et al., 1985). Environments and programs can be designed to minimize some of these difficulties and to maximize performance. As noted by Grimm and Bleiberg (1986), environmental modifications may obviate the need for most or all new learning on the part of the brain injured individual. Having a routine schedule, for example, can significantly reduce confusion and anxiety about what to expect (e.g., Cohen, Joyce, Weider Rhoades, & Welks, 1985) and thereby improve overall behavior and performance. In some settings, providing written lists and cues can also facilitate independent functioning even if the child or adolescent has severe memory problems or difficulty completing tasks. The following case study suggests how a combination of social, behavioral, and physiological problems can be addressed effectively in a prevocational setting through environmental modifications and careful selection of prevocational tasks (Deaton, Poole, & Long, in press).

> Anne, a 16-year-old, sustained a brain injury as a result of a brain tumor and the subsequent surgery required to remove it. She had temporal lobe, pituitary, hypothalamic, frontal lobe, and limbic system damage as a result. Although Anne was very verbal and performed in the borderline range on intelligence measures, she learned new information with difficulty and only after much repetition. Anne had ongoing problems with sudden sleep onset. She also had severe visual deficits, tended to give up at the first sign of difficulty, and was easily sidetracked. Resources included Anne's responsiveness to positive feedback and her willingness to attempt new tasks. To minimize the impact of her sleep disorder on work performance, Anne was assigned tasks that were active in nature, requiring her to go from office to office rather than staying in one place and, inevitably, falling asleep. Moving about was difficult for Anne, however, because she was easily distracted from what she was doing and also because her visual limitations made finding the offices difficult. To deal with these problems, Anne's route was the same each day so that she could establish a visual scanning routine as well as an internal map of where she needed to go. When the effectiveness of these interventions was evaluated, Anne performed well in her daily tasks but did not generalize her compensatory skills to novel tasks, indicating the need for changes in her routine to facilitate generalization. With these changes, Anne's irritability and frustration returned, as did the episodes of sudden sleep onset. She was returned to her original route to reestablish an acceptable level of functioning. Recommendations were made for a highly structured sheltered school and work setting with established routines for work completion.

CONCLUDING REMARKS

Brain injury in children is commonly associated with a host of behavioral problems; some are a direct result of the injury, some are related to the child and family's reduced ability to cope following the injury, and others are exacerbations of preinjury behavioral predispositions. These behavioral difficulties often severely impact outcome, even when cognitive and motor skills are relative strengths. Traditional behavioral change strategies can be effective with brain injured children and adolescents as long as they are modified to address the unique strengths and impairments of this population. These techniques can be effective in decreasing specific problem behaviors, teaching strategies for compensation, and helping to increase adaptive skills such as eating or socializing. Behavioral difficulties can often be prevented by structuring the brain injured person's environment to ensure success, which may, in turn, contribute to the redevelopment of self-esteem following a brain injury. Finally, when the brain injured child's behavior is acceptable and effective in one situation, it is often possible to facilitate gradual generalization to other settings. The child who has the ability and the professional help to negotiate this change process has taken a giant step toward regaining control and independence.

REFERENCES

Auerbach, S.H. (1986). Neuroanatomical correlates of attention and memory disorders in traumatic brain injury: An application of neurobehavioral subtypes. *The Journal of Head Trauma Rehabilitation, 1*, 1–12.

Barin, J.J., Hanchett, J.M., Jacob, W.L., & Scott, M.B. (1985). Counseling the head injured patient. In M. Ylvisaker (Ed.), *Head injury rehabilitation: Children and adolescents* (pp. 361–379). San Diego: College-Hill.

Ben-Yishay, Y. (Ed.). (1980). *Working approaches to remediation of cognitive deficits in the brain damaged. Supplement to the Eighth Annual Workshop for Rehabilitation Professionals.* New York: New York University.

Brooks, N.D. (Ed.). (1984). *Closed head injury: Psychological, social, and family consequences.* New York: Oxford University Press.

Brown, G., Chadwick, O., Shaffer, D., Rutter, M., & Traub, M. (1981). A prospective study of children with head injuries. III. Psychiatric sequelae. *Psychological Medicine, 11*, 63–78.

Cohen, S.B., Joyce, C.M., Weider Rhoades, K., & Welks, D.M. (1985). Educational programming for head injured students. In M. Ylvisaker (Ed.), *Head injury rehabilitation: Children and adolescents* (pp. 383–410). San Diego: College-Hill.

Dean, R.S. (1986). Neuropsychological aspects of psychiatric disorders. In J.

Obrzut & G.W. Hynd (Eds.), *Child neuropsychology* (Vol. 2, pp. 83–112). New York: Academic Press.

Deaton, A.V. (1986, August). *Self-assessment group: An intervention strategy for head injured adolescents.* Paper presented at the Annual Meeting of the American Psychological Association, Washington, DC.

Deaton, A.V., Poole, C.P., & Long, D. (in press). Improving the work potential of brain-injured adolescents and young adults: A model for evaluation and individualized training. *Occupational Therapy in Health Care.*

Divack, J.A., Herrie, J., & Scott, M.B. (1985). Behavior management. In M. Ylvisaker (Ed.), *Head injury rehabilitation: Children and adolescents* (pp. 347–360). San Diego: College-Hill.

Dunn, L.M. (1965). *Expanded manual for the Peabody Picture Vocabulary Test.* Minneapolis: American Guidance Service.

Eames, P., & Wood, R. (1985). Rehabilitation after severe brain injury: A special unit approach. *International Rehabilitation Medicine, 7*(3), 130–133.

Gelfand, D.M., & Hartmann, D.P. (1984). *Child behavior analysis and therapy.* New York: Pergamon.

Goethe, K.E., & Levin, H.S. (1984). Behavioral manifestations during the early and long-term stages of recovery after closed head injury. *Psychiatric Annals, 14*(7), 540–546.

Grimm, B.H., & Bleiberg, J. (1986). Psychological rehabilitation in traumatic brain injury. In S. Filskov & T. Boll (Eds.), *Handbook of clinical neuropsychology* (pp. 495–560). New York: Wiley.

Heaton, R.K., & Pendleton, M.G. (1981). Use of neuropsychological tests to predict adult patients' everyday functioning. *Journal of Consulting and Clinical Psychology, 49*, 807–821.

Helffenstein, D.A., & Wechsler, F. (1982). The use of Interpersonal Process Recall (IPR) in the remediation of interpersonal and communication skill deficits in the newly brain injured. *Clinical Neuropsychology, 4*(3), 139–143.

Horton, A.M., & Sautter, S.W. (1986). Behavioral neuropsychology: Behavioral treatment for the brain-injured. In D. Wedding, A.M. Horton, & J. Webster (Eds.). *The neuropsychology handbook: Behavioral and clinical perspectives* (pp. 259–277). New York: Springer.

Jacobs, H. (1987, March). *Behavior problems.* Workshop presented at the National Head Injury Foundation Annual Conference, Crystal City, VA.

Jennett, B., & Teasdale, G. (1981). *Management of head injuries.* Philadelphia: F.A. Davis.

Lezak, M.D. (1987). Relationships between personality disorders, social disturbances and physical disability following traumatic brain injury. *The Journal of Head Trauma Rehabilitation, 2*, 57–69.

Malec, J. (1984). Training the brain-injured client in behavioral self-management skills. In B.A. Edelstein & E.T. Couture (Eds.), *Behavioral assessment and rehabilitation of the traumatically brain damaged* (pp. 121–150). New York: Plenum.

McGuire, T.L., & Rothenberg, M.B. (1986). Behavioral and psychosocial sequelae of pediatric head injury. *Journal of Head Trauma Rehabilitation, 1*(4), 1–6.

Oddy, M. (1984). Head injury during childhood: The psychological implications. In D.N. Brooks (Ed.), *Closed head injury: Psychological, social, and family consequences* (pp. 177–194). New York: Oxford University Press.

Prigatano, G.P. (1986). *Neuropsychologi-*

cal rehabilitation after brain injury. Baltimore: Johns Hopkins University Press.

Rey, A. (1964). *L'examen clinique en psychologie.* Paris: Presses Universitaires de France.

Rivara, F.P., & Mueller, B.A. (1986). The epidemiology and prevention of pediatric head injury. *Journal of Head Trauma Rehabilitation, 1*(4) 7–15.

Rutter, M. (1981). Psychological sequelae of brain damage in children. *American Journal of Psychiatry, 138,* 1535–1544.

Sand, P.L., Trieschmann, R.B., Fordyce, W.E., & Fowler, R.S. (1970). Behavior modification in the medical rehabilitation setting. *Rehabilitation Research and Practice Review, 1,* 11–24.

Savage, R.C. (1987). Educational issues for the head-injured adolescent and young adult. *Journal of Head Trauma Rehabilitation,* 2(1), 1–10.

Tynan, W.D., Pearce, B.A., & Royall, K.W. (1986, November). *Comprehensive behavioral treatment of self injurious behavior in a head injured adolescent.* Paper presented at the 20th Annual Convention of the Association for the Advancement of Behavior Therapy, Chicago.

Vredevoogd, M.J. (1986, August/September). *Suggestions for working with the difficult to handle closed head injured person.* Ditty, Lynch, and Associates, A Newsletter/Updater (Available from Ditty, Lynch, and Associates, Inc., Bloomfield Medical Village, 6405 Telegraph Rd., Suite K, Birmingham, MI 48010).

Wood, R.L. (1984). Behavior disorders following severe brain injury: Their presentation and psychological management. In D.N. Brooks (Ed.), *Closed head injury: Psychological, social, and family consequences* (pp. 195–219). New York: Oxford University Press.

11

Management of Academic and Educational Problems in Traumatic Brain Injury

CATHY F. TELZROW

Returning to school following a major catastrophe such as a cerebral trauma represents an important step along the path to recovery. For parents and affected children alike, resuming school attendance heralds a return to normalcy. Very often, however, these feelings of optimism are dashed when the traumatically brain injured (TBI) child encounters new and unexpected difficulties in the school environment, and the sense that the student is now "well" is replaced with recognition of additional limitations.

This chapter briefly summarizes data on the educational outcome for populations of TBI children and describes the educationally relevant sequelae of pediatric head injury. In addition, this discussion reviews several systematic deterrents to successful school re-entry, together with suggestions for eliminating or mitigating such obstacles. Finally, characteristics associated with quality educational programs for TBI children are described.

REVIEW OF EDUCATIONAL OUTCOME IN CHILDREN WITH HEAD INJURIES

Studies of the longitudinal outcome of children with head injuries indicate that there is often profound impact on the educational adjustment of children returning to school. In a review of the intellectual and academic outcomes for children with traumatic cerebral injury, Goldstein and Levin (1985) concluded, "head injury leads to impressive cognitive and academic difficulties" (p. 201). Several indicators of educational difficulty have been described, including the need for special education or related services, grade repetition, poor academic performance, and interpersonal adjustment difficulties.

Klonoff and Paris (1974) conducted a longitudinal study of 231 TBI children in which TBI was defined as consecutive hospital admissions with head injury diagnoses. Although severity levels were not specified, most appeared to be mild injuries, as the overall incidence of unconsciousness was 60%, with only 8% of the total sample experiencing unconsciousness for more than 24 hours. While all school-aged children were reported to be attending regular education programs after 1- and 2-year intervals, the incidence of academic difficulties for the older students (ages 9–16) increased from 11% 1 year subsequent to trauma to 17% 2 years later. Complaints of physical and psychological symptoms, including personality changes, learning difficulties, and problems with memory and concentration, were reported for 56% of the group 1 year and 44% 2 years following head trauma. Klonoff, Low, and Clark (1977) followed this group to 5 years postinjury. They reported 15.4% of the younger group and 17.9% of the older group had experienced grade failure, although they still attended regular classes. Special/remedial education was required by 10.3% of the younger and 2.6% of the older subjects. A sizable minority (12.8%) of the older students had experienced successive school failures or had withdrawn from school.

Even more pessimistic findings were reported by Brink, Garrett, Hale, Woo-Sam, and Nickel (1970), who followed 52 patients (ages 2–18) with severe head injury. All children in their sample experienced at least 1 week of coma; modal length of coma was 4 weeks. Of the 34 patients who had returned home, at the time of follow-up, only 8 (24%) were enrolled in regular education classes, and some of these were described as performing below expectancy levels derived from measured intellectual ability. The majority of students in special education (56%) were enrolled in classes for students with physical handicaps, with most others in programs for children with mild to profound levels of mental retardation.

Mahoney et al. (1983) described outcome at follow-up (9 months to 4 years; mean length of follow-up was 21 months) for 34 survivors of severe pediatric head trauma (average length of coma was 15.5 days). Nine percent of the group had severe handicaps (e.g., mental retardation, severe motor disability), and 9% were described as having moderate motor difficulties in conjunction with normal intelligence. More than half (53%) of the group had "mild cognitive dysfunction," characterized by essentially normal intelligence, but evidence of learning and behavior problems, some of which were reported to have been present premorbidly as well. Fewer than one-third of this population (29%) were described as attending regular schools and essentially "normal." It is noteworthy that Mahoney et al. (1983) defined normal intelligence as IQ scores above 80, suggesting the possibility that many of these "normal" children had incurred significant intellectual deficits that might be reflected in greater academic difficulties after a longer follow-up period.

The studies just reviewed indicate there is an adverse effect on educational adjustment for the majority of children with head injuries. Many of these students required some type of significant instructional modifications, such as special education or an adjusted school program. Even children whose school re-entry resulted in a regular classroom assignment often encountered significant adjustment problems, such as grade repetition or learning or behavior problems.

OVERVIEW OF EDUCATIONALLY RELEVANT SEQUELAE OF HEAD INJURIES IN CHILDREN

Each head injured child displays a unique pattern of recovery. Although studies of groups of children indicate it is possible to identify predictors of good or poor outcome (e.g., Brink, Imbus, & Woo-Sam, 1980; Stover & Zeiger, 1976), establishing a course of recovery for individual children often is quite difficult. Nevertheless, it is possible to describe general categories of residual deficits that may affect, to a greater or lesser extent, the educational performance of survivors of cerebral trauma suffered during childhood.

Cognitive Impairment

Most children with severe head injuries display some degree of decline in intellectual functioning relative to premorbid levels (Chadwick, Rutter, Brown, Shaffer, & Traub, 1981; Goldstein & Levin, 1985; Klonoff, Crockett, & Clark, 1984; Levin, Benton, & Grossman, 1982), and such deficits have been reported to produce greater levels of dependence among survivors (Eiben et al., 1984). There is less consensus about deficits in intellectual performance following mild head injury (e.g., Chadwick, Rutter, Brown, Shaffer, & Traub, 1981; Rutter, 1981; Rutter, Chadwick, & Shaffer, 1983), although unique cognitive problems not reflected on formal intellectual measures may be present. Recovery of at least some degree of intellectual functioning may occur fairly soon following injury (Chadwick, Rutter, Brown, Shaffer, & Traub, 1981). There is some evidence that children without residual neurologic effects may not be distinguishable from control subjects on measures of intellectual functioning after several years (Klonoff et al., 1977), although other investigators have reported that cognitive deficits may persist even when neurologic signs disappear (Fuld & Fisher, 1977).

Because of the typically diffuse nature of traumatic head injuries in children, as well as age-related aspects of lateralization, it generally is not possible to identify unique neuropsychological performance patterns of localizing significance (e.g., Verbal-Performance differences on the Wechsler scales) (Chadwick, Rutter, Thompson, & Shaffer, 1981). However, there is some evidence from selected studies that the types of tasks associated with the Wechsler Intelligence Scale for Children–Revised (WISC-R; Wechsler, 1974) Performance scale may be more sensitive to the neuropsychological sequelae of head injuries (Bawden, Knights, & Winogron, 1985; Chadwick, Rutter, Brown, Shaffer, & Traub, 1981). This phenomenon may be attributed to the speeded, visual-motor nature of these tasks (Chadwick, Rutter, Brown, Shaffer, & Traub, 1981). Another possibility is that the Performance subtests tap fluid intellectual abilities to a greater degree than the Verbal tasks, and such abilities are more directly linked to physiological substrates of intelligence (Sattler, 1982).

For educators, the implications of cognitive impairment in TBI children are profound. For a given child who returns to school following a head trauma, there may be marked differences in the degree of general comprehension and problem-solving ability displayed. Children may demonstrate regressions in achievement skills from previous levels, and may appear to be unaware of these losses. For example, a youngster who previously had mastered two-digit subtraction with regrouping may, 3 months later, upon returning to school, be completely unfamiliar with this procedure. The acquisition of new learning, in addition, may be unusually difficult for the child (Henry, 1983). The youngster may appear more immature and "childlike" than previously.

In understanding the neuropsychological sequelae of cognitive impairment in children with head injuries, it is important to note that many children display marked variations in intellectual abilities in different areas. A single index of ability such as IQ cannot capture the range of actual performance levels displayed by head injured children (e.g., Chance, 1986). Although "preserved abilities," such as general information and vocabulary, give the impression of a higher level of functioning, the child may be incapable of reasoning and problem solving at an equivalent level.

A final note of relevance to this discussion of cognitive deficits subsequent to head injury is that formal measures of intellectual ability may not provide a good estimate of future performance (Cohen, Joyce, Rhoades, & Welks, 1985; Cohen & Titonis, 1985). Because these measures are administered in highly controlled settings, they may overestimate a TBI individual's actual level of functioning in the classroom, where demands and distraction are greater. In addition, measures of intellectual ability are circumscribed in terms of the types of neuropsychological abilities they assess, and even students who perform within normal limits on intellectual scales may demonstrate serious impairments in other areas (Levin, Benton, & Grossman, 1982; Shaffer, Bijur, Chadwick, & Rutter, 1980).

Language Deficiencies

Although language skills are among those neuropsychological abilities that often display significant recovery in head injured children (Ewing-Cobbs, Fletcher, & Levin, 1985; Levin, Benton, & Grossman, 1982), residual language-related problems sometimes are apparent in a given student. Among the signs of speech-language difficulties that may persist at the time of school re-entry are *dysnomia* (difficulty in retrieving a specific name of an item or individual, particularly during a demanding situation) and *dysarthria* (slow, poorly articulated speech). Written language skills may be impaired because of underlying language deficits or because of motor difficulties.

The educational implications of language-related deficits are dependent upon the nature and degree of the residual difficulties. In most cases, it is prudent for educators to avoid situations, such as confrontational naming tasks, that may exacerbate the display of dysnomic symptoms. If dysarthria is a factor, teachers may wish to sensitize other students to the nature of this disorder in order to avoid teasing. Permitting ample time for responses, or if the condition is severe, permitting alternative methods of communication, also might be considered. For students who have residual speech-language difficulties, subsequent to a head injury, the option of services of a speech-language pathologist, either on a consultative or therapeutic basis, should be explored.

Impairment of Motor Functioning

Motor skills often recover to a point where normal independent functioning is possible following a head injury (Brink et al., 1980; Stover & Zeiger, 1976). However, in some students, significant motor sequelae, such as ataxia, tremor, hemiparesis, or spasticity, may be evident. Brink et al. (1970) reported that 93% of their sample exhibited spastic symptoms of a minimal, moderate, or severe degree, and Brink et al. (1980) reported that 38% of their sample showed spastic signs, with 39% showing a combination of spasticity and ataxia. Sixty percent of Brink et al.'s (1970) sample exhibited some degree of ataxia. In their analysis of the predictors of subsequent quality of life in TBI patients aged 17 to 40 at the time of injury, Klonoff, Costa, and Snow (1986) suggested that motor disability may adversely affect quality of life. For young people, whose sense of self may be a direct result of body image and athletic proficiency, residual motor impairment can be a particularly negative variable.

The educational management of residual deficits in motor functioning is specific to the nature of the impairment. Severe motor impairments may necessitate the use of adaptive equipment such as wheelchairs, walkers, head pointers, or technological devices such as computers or electronic switches. Assistance from educational attendants for basic functions such as feeding and toileting may be necessary for some severely motorically involved children. Thorough evaluations of motor skills by physical (PT) and occupational (OT) therapists are recommended prior to the TBI student's school re-entry, so that specific suggestions about educational adjustments can be provided.

Memory and Attention Deficits

Memory and attention deficits have been identified as among the more lasting and pervasive of neuropsychological sequelae of head injuries in adults (Grimm & Bleiberg, 1986; Wood, 1984). Although memory deficits have been less widely investigated in children (Ewing-Cobbs et al., 1985; Levin, Benton, & Grossman, 1982), available data suggest that neuropsychological disorders of memory and associated attention deficits may be significant in children who have suffered head injuries (Eiben et al., 1984; Ewing-Cobbs et al., 1985; Levin, Eisenberg, Wigg, & Kobayashi, 1982).

These deficits have direct impact on the educational management of head injured children, since learning is so adversely affected. Old learning is sometimes lost, and new learning becomes a long, slow process (Henry, 1983). Occasionally children not only do not remember a specific procedure in math or the list of continents in geography, but *do not recall having had such a learning experience.*

Memory deficits affect the child's adjustment to noninstructional components of school as well. For example, the youngster may not remember the day's schedule, may not be able to locate different rooms when changing classes, or may not recall sequences of procedures, such as how to move through a cafeteria line or organize a notebook. This bombardment of failures in routine, automatic activities of daily living often compounds the adjustment difficulties of the TBI child returning to school.

Behavior and Personality Changes

Perhaps more than any other head injury sequelae, those related to behavior and personality reinforce the truth of the slogan of the National Head Injury Foundation: "Life after head injury is never the same." The behavior of head injured children may be dramatically different following the insult, and in some cases these changes represent the most distinctive feature of the injury (Klesges & Fisher, 1981; Klonoff & Paris, 1974). Some investigators have reported a significant increase in the incidence of psychiatric disorders in children who sustained severe, but not mild head injuries (Brown, Chadwick, Shaffer, Rutter, & Traub, 1981). Boll (1983) believes that even mild injuries are characterized by behavior and personality changes. There is some evidence that the expression of these sequelae is age related, with younger children displaying hyperactivity, attention deficits, and aggressiveness, and older children demonstrating poor impulse control and difficulty in self-monitoring (Brink et al., 1970). Klonoff et al. (1984) described irritability and personality changes as the major neurologic sequelae for the younger children in their sample, whereas cognitive deficits such as problems with learning and memory tended to plague the older children.

Personality changes in TBI children are sometimes marked, and the dramatic nature of these behaviors may produce feelings of anxiety and confusion in parents and teachers, complicating home and school management (Barin, Hanchett, Jacob, & Scott, 1985). Among the head injured children evaluated by the author within the past few months, for example, was a 12-year-old girl who was transformed by her head trauma from a sweet, compliant honor student to a loud, complaining youngster who made overt racist statements about black students and faculty. Imagine her parents' concern when their intake conference for educational placement was coordinated by a black principal! Sometimes these behavior and personality changes are the only neuropsychological indicators of the head injury. For example, a 17-year-old girl who had sustained a head injury was evaluated by the author 2 months postinjury. All formal cognitive, achievement, and neuropsychological test results were within normal limits. Yet her mother reported that it was as if her daughter had regressed to the level of an 11-year-old, as evidenced by her insistence on having with her a small stuffed tiger during the evaluation. Contradictions in behavior and personality among TBI children often are apparent. For example, this same young lady, who in many ways acted the part of a preteen, also exhibited extremely poor social judgment and self-monitoring, and described her sexual experiences to the examiner during the first few moments of interaction.

Another significant variable in the expression of psychiatric sequelae in TBI children is the nature of premorbid psychological functioning (Brown, Chadwick, Shaffer, Rutter, & Traub, 1981; Levin, Benton, & Grossman,

1982). Several studies have suggested that children with premorbid adjustment problems exhibit a greater degree of psychosocial problems following head injury (Brown et al., 1981). Rutter et al. (1983), for example, reported that "whereas only a quarter of the group with normal preaccident behavior developed disorder by the time of 1-year follow-up, over half of those with pre-injury abnormalities did so" (p. 102). Such reports suggest that traumatic brain injury may exacerbate premorbid adjustment problems.

Educational management of these behavior and personality changes is quite difficult for teachers, who often are ill-prepared to cope with an unpredictable, emotionally labile child. Traditional approaches to problem behavior (e.g., behavior management techniques) may be unsuccessful with TBI children because of cognitive and social perceptual deficits (Cohen et al., 1985; Gianutsos & Grynbaum, 1983). Furthermore, it is critical to recognize the complex interplay between neuropsychological deficits and environmental demands, particularly with regard to how these may mitigate or exacerbate personality and behavior problems (Fuld & Fisher, 1977; Long, Gouvier, & Cole, 1984).

MAJOR SYSTEMIC DETERRENTS TO SUCCESSFUL RE-ENTRY IN EDUCATIONAL AGENCIES

Traditional educational agencies such as public schools are characterized by many entrenched practices and policies, some of which are the result of regulations promulgated by federal and state legislatures; some are reflections of local board of education policy; others are simply custom. Although most practices and procedures implemented by public schools typically serve the average pupil well, some represent obstacles for the TBI child returning to school. This section outlines several of the systemic problems that interfere with successful school re-entry for children who have sustained head injuries.

Conflict Between Hospital/Rehabilitation Center and Educational Agency

The Problem. Agencies that treat the TBI child during the acute stages following the trauma, such as hospitals and rehabilitation centers, can play an important role in facilitating the youngster's return to school. To do so, key personnel in these agencies, such as social workers and therapists, must be cognizant of and responsive to the unique requirements and procedures under which public schools must operate. Too often, the failure of both treatment center and school personnel to recognize the differences in their orientations and to work together to ensure a smooth transition results in delay and frustration for all concerned.

One area of conflict arises when personnel in treatment centers assume a militant advocacy role for TBI children and their parents without adequate understanding of school district policies. For example, insisting upon a specific type and level of "special education" placement without knowledge of eligibility requirements places school personnel in the unpopular position of informing parents their child does not qualify for services that a trusted advocate indicates are essential to recovery. Assessment activities represent another arena where unnecessary complications sometimes occur between treatment center and school personnel. In order to determine eligibility for special education, specific types of evaluations are prescribed by state and federal law. Sometimes treatment facilities have conducted recent assessments in these areas for their own therapeutic and research purposes, and yet neglect to inform school personnel of such activities. Evaluations may be duplicated and sometimes invalidated as a result. In addition, in some states, when treatment facilities administer intellectual tests for research purposes, credentialing requirements (e.g., certification or licensure) do not apply, and noncredentialed agency personnel may be involved. School officials cannot utilize data obtained under these circumstances for clinical decision making, and yet cannot validly readminister the tests. A third problem in complicating transfers from the treatment center to school relates to time lines and expectations. School districts, particularly in major cities, where bureaucracies tend to have more layers, usually require several weeks of "lead time" in order to complete the necessary evaluations and planning activities for a TBI child's re-entry into school. Treatment centers, by their very nature, operate on a more immediate schedule, and may notify school officials of a pending transfer only a week or two in advance. Understandably, the personnel in these agencies become frustrated and annoyed when school districts are not prepared to accommodate children in school at the time of discharge.

The Solution. The essence of all of these conflicts is communication and mutual respect for the institutionalized demands of diverse systems. It behooves personnel in sending agencies (e.g., hospitals and rehabilitation centers) to identify appropriate contact persons within local educational agencies (LEAs) and to develop cooperative working relationships to avoid snags such as the ones described above (e.g., Stonnington, 1986). It is helpful for both the treatment center and the LEA to assign a "case manager" for each child for whom transfer to school is planned (Cohen & Titonis, 1985). By assuming responsibility for coordinating data and communication about a given youngster within their respective systems, these individuals can facilitate school re-entry.

Lack of Appropriate Adjusted Programs

The Problem. As has been demonstrated in earlier sections, most TBI children who return to school require modified programming because of a variety of pervasive neuropsychological sequelae that impair learning and behavior. However, alternatives to regular education that exist in most school systems, primarily programs for handicapped children and federally funded remedial classes for low-achieving economically disadvantaged students (e.g., Chapter I programs), are not appropriate for the majority of children with head injuries. Thus school personnel find themselves in the untenable position of choosing among a few poor alternatives for program placement for TBI children.

Special education programs often are selected as the modification of choice for head injured students. There are several advantages of special education placement, including guaranteed rights for multifactored evaluation to determine educational needs; formalized parent participation in program planning; lower adult-pupil ratios; individually designed instruction, including necessary related services, such as therapies; and annual program reviews. Despite the apparent attractiveness of special education for TBI children as it is traditionally implemented, this option has several limitations. Many head injured children do not qualify for special education services as described in federal and state regulations. The handicapping conditions recognized by P.L. 94-142 (*Federal Register*, 1977), the Education of the Handicapped Act, are deaf, deaf-blind, hard of hearing, mentally retarded, multihandicapped, orthopedically impaired, other health impaired, seriously emotionally disturbed, specific learning disability, speech impaired, and visually handicapped. Examination of the definitions of these conditions illustrates that except for TBI children who have significant intellectual impairment or pervasive sensory or motor deficits, few would meet the eligibility requirements for most special education categories. In the case of specific learning disabilities (SLD), for example, few head injured children exhibit a severe discrepancy between intellectual ability and achievement ("Assistance," 1977), since formal educational skills may be fairly well preserved. This frequently results in a profile where achievement test scores are *higher* than measured intellectual ability.

Even when a multifactored evaluation (MFE) team determines that a TBI child is eligible for a particular category of special education, the appropriateness of placement in such programs is open to serious question. To illustrate, most programs for SLD students are directed toward remediation of specific academic skills, such as reading or math. They are not, with perhaps a few exceptions, designed to provide intensive cognitive rehabilitation of the sort necessary for head injured children. Similar objections can be raised about placement of TBI children in other traditional special education programs. For example, most programs for children with health impairments are designed for youngsters who are confined to wheelchairs, require assistance for ambulation, or who have serious medical conditions, often progressive in nature, which limit their vitality and stamina (e.g., cancer, heart disorders). The integration of most TBI children, many of whom are fully ambulatory and have behavior problems such as aggressiveness and poor impulse control, into such programs, does not appear reasonable for either the TBI children or the other youngsters in these units. Another special education category that is sometimes considered for children who are returning to school after suffering a head injury is that for seriously emotionally disturbed children. However, TBI children often do not meet eligibility criteria because of the requirement for specific deficits to be demonstrated "over a long period of time" and because of exclusionary criteria stating that the inability to learn cannot be due to intellectual or health factors. Even in cases in which the TBI child meets eligibility criteria, it is doubtful that the focus of these programs would be appropriate.

In summary, a major systemic deterrent to the successful school re-entry of TBI children is the absence of appropriate alternatives to regular education. Special education, with its requirements for individually designed programming and periodic reviews of progress, initially appears to be a viable option, but closer examination of the categories of special education available through federal legislation suggests that as currently defined and operated, these are not appropriate for most head injured children. The unique expression of learning and behavioral deficits subsequent to acquired cerebral trauma results in an adverse effect on educational performance that is unlike those conceptualized in the established special education categories.

The Solution. In this author's judgment, the rights and privileges of P.L. 94-142 can be extended to TBI children appropriately through the category "other health impaired" ("... limited ... alertness, due to chronic or acute health problems ... which adversely affects a child's educational performance") (*Federal Register*, 1977, p. 42478). To avoid the difficulties of inappropriate grouping with children who are frail or confined to wheelchairs or whose educational objectives are quite different, a designated other health impaired unit for TBI children can be developed cooperatively on a regional basis. The organization and structure of this unit can be designed with the unique needs of TBI children in mind, as is described in a later section. Excess costs for the operation of such programs can be charged back to sending school districts.

Inadequacy of School Calendar

The Problem. With few exceptions, public schools follow schedules that date back to an agrarian society, with an extended vacation during the summer months. It has been argued that this design runs counter to what we know about the learning process in most youngsters. For TBI children, an extended vacation such as that imposed by the summer hiatus can be particularly detrimental. Research on cognitive rehabilitation with head injured students emphasizes the importance of massed practice, of repetition, and of continuity. None of these is possible for a head injured student whose critical period of cognitive rehabilitation is interrupted by a 3-month vacation.

The issue of an extended school year for handicapped students is one that has been considered by the courts (Bersoff, 1982; Slenkovich, 1987). The most conservative interpretation of these decisions is that few (generally severely handicapped) students would be eligible for extended programming. Such extended programming must be *necessary,* not merely beneficial, as determined by the criterion that without it the student would experience such severe regression that recoupment would not be possible, resulting in a failure to attain goals and objectives and ultimately resulting in a lesser degree of self-sufficiency (Slenkovich, 1987). While there is evidence that a number of handicapped children (e.g., 12,000 to 20,000 in New York State; "New York," 1987) do receive year-round schooling, the degree to which TBI populations are eligible depends upon whether or not the child is identified as handicapped, a difficult matter in itself, as was discussed in the previous section. Even then, compelling a given school district to provide an appropriate special education program through the summer months may require time-consuming litigation, during which the student's needs remain unmet.

The Solution. Hard problems demand creative solutions. The traditional school calendar, particularly with regard to the extended summer vacation, must be modified to permit continuation of intensive services for TBI children at critical stages of cognitive rehabilitation. To do otherwise would appear to deny a major tenet of P. L. 94-142: requiring individual programming (Bersoff, 1982). Even the most conservative position suggests that extended programming may be required for students who, without such intervention, would regress so severely that recoupment is not possible, that goals and objectives could not be met, and that a lower degree of self-sufficiency would occur (Slenkovich, 1987). While it is never possible to prove this inevitability, since a given student cannot experience both treatment and no-treatment conditions simultaneously, many experts would argue that these conditions do apply to TBI students during critical stages of recovery. Models for extended schooling exist in special education (e.g., "New York," 1987), and should be applied to TBI children when determined to be appropriate.

Complications of School Schedules and Noninstructional Practices

The Problem. Most school schedules and noninstructional practices are not conducive to optimal learning for TBI children. Consider for a moment the types of environmental stimulation encountered by a child during the course of a school day. Examples are school buses or public transportation, class changes, the variable and sometimes conflicting demands of as many as 10 different teachers during the week, combination locks, restroom etiquette, physical education, cafeteria lines, and countless interpersonal encounters with fellow students and adults. To head injured children, who have difficulty sorting and prioritizing environmental stimuli, many of these rather ordinary tasks represent obstacles to successful school re-entry (Cohen et al., 1985). Even educators who are sensitive to the unique programmatic needs of TBI children may not have considered that noninstructional variables may sabotage the youngster's school adjustment, often provoking or exacerbating psychological disturbances such as anxiety or depression (e.g., Atteberry-Bennett, Barth, Loyd, & Lawrence, 1986; Fuld & Fisher, 1977; Long et al., 1984).

The Solution. Organization of the entire school experience must be carefully controlled for returning TBI children. Potential problems must be anticipated and the environment structured accordingly to incorporate systematic reorientation to the countless noninstructional experiences (Fuld & Fisher, 1977). Specific suggestions with regard to implementing these objectives are provided below.

CHARACTERISTICS OF QUALITY EDUCATIONAL DELIVERY SYSTEMS FOR TBI CHILDREN

Using as a foundation the description of educationally relevant sequelae of head injuries provided above, as well as the major systemic deterrents to successful school re-entry in the immediately preceding section, it is possible to design optimal educational programs for TBI children. While the development and implementation of such programs may require significant changes in the ways education traditionally has been conceptualized and delivered, such modifications may be necessary in order for appropriate educational services to become available for this population.

1. Maximally Controlled Environment

Rehabilitation programs generally are characterized by engineered environments designed to reduce stress for impaired individuals (Grimm & Bleiberg, 1986). Within the context of the educational agency, this objective can be met by a self-contained classroom unit model where adults, expectations, and the surroundings remain constant.

The self-contained unit model is not widely employed for most "typical" students. Even very young children often receive "special" instruction (e.g., art, music, physical education) from teachers other than their "classroom teacher," and many elementary buildings are even more departmentalized, such that youngsters change classes several times each day. Inherent in such a model is a host of problems for TBI students, including difficulties in recalling schedules, locating classrooms, organizing books and materials, and adjusting to diverse teaching styles and behavioral expectations. One TBI girl known to the author returned to a large high school with an unadjusted program several weeks following a head injury, and was promptly suspended because she was consistently late for her classes and could not remember which was her assigned seat each time she entered a different classroom.

Ideally, a program for TBI students would be based in a self-contained classroom unit, where the re-entering youngster initially would spend 100% of his or her time while in school. Such a model facilitates control of the environment so that the variables confronted by recovering children are within their range of coping ability (Fuld & Fisher, 1977; Long et al., 1984). Integration into other school activities outside of the self-contained unit could be introduced in a gradual and systematic fashion, depending upon the unique characteristics of each student (Haarbauer-Krupa, Henry, Szekeres, & Ylvisaker, 1985).

2. Low Pupil-Teacher Ratio

Data on the most successful cognitive rehabilitation programs indicate that the ratio of instructors to clients may be as low as 2:1 (Ben-Yishay, 1985). For head injured students, a similarly low adult-pupil ratio is recommended because of the need for individual instruction and direct personal feedback. Ideally, adults with a variety of training and credentials would be involved in providing instruction, including teachers, therapists, and instructional aides. A coordinating or master teacher might assume responsibility for a student's program, although other specialists and aides would interact with the student in the unit.

3. Intensive and Repetitive

The injured brain is impaired in its ability to learn. Thus for learning to occur intensive instruction, characterized by repetition and practice, is necessary (Miller, 1980; Szekeres, Ylvisaker, & Holland, 1985). For the TBI child this translates into a requirement for more time needed to learn (Carroll, 1984; Gettinger, 1984; Kavale & Forness, 1986). Since time is a variable with an inherent ceiling—we all have the same amount and we all have all there is—some modifications in the delivery of educational services for TBI children are necessary in order to "borrow" time so that the time needed to learn can be provided.

Two major mechanisms for providing necessary time for learning for TBI students exist. The first is to reduce time devoted to noninstructional activities to a minimum. Research on time and school learning has revealed that more than one-third of the school day is passed in transitional and noninstructional activities (Burns, 1984). By designing programs for TBI students in a self-contained format where adult-pupil ratios are low, time spent in direct instructional activities is maximized. In addition, it is suggested there be limited exposure, especially during critical phases of cognitive retraining, to nonacademic or "special" classes such as physical education, music, art, and extracurricular activities. Although it can be argued that these pursuits are therapeutic and personally rewarding, it is suggested that the student's rehabilitation is enhanced when initial emphasis is given to cognitively based activities instead. Later, these activities should be delivered in an integrated fashion, which reduces the amount of time in transitional, noninstructional activities as well.

A second means of increasing time for learning is to lengthen the school year. This admittedly controversial recommendation is based on evidence that continuous repetition and practice may be necessary for optimal recovery in TBI students (Miller, 1980). Altering the school calendar to sustain intervention efforts throughout the summer vacation period for pupils whose rehabilitation is at a critical phase is likely to be reflected in noteworthy gains for this population.

4. Emphasis on Process

Unlike most educational programs, which emphasize specific academic content, interventions for TBI children should focus on learning processes (Cohen, 1986; Henry, 1983; NHIF, 1985). Increasing sustained attention, developing and following a plan of study, and applying memory cues are examples of cognitive processes that might be incorporated into an educational program for children who have sustained head injuries. Key ingredients in process training for TBI children are the careful assessment of neuropsychological strengths and weaknesses and a well-matched intervention plan that emphasizes the development of compensatory skills when appropriate (Grimm & Bleiberg, 1986; Henry, 1983; Telzrow, 1985).

5. Behavioral Programming

Cognitive retraining of TBI students is most successful when behavioral instructional strategies are employed. Such interventions are characterized by a careful task analysis of desired outcomes, with instruction progressing in a systematic fashion from mastery of the earliest component skills to the end goal (Adamovich, Henderson, & Auerbach, 1985; Grimm & Bleiberg, 1986). Henry (1983) provides a useful list of questions that can assist educators in evaluating performance of students in a number of key areas such as attention, problem solving, reasoning, and memory. Specific suggestions for developing component skills within each area are included.

6. Integrated Instructional Therapies

Ben-Yishay, recognized as a leader in cognitive retraining of TBI individuals, notes that many of his clients have "passed rehabilitation, but failed real life" (Ben-Yishay, 1985). He contends that one of the reasons for the poor transfer of skills from rehabilitation programs to daily life is the segregated model of therapeutic services. Ben-Yishay maintains that an integrated program, where services pertinent to speech-language, OT, PT, and other areas can be incorporated into the client's rehabilitation plan, is preferable to a model of segregated services.

This observation is relevant to educational programs for TBI students as well. An analogous model, which resembles what Rourke, Bakker, Fisk, and Strang (1983) refer to as a "dynamic interactive milieu intervention," is conceptualized in the following manner. All necessary related services, such as speech therapy, occupational therapy, and physical therapy, are integrated into the student's primary instructional setting rather than delivered via a "pull out" design. Specialists may work directly with students, along with other instructors, or provide consultative services to these instructors, or both. Such an approach is consistent with several of the characteristics of quality educational intervention programs outlined above, such as low pupil-staff ratios and the need for intensive training. Rourke et al. (1983) noted some potential difficulties associated with such an integrated model, but they identify this approach as a particularly well-suited intervention strategy for head injured children. One important effect of an integrated model of related services is that it facilitates transfer and generalization. For TBI students, who have unique difficulty accomplishing application skills, this is an important advantage.

7. Simulation Experiences

Because of the problem of transfer, successful intervention programs for TBI students should incorporate a broad variety of simulation experiences. Examples of simulations include preparing a student to give an oral presentation or simulating appropriate resolution of a confrontation with another student. Simulations may be conducted through the use of adult or peer demonstrations, or may involve the use of self-modeling via videotaped technology (e.g., Cohen, 1986; Haarbauer-Krupa et al., 1985). Even when employing simulations, unanticipated problems may arise when transitions to the actual situation occur, and ongoing assessment of obstacles and planning for resolution are necessary (e.g., Gianutsos & Grynbaum, 1983).

8. Cuing, Fading, and Shadowing

In retraining the injured brain, basic learning principles such as cuing and fading should be emphasized (Divack, Herrle, & Scott, 1985; Grimm & Bleiberg, 1986; Szekeres et al., 1985). To a much greater extent than average pupils, students who have suffered head injuries require the use of environmental cues in the process of encoding, storing, and recalling information. Such cues should be an integral part of the educational program for TBI students (Adamovich et al., 1985; Wood, 1984). Fading of externally controlled cues, together with the development of independently generated cues, should be encouraged as recovery progresses (Cohen et al., 1985; Henry, 1983).

Shadowing experiences are widely employed in vocational training programs. The shadowing experience, in which an adult provides close and direct supervision during a student's early trials at displaying a specific skill, can be adapted successfully to a wide variety of learning and behavior skill training sessions for TBI students. Shadowing might be provided, for example, when a TBI student leaves the self-contained unit to change classes for the first time. To minimize student anxiety and avoid possible problems such as tardiness, an adult "shadow" can accompany the student, providing direction and feedback as appropriate.

9. Readjustment Counseling

In his work with TBI adults, Ben-Yishay (1985) argues cogently that successful rehabilitation depends upon the restructuring of the ego so that the impaired individual relinquishes the premorbid sense of self and redefines personal goals and aspirations in light of the new circumstances imposed by the head injury. The implication of this observation is that educational programs for TBI students should incorporate readjustment counseling. Delivered in an integrated rather than a pull-out fashion, consistent with the recommendation offered above, such services could focus not only on readjustment but also on presenting psychological problems of students, such as anxiety, acting-out behavior, or depression (Barin et al., 1985; Cohen et al., 1985).

10. Home-School Liaison

Beginning at the moment of the trauma, parents of TBI children board a roller coaster of emotional highs and lows. Initial shock and fear of death are replaced by relief and joy because the youngster will survive. By the time the child is sufficiently recovered to re-enter school, parents frequently are numbed or depressed by the realization that their child requires a dramatically modified educational program, and that a new set of activities the child can't accomplish is being defined (Polinko, Barin, Leger, & Bachman, 1985).

Significant others in the TBI child's life are critically important to the recovery process (Grimm & Bleiberg, 1986). A number of experts have described these relationships (e.g., Lezak, 1978; Long et al., 1984). School officials can maximize the positive influence of parents on the recovery process by establishing a formal communication system for families of TBI children, including a mechanism for providing information, personal progress reports, and peer support.

SUMMARY

The evidence reviewed in this article and elsewhere in this book indicates that children who have sustained traumatic head injuries typically have significant physical, cognitive, and behavioral sequelae that adversely affect their educational performance. Once TBI children have left the rehabilitation setting and have returned to school, the educational agency becomes the primary vehicle for facilitating ongoing recovery. Appropriate educational management of TBI children requires recognition of the major systemic variables that impede successful school re-entry, and commitment to developing reasonable solutions to these problems. Ten characteristics associated with quality educational delivery systems were outlined. These features were derived from data on successful rehabilitation programs for TBI persons, and are intended to provide a carefully engineered environment that can manage residual cognitive and behavioral weaknesses while retraining neuropsychological processes and developing compensatory skills.

REFERENCES

Adamovich, B.B., Henderson, J.A., & Auerbach, S. (1985). *Cognitive rehabilitation of closed head injured patients. A dynamic approach.* San Diego: College-Hill.

Assistance to states for education of handicapped children: Procedures for evaluating specific learning disabilities. (1977, December 19). *Federal Register, 42*(250).

Atteberry-Bennett, J., Barth, J.T., Loyd, B.H., & Lawrence, E.C. (1986). The relationship between behavioral and cognitive deficits, demographics and depression in patients with minor head injuries. *The International Journal of Clinical Neuropsychology, 8*, 114–117.

Barin, J.J., Hanchett, J.M., Jacob, W.L., & Scott, M.B. (1985). Counseling the head injured patient. M. Ylvisaker (Ed.), *Head injury rehabilitation: Children and adolescents* (pp. 361–379). San Diego: College-Hill.

Bawden, H.N., Knights, R.M., & Winogron, H.W. (1985). Speeded performance following head injury in children. *Journal of Clinical and Experimental Neuropsychology, 7*, 39–54.

Ben-Yishay, Y. (1985, October). *Holistic neuropsychological rehabilitation program for chronic, traumatically head injured individuals.* Workshop presented at the meeting of the National Academy of Neuropsychologists, Philadelphia.

Bersoff, D.N. (1982). From courthouse to schoolhouse: Using the legal system to secure the right to an appropriate education. *American Journal of Orthopsychiatry, 52*, 506–517.

Boll, T.J. (1983). Minor head injuries in children: Out of sight but not out of mind. *Journal of Clinical Child Psychology, 12*, 74–80.

Brink, J.D., Garrett, A.L., Hale, W.R., Woo-Sam, J., & Nickel, V.L. (1970). Recovery of motor and intellectual function in children sustaining severe head injuries. *Developmental Medicine and Child Neurology, 12*, 565–571.

Brink, J.D., Imbus, C., & Woo-Sam, J. (1980). Physical recovery after severe closed head trauma in children and adolescents. *The Journal of Pediatrics, 97*, 721–727.

Brown, G., Chadwick, O. Shaffer, D. Rutter, M., & Traub, M. (1981). A prospective study of children with head injuries: III. Psychiatric sequelae. *Psychological Medicine, 11*, 63–78.

Burns, R.B. (1984). How time is used in elementary school: The activity structure of classrooms. In L.W. Anderson (Ed.), *Time and school learning* (pp.

91–127). New York: St. Martin's Press.

Carroll, J.B. (1984). The model of school learning: Progress of an idea. In L.W. Anderson (Ed.), *Time and school learning* (pp. 15–45). New York: St. Martin's Press.

Chadwick, O., Rutter, M., Brown, G., Shaffer, D., & Traub, B. (1981). A prospective study of children with head injuries: II. Cognitive sequelae. *Psychological Medicine, 11*, 49–61.

Chadwick, O., Rutter, M., Thompson, J., & Shaffer, D. (1981). Intellectual performance and reading skills after localized head injury in childhood. *Journal of Child Psychology and Psychiatry, 22*, 117–139.

Chance, P. (1986, October). Life after head injury. *Psychology Today,* pp. 62–69.

Cohen, S.B. (1986). Educational reintegration and programming for children with head injuries. *Journal of Head Trauma Rehabilitation, 1*(4), 22–29.

Cohen, S.B., Joyce, C.M., Rhoades, K.W., & Welks, D.M. (1985). Educational programming for head injured students. In M. Ylvisaker (Ed.), *Head injury rehabilitation: Children and adolescents* (pp. 383–409). San Diego: College-Hill.

Cohen, S.B., & Titonis, J. (1985). Head injury rehabilitation: Management issues. In M. Ylvisaker (Ed.), *Head injury rehabilitation: Children and adolescents* (pp. 429–443). San Diego: College-Hill.

Divack, J.A., Herrle, J., & Scott, M.B. (1985). Behavior management. In M. Ylvisaker (Ed.), *Head injury rehabilitation: Children and adolescents* (pp. 347– 360). San Diego: College-Hill.

Eiben, C.G., Anderson, T.P., Lockman, L., Matthews, D.J., Dryja, R., Martin, J., Burrill, C., Gottesman, N., O'Brien, P., & Witte, L. (1984). Functional outcome of closed head injury in children and young adults. *Archives of Physical Medicine Rehabilitation, 65,* 168–170.

Ewing-Cobbs, L., Fletcher, J.M., & Lewis, H.S. (1985). Neuropsychological sequelae following pediatric head injury. In M. Ylvisaker (Ed.), *Head injury rehabilitation: Children and adolescents* (pp. 71–89). San Diego: College-Hill.

Federal Register. (1977, August 23). Education of handicapped children, *42*(163).

Fuld, P.A., & Fisher, P. (1977). Recovery of intellectual ability after closed head-injury. *Developmental Medicine and Child Neurology, 19*, 495–502.

Gettinger, M. (1984). Measuring time needed for learning to predict learning outcomes. *Exceptional Children, 51,* 244–248.

Gianutsos, R., & Grynbaum, B.B. (1983). Helping brain-injured people to contend with hidden cognitive deficits. *International Rehabilitation Medicine, 5*, 37–40.

Goldstein, F.C., & Lewis, H.S. (1985). Intellectual and academic outcome following closed head injury in children and adolescents: Research strategies and empirical findings. *Developmental Neuropsychology, 1*, 195–214.

Grimm, B.H., & Bleiberg, J. (1986). Psychological rehabilitation in traumatic brain injury. In S.B. Filskov & T.J. Boll (Eds.), *Handbook of clinical neuropsychology* (Vol. 2, pp. 495–560). New York: Wiley.

Haarbauer-Krupa, J., Henry, K., Szekeres, S.F., & Ylvisaker, M. (1985). Cognitive rehabilitation therapy: Late stages of recovery. In M. Ylvisaker (Ed.), *Head injury rehabilitation: Children and adolescents* (pp. 311–343). San Diego: College-Hill.

Henry, K. (1983). Cognitive rehabilitation and the head-injured child. *Journal of Children in Contemporary Society, 16,* 189–205.

Kavale, K.A., & Forness, S.R. (1986). School learning, time and learning disabilities: The disassociated learner. *Journal of Learning Disabilities, 19,* 130–138.

Klesges, R.C., & Fisher, L.P. (1981). A multiple criterion approach to the assessment of brain damage in children. *Clinical Neuropsychology, 3*(4), 6–11.

Klonoff, P.S., Costa, L.D., & Snow, W.G. (1986). Predictors and indicators of quality of life in patients with closed-head injury. *Journal of Clinical and Experimental Neuropsychology, 8,* 469–485.

Klonoff, H., Crockett, D.D., & Clark, C. (1984). Head injuries in children: A model for predicting course of recovery and prognosis, In R.E. Tarter & G. Goldstein (Eds.), *Advances in clinical neuropsychology* (Vol. 2, pp. 139–157). New York: Plenum Press.

Klonoff, H., Low, M.D., & Clark, C. (1977). Head injuries in children: A prospective five year follow-up. *Journal of Neurology, Neurosurgery, and Psychiatry, 40,* 1211–1219.

Klonoff, H., & Paris, R. (1974). Immediate, short-term and residual effects of acute head injuries in children: Neuropsychological and neurological correlates. In R.M. Reitan & L.A. Davison (Eds.), *Clinical neuropsychology* (pp. 179–210). Washington, DC: Hemisphere.

Levin, H.S., Benton, A.L., & Grossman, R.G. (1982). *Neurobehavioral consequences of closed head injury,* New York: Oxford University Press.

Levin, H.S., Eisenberg, H.M., Wigg, N.R., & Kobayashi, K. (1982). Memory and intellectual ability after head injury in children and adolescents. *Neurosurgery, 11,* 668–673.

Lezak, M.D. (1978). Living with the charaterologically altered brain injured patient. *Journal of Clinical Psychiatry, 39,* 592–598.

Long, C.J., Gouvier, W.D., & Cole, J.C. (1984). A model of recovery for the total rehabilitation of individuals with head trauma. *Journal of Rehabilitation, 50,* 39–45.

Mahoney, W.J., D'Souza, B.J., Haller, J.A., Rogers, M.C., Epstein, M.H., & Freeman, J.M. (1983). Long-term outcome of children with severe head trauma and prolonged coma. *Pediatrics, 71,* 756–762.

Miller, E. (1980). The training characteristics of severely head-injured patients: A preliminary study. *Journal of Neurology, Neurosurgery, and Psychiatry, 43,* 525–528.

National Head Injury Foundation (NHIF). (1985). *An educator's manual: What educators need to know about students with traumatic brain injury.* Framingham, MA: Author.

New York revamps 12-month program for severely handicapped students. (1987, February 18). *Education of the Handicapped,* pp. 1–2.

Polinko, P.R., Barin, J.J., Leger, D., & Bachman, K.M. (1985). Working with the family. In M. Ylvisaker (Ed.), *Head injury rehabilitation: Children and adolescents* (pp. 91–115). San Diego: College-Hill.

Rourke, B.P., Bakker, D.J., Fisk, J.L., & Strang, J.D. (1983). *Child neuropsychology.* New York: Guilford.

Rutter, M. (1981). Psychological sequelae of brain damage in children. *American Journal of Psychiatry, 183,* 1533–1542.

Rutter, J., Chadwick, O., & Shaffer, D. (1983). Head injury. In M. Rutter (Ed.), *Developmental neuropsychiatry* (pp. 83–111). New York: Guilford.

Sattler, J.M. (1982). *Assessment of chil-*

dren's intelligence and special abilities. Boston: Allyn & Bacon.

Shaffer, D., Bijur, P., Chadwick, O., & Rutter, M. (1980). Head injury and later reading disability. *Journal of American Academy of Child Psychiatry, 19,* 592–610.

Slenkovich, J.E. (1987, February). Extended school year: When is it really required? *The Schools' Advocate,* 65–66, 68–71.

Stonnington, H.H. (1986). Traumatic brain injury rehabilitation. *American Rehabilitation, 12,* 4–5, 19–20.

Stover, S.L., & Zeiger, H.E. (1976). Head injury in children and teenagers: Functional recovery correlated with the duration of coma. *Archives of Physical Medicine and Rehabilitation, 57,* 201–205.

Szekeres, S.F., Ylvisaker, M., & Holland, A.L. (1985). Cognitive rehabilitation therapy: A framework for intervention. In M. Ylvisaker (Ed.), *Head injury rehabilitation: Children and adolescents* (pp. 219–246). San Diego: College-Hill.

Telzrow, C.F. (1985). The science and speculation of rehabilitation in developmental neuropsychological disorders. In L.C. Hartlage & C.F. Telzrow (Eds.), *Neuropsychological aspects of individual differences: A developmental perspective* (pp. 271–307). New York: Plenum Press.

Wechsler, D.A. (1974). *Manual for the Wechsler intelligence scale for children–Revised.* New York: Psychological Corp.

Wood, R.L. (1984). Management of attention disorders following brain injury. In B.A. Wilson & N. Moffat (Eds.), *Clinical management of memory problems* (pp. 148–170). Rockville, MD: Aspen Systems.

12

Recovery and Cognitive Retraining After Cognitive Brain Injury

GEORGE P. PRIGATANO

There has been in recent years an explosion of interest and activity in developing cognitive remediation or cognitive retraining activities for traumatic brain injured patients. Unfortunately, this has not been paralleled by new scientific insights that would allow us to make a bad memory good (Schacter & Glisky, 1986), reverse the effects of severe visual-spatial deficits (Diller & Weinberg, 1986), or substantially improve abstract reasoning and problem solving skills (Goldstein & Levin, 1987) Yet, *some* patients who suffer craniocerebral trauma make substantial progress in their recovery and it would seem that retraining or educational/therapeutic activities might facilitate the rate and/or level of recovery. Moreover, for a subgroup of patients who are relatively self-sufficient in terms of activities of daily living, intensive neuropsychologically oriented rehabilitation can substantially improve their level of psychosocial adjustment (Ben-Yishay et al., 1985; Prigatano and Others, 1986).

Clinicians and researchers involved in the re-education of brain damaged patients have emphasized the importance of teaching patients to be realistically aware of residual deficits. They also emphasize helping patients learn compensatory techniques to circumvent functional disabilities and to attain eventual acceptance of the consequences of permanent changes in higher cerebral (or subcortical) function (e.g., Ben-Yishay & Prigatano, in press; Diller & Weinberg, 1986; Prigatano and Others, 1986).

The terms *rehabilitation, remediation,* or *retraining* connote to some individuals the idea of regaining lost function. It is doubtful, however, that our present teaching methods will allow us to do this (see chap. 4, Prigatano and Others, 1986). Yet, we are faced with many paradoxes as we observe the recovery of individuals following traumatic brain injury. Most patients with mild injuries (i.e., Glasgow Coma Scale scores [GCS] at admission of 13 through 15) show substantial recovery and are often back to work within 3 to 6 months postinjury (Prigatano, Klonoff, & Bailey, 1987). Patients with moderate injuries (GCS between 9 and 12 at admission) and severe injuries (GCS of 3 to 8) are quite *variable* in their recovery course.

The factors that determine good versus poor recovery are still not understood, but certainly the type of lesion and the amount of structural brain damage seem to be quite important (e.g., Chapman & Wolff, 1959; Uzzell, Dolinskas, Wiser, & Langfitt, 1987). The recent report by Uzzell et al. (1987) shows different recovery patterns after traumatic brain injuries depending on the nature of computerized axial tomography (CT) findings at admission or shortly after injury. Patients who show only diffuse swelling on CT examination have a better level of neuropsychological recovery than those who evidence diffuse axonal injury. Yet even in this study, individual differences in both level and rate of recovery occurred. Clearly, both neurological and non-neurological factors seem to contribute to the overall recovery process (Prigatano, 1987, in press).

HISTORICAL CONTRIBUTIONS TO COGNITIVE RETRAINING

In 1897, John Hughlings Jackson delivered a lecture to the British Neurological Society. Published in *Lancet* in January of 1898, "Relations of Different Divisions of the Central Nervous System to One Another and to Parts of the Body" revealed how Darwin's theory of evolution had influenced Jackson's thought about the nervous system (Prigatano, 1986). Jackson believed that the higher cerebral functions (which present-day cognitive retraining activities attempt to address) were actually less complex in their structural organization than so-called lower brain functions. Consequently, higher cerebral functions may actually be more modifiable than previously considered. Jackson had the following to say about this paradox of the higher functions being less complex:

> It is necessary here to remark that such an expression as "high organization" is not, when used with regard to the nervous system, synonymous with most

> complex ... Indeed, the most complex, nervous arrangements, centers and levels are the least organized; the most simple are the most organized. Thus the centers of the lowest levels are much more strongly organized than those of the highest level are. It is very important to bear this in mind. A man deeply comatose from sucking raw spirits out of a cask and whose highest level, or presumably most of it, is rendered quite functionless by much alcohol rapidly taken, recovers because the "vital" centers of his lowest level are very strongly organized and go on working although imperfectly, when the comparatively weakly organized centers of the highest level have "given out." If the "vital" centers of the lowest level were not strongly organized at birth life would not be possible; if centers of the highest level "mental centers" were not little organized and therefore very modifiable, we could only with difficulty and imperfectly adjust ourselves to new circumstances and should make few new acquirements. (Jackson, 1898, pp. 84–85)

This theoretical model perhaps predicted the earlier experimental findings of Flourens and later work of Lashley (cited in Prigatano, 1986). In 1824 Flourens reported on the recovery of higher cerebral functions in pigeons subject to cerebral ablations. In 1927 Lashley reported on the ability of rats to learn mazes after serial ablations to the cerebral hemispheres. In both instances, the researchers were struck with the degree of *recovery* rather than the *lack of it*. These findings and many others (Bach-y-Rita, 1986) suggest that the *potential* for recovery of higher cerebral function may be greater than for any other functions mediated by the central nervous system.

On the other hand, not all early investigators shared these optimistic theoretical notions. Other explanations regarding recovery are equally plausible. In 1914, Von Monakow (cited in Prigatano, 1986) emphasized that what looked like recovery was actually the process of uninjured brain systems reassuming normal function following the phenomenon of diaschisis. Also, clinicians working with brain injured soldiers (e.g., Goldstein, 1942; see also Prigatano, 1986) argued that true recovery of function after brain injury resulted only from the restoration of an anatomical substrate. Since this does not actually occur (neurons do not regenerate), apparent recovery is simply a readjustment—a getting along with a lost function.

Lashley (1938) argued, however, that several mechanisms may account for recovery or lack of it: "functional loss may be secondary to destruction of essential neurostructures, temporary disruption of existing pathways, diaschisis, metabolic disturbances, or a lower tonic level of activity" (p. 735).

Luria's early work (1963) suggested that partial restoration of higher cerebral functions could be achieved because these higher cerebral functions were the result of overlapping and interconnected functional systems or subsystems. In the case of localized cerebral destruction, a new subsystem or a new subroutine could theoretically be established by retraining methods and pharmacological treatment. Theoretically, both methods would deblock states of brain inhibition following Von Monokow's earlier ideas concerning the hypothesized phenomena of diaschisis.

In the mid-sixties, a considerable amount of work was done to re-educate language function in aphasic patients (Vignolo, 1964). By the late seventies, research emerged that clearly documented for the first time that language skills in aphasic patients could be improved by rehabilitation even though complete restoration of the deficit areas was not possible (Basso, Capitani, & Vignolo, 1979). Thus, a sophistication in the broad field of cognitive remediation began to appear. Some functions can be modestly or even moderately helped, but the overall outcome is seldom, if ever, a return to normality. To better appreciate this, some understanding of the natural recovery process is necessary.

RECOVERY OF HIGHER CEREBRAL DEFICITS AFTER CRANIOCEREBRAL TRAUMA: A FEW EXAMPLES

The major problem in studying recovery phenomena after traumatic brain injury is that there is *great variability* in the type and severity of actual brain pathology associated with these injuries. This point has been made by several authors (Hagen, 1982; Jennett & Teasdale, 1981; Levin, Benton, & Grossman, 1982). Also, there are, in all likelihood, equally great differences in preexisting intelligence, memory, and personality characteristics of patients who suffer these injuries. Thus, where patients start off, how badly they were injured, and what they are willing to try to do about it all seem to contribute to the level and possible course of recovery.

Data on changes in IQ scores following trauma are sparse, but the work of Bond (1975) is informative. Using the period of posttraumatic amnesia (PTA) as the measure of severity of injury (GCS scores were not available at that time), he reported on the relationship of Wechsler IQ scores to the severity of injury over time. As Figure 12.1 illustrates, Verbal IQ seems to improve quickly if the PTA is less than 7 weeks. A similar pattern is noted for Performance IQ scores, except improvement takes place for a longer period of time. If PTA is longer than 12 weeks, the recovery curve is not promising. Bond (1975) reported that the "most rapid period of recovery is during the first 6 months, but this is followed by a slower rate of improvement which continues steadily, and, although not shown [in this figure], reaches a maximum 24 months after injury (p. 151).

While the Bond (1975) results are hampered by the methodological problem that his data are based on different groups of patients assessed in a cross-sectional design versus a longitudinal study of the same patients, his conclusions have been readily accepted by clinicians working in the field.

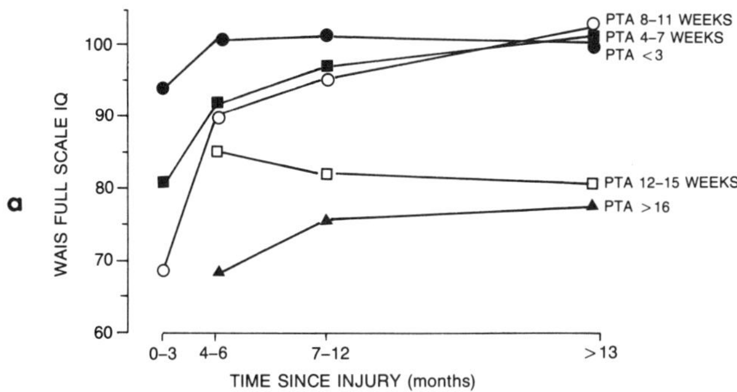

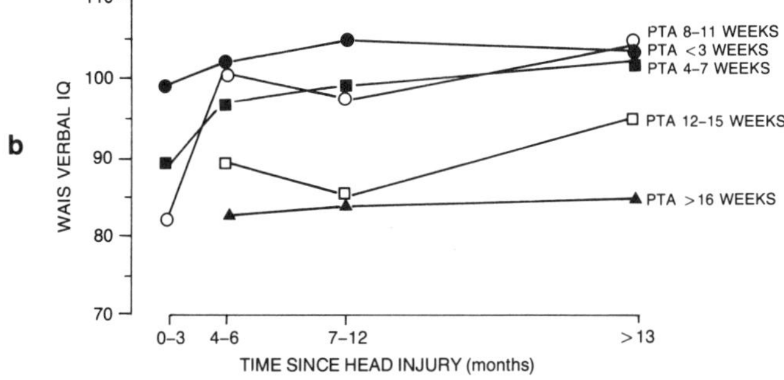

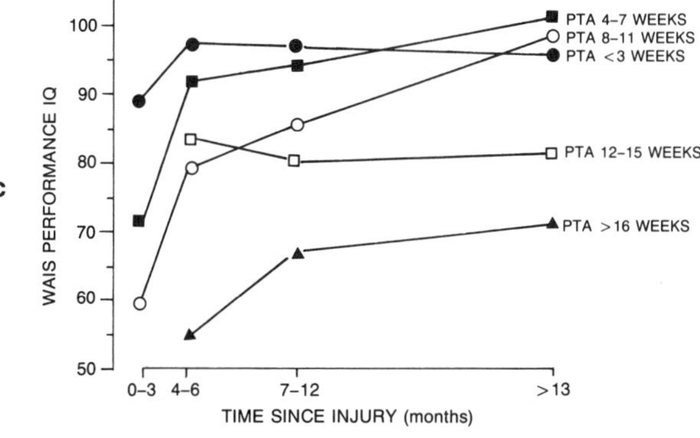

Figure 12.1. The relation of the recovery of cognitive ability—*(a)* WAIS Full scale, *(b)* WAIS Verbal scale, *(c)* WAIS Performance scale—to time from injury and the duration of post-traumatic amnesia: ●, less than 3 weeks; ■, 4–7 weeks; ○, 8–11 weeks; □, 12–15 weeks; ▲, more than 16 weeks. *Note:* From "Assessment of the Psychosocial Outcome After Severe Head Injury" by M.R. Bond, 1975. In Ciba Foundation Symposium, *Outcome of Severe Damage to the Central Nervous System* (pp. 141–157). New York: American Elsevier/ Excerpta Medica/North-Holland. Reprinted by permission of author.

Verbal skills (Verbal IQ included) seem to show the most rapid improvement over the first 6 months following injury. Nonverbal skills (e.g., visual/spatial problem solving and speed of information processing) are slower to recover and may show the most dramatic improvement about 1 year postinjury. Yet continued improvement is often seen 2 years postinjury. Even past 2 years, some improvement can be seen, but is often not described as dramatic. For example, Von Zomeren and Deelman (1978) reported improvement in reaction time several months posttrauma. There have also been case reports of continued improvement in selected areas of function several years posttrauma, particularly when the person was an adolescent or young adult at the time of injury (e.g., Brown, 1975). These findings suggest that as long as the brain is alive, it can continue to learn and readapt. However, the degree of recovery in higher cerebral functioning possible for a given individual continues to be both a clinical and scientific guessing game. Recovery of various aspects of higher cerebral functions may indeed be differentially determined and resistant or responsive to different rehabilitation experiences.

For example, some memory phenomena may rapidly improve while other aspects of memory function may be relatively resistant to improvement. Complex personality characteristics can also vary in their recovery course. In reviewing the literature on memory functioning after closed head injury, Schacter and Crovitz (1977) reported on the paucity of systematic findings on the time course of memory recovery. They noted that different components of memory function may, in fact, recover at different time periods. Brooks (1976), using a cross-sectional design, concluded that recovery of memory may take place very early after injury as measured by portions of the Wechsler Memory scale. In groups matched on age and PTA over three time periods (1 to 4 months; 5 to 12 months; and 13 months or longer postinjury), paired associate learning scores were not significantly different between the groups. Lezak (1979) studied traumatic brain injuries in patients over time. She reported improvement on several measures of memory between 6 months and 12 months postinjury, but no significant change in positive direction after that. Interestingly, she reported that on some measures, patients actually *declined* in their performance several months posttrauma. This may be attributable to actual deterioration of function or other factors contributing to test performance (i.e., increased psychiatric or coping problems). The same phenomenon has been seen in traumatic brain injured patients who have been involved in our neuropsychological rehabilitation programs. For example, the patient D.R. shows an interesting pattern of results that is frequently reported in the literature (see Table 12.1). Performance IQ scores improved from 5 months to 27 months postinjury. Verbal IQ remained the same and again supported the Bond (1975) data. The Wechsler Memory Quotient declined between 27 months postinjury and 42 months. Other measures of memory, such as the Rey Complex figure, show some modest improvement. There was

TABLE 12.1
Case D.R.

Age: 27
Educ: HS + 1 yr degree (Mortician)
Hand: Right
D.O.I. 7/23/83
DX: Traumatic Brain Injury
GCS: Not available, but LOC = 16 days
CT: L-side: hematomas on convexity, insula, & frontal lobe; R-side: deep hemorrhage in thalamic or subthalamic region.

Test	TIME OF FOLLOW-UP (5 mos) 12/27/83	(27 mos) 10/28/85	(42 mos) 02/09/87
WAIS-R:			
VIQ	95	97	92
PIQ	75	87	88
FSIQ	84	92	89
Information	7	9	8
Digit Span	12	12 (7/6)	9 (5/5)
Comprehension	11	—	—
Vocabulary	10	10	9
Arithmetic	6	7	8
Similarities	9	12	12
Picture Completion	6	11	11
Picture Arrangement	10	8	8
Block Design	7	7	7
Object Assembly	5	—	—
Digit Symbol	4	6	7
Wechsler Memory Scale:			
Memory Quotient	N/A*	100	86
Logical Mem. (immed/delay)	N/A*	11/8	9/3
Visual Rep. (immed/delay)	N/A*	9/9	9/9
Paired Assoc: Easy	N/A*	5-6-6	5-6-6
		1-4-2	0-1-1
Rey Complex Figure:			
Copy/Delay (30 min)	N/A*	20%/20%	30%/30%
Buschke Selective Reminding			
Trial 1/Trial 12	7/5	—	8/7
Test Behavior:	LVF Neglect	LVF Neglect (Occasional)	(LVF Neglect NOT noted)

N/A* = Not Administered. *Note.* D.O.I. = date of injury; DX = diagnosis; GCS = Glasgow Coma Score; LVF = left visual field.

no substantial improvement on other measures of memory such as the Buschke Selective Reminding Test (see Lezak, 1983, for a description of these tests). These data emphasize that the recovery course is indeed variable and that memory functions in particular may show different patterns in rate and level of recovery.

While personality problems are exceedingly complex and their recovery course is not well understood, the reports in the literature do suggest that some personality difficulties improve with time, while others deteriorate. In a rare long-term follow-up study, Thomsen (1984) reported on patients' personal adjustment 10 to 15 years posttrauma. She reported that the problem of childishness actually declined as reported by relatives of these patients several years posttrauma. However, sensitivity to distress and loss of interest in environment may actually increase (see Table 12.2).

Levin (1985) has recently summarized many aspects of neurobehavioral recovery after traumatic brain injury. Yet, as his paper illustrates, there are many notable gaps in our understanding about the return of higher cerebral functions after traumatic brain injuries. Patients generally improve, but the course is variable and some patients actually show deterioration of performance on some abilities with the passage of time.

PRESENT-DAY COGNITIVE REMEDIATION ACTIVITIES AND GUIDELINES

What are the present approaches to cognitive remediation, do they make sense, and what is their efficacy? Diller and Weinberg's (1986) early reports on training right hemisphere cerebral vascular accident (CVA) patients to pay attention to the left side of space were the first and best studies on how to use specific training procedures to facilitate adaptation following a sensory/perceptual deficit (see Diller & Weinberg, 1986, for review and references). Following this work, Ben-Yishay and Diller and their colleagues produced a number of monographs describing specific modular training procedures to deal with various cognitive/perceptual deficits (e.g., Working Approaches to Remediation of Cognitive Deficits in the Brain Damaged, Institute of Rehabilitative Medicine, New York University Medical Center, 1978). More recently, Ben-Yishay, Piasetsky, and Rattok (1987) reported on the effectiveness of what they termed the Orientation Remedial Module (ORM) for ameliorating deficits of basic attention. This training procedure, which was part of their intensive outpatient day program, was shown to improve test performance over time, and the effects were generally maintained 6 months

TABLE 12.2
Problems at First and Second Follow-up*

Problem	2 to 5 years	10 to 15 years
Poor Memory	80%	75%
Changes in personality and emotion	80%	65%
childishness	60%	25%
emotional lability	40%	35%
irritability	38%	48%
restlessness	25%	38%
disturbed behavior	23%	20%
Poor concentration	73%	53%
Slowness	65%	53%
Loss of social contact	60%	68%
Aspontaneity	43%	53%
Tiredness	28%	50%
Sensitivity distress	23%	68%
Lack of interest	20%	55%

*These data, taken from Thomsen's (1984) research, show how relatives' ratings of personality characteristics of brain injured patients changed from 2 to 5 years postinjury to 10 to 15 years postinjury. Percentages refer to percentage of frequency reported by relatives.

posttraining. The authors pointed out, however, that patients varied considerably as to the magnitude of functional change and its practical significance. Yet, their work suggests that brain injured patients can improve on tasks with practice. This observation has been noted by others (Miller, 1984). Moreover, as they improve there may be some modest effect on test scores and ability to adapt. Ben-Yishay and his colleagues (Ben-Yishay et al., 1985) and others (Prigatano and Others, 1986) suggested that such retraining activities helped the patients use *residual* cognitive/perceptual skills more efficiently rather than truly retraining lost functions. Ben-Yishay et al. (1985) summarized their findings and observations as follows:

> Based on the preliminary group analyses, we tentatively conclude that the improvements in the cognitive function are attributable mainly to a generalized improvement in the ability to maintain focused attention and an enhanced ability to process information more efficiently. The results strongly suggest that, in the main, gains achieved by the patients in the cognitive domain through their participation in a program of systematic remedial interventions represent an improvement in the effective functional application of residual cognitive skills, rather than an increase in the capacity levels of these underlying cognitive abilities per se. (pp. 257–258)

In addition to the work done on perceptual retraining and enhancing attentional skills, considerable work has been conducted on so-called memory retraining. Schacter and Glisky (1986) have recently reviewed the literature on memory remediation. Their conclusion is that memory is not like a muscle. More exercise does not necessarily improve its functional capacity or make it stronger. However, even patients with significant memory disturbance can be taught to learn or carry out complex tasks. Under the rubric of domain specific knowledge, Schacter and Glisky (1986) suggested that perhaps patients with memory disorder can be taught to use complex compensational devices (such as using and programming a microcomputer) to organize their day and carry out various tasks. Thus the earlier concept of Goldstein (1942) of learning to compensate for behavioral deficits continues to find support in modern research on memory remediation. In this regard, Wilson (1987) has recently provided a useful text to guide clinicians in managing memory problems of brain damaged patients. It should be clear that the emphasis is on management and effective use of residual skills versus a reversing of an underlying generic cognitive deficit (Ben-Yishay & Prigatano, in press).

Scholarly summaries and reviews of what might be called cognitive or neuropsychological aspects of rehabilitation have recently been provided by Newcombe (1985) and Miller (1984). These papers reinforce the idea that retraining or remediation seems to enhance the effective use of residual skills with the possibility of mild improvement in some impaired functions (like attention and speed of information processing).

Given these observations, what should actually be done in present-day cognitive retraining activities? It is noted elsewhere (Prigatano and Others, 1986) that the answer depends on many variables, including the severity of brain injury and resultant neuropsychological deficits, as well as the skill and theoretical orientation of the clinician or therapist. There are, however, ideas that have emerged from Luria's work (Luria, Naydin, Tsvetkova, & Vinarskava, 1969), Ben-Yishay and Diller's work (1983), and our own work (Prigatano and Others, 1986) suggesting some practical guidelines that might be used in many different settings of cognitive retraining. My own interpretations of previous contributions have led to the suggestion of some possible clinical guidelines for conducting cognitive retraining activities.

1. Never underestimate the severity of a cognitive deficit. Even so-called mild problems can greatly impact the day-to-day behavior of a patient. Frequently, psychological tests underestimate the actual severity of the problem.

2. Assume (until proven otherwise) that the patient does not fully recognize the severity or impact of a residual cognitive (or personality) deficit. This lack of awareness can be organically based even though denial of deficits and their severity can have a psychiatric basis.

3. Approach the patient on any cognitive retraining task with a spirit that you and he or she will learn together the nature of the problems. Retraining activities will also help clarify if treatment will improve the deficits, and, if not, both parties can brainstorm as to how to compensate for the deficits.

4. After the patient records and observes his or her own behavior, encourage and allow the patient to examine the therapist on the same task. Only by revealing his or her own strengths and weaknesses will the therapist establish the necessary working alliance with the patient to influence the patient's recognition and eventual acceptance of the neuropsychological situation.

5. Don't lecture the patient as to his or her deficits or need to compensate for them. Show the patient that compensation improves performance by carrying out the activity with the patient, who needs to recognize this with very little lecturing.

6. Carefully record training activities and measure behavioral outcome. This presents hard data that the patient and therapist can relate to and base their decisions on. Training materials have to be interesting and appropriate to the patient's background and interests. Here the microcomputer can be helpful. But remember, it is doubtful that the computer or program retrains anything. Such devices only provide interesting tasks and a way of measuring performance on those tasks.

7. Do not limit cognitive retraining activities to one-on-one tasks. The cognitive deficits must be worked with as they emerge in the interpersonal situation. If a patient, for example, has attentional problems or memory problems, the problems should not be worked with just individually. The problems should be worked with as they emerge in interpersonal interactions (as patients talk to one another; as they relate to family members, staff, etc.). Learning to compensate for the deficit means that one is able to compensate for it as it emerges in an interpersonal setting.

8. Remember, cognitive retraining will stimulate an affective reaction! Boredom and interest are the two most obvious responses. Also, the catastrophic reaction can be easily stimulated by cognitive retraining activities. Generally speaking, this should be avoided so that the patient can work on tasks that he or she can perform and only slowly and progressively be asked to do more difficult tasks. If the catastrophic reaction emerges, it is important

for the therapist to understand this reaction and to warn the patient ahead of time so that the problem can be addressed in other therapeutic hours (Prigatano & Klonoff, 1988).

9. Provide an abundance of practice. The patient needs a tremendous amount of practice, which should be done in as many settings as possible. This is obvious to any clinician and is what Luria et al. (1969) referred to as extended programming.

10. Work with the patient not only to remediate cognitive deficits, but also to alleviate personality problems. This is best accomplished within the context of holistic or milieu oriented neuropsychological rehabilitation programs, which are described below. Simple modular training seldom, if ever, accomplishes anything of major significance for the patient.

CLINICAL EXAMPLES OF EFFECTIVE AND INEFFECTIVE COGNITIVE RETRAINING ACTIVITIES

Elsewhere (Prigatano and Others, 1986), a detailed case example has been presented on how a modular approach to memory retraining was thought to initially help the patient. Later, the approach was discovered to have no practical impact. If anything, it gave the patient and the family a false sense of security about the nature of the deficits and their compensation. In that particular case, a man who had a lesion of the corpus callosum was trained on a series of visual imagery tasks in the hope that it would improve his verbal recall. It was demonstrated on psychometric testing that, in fact, paired associate learning was improved by this procedure. Several years later, the individual was able to use the visual imagery retraining to aid his recall of paired-associate words. In day-to-day activities, however, the individual was presented tasks that could not be easily recalled via visual imagery. It was naively thought that the patient would automatically use this procedure to help him in his day-to-day memory. Without having adequately considered the severity of the problem and the limits of the compensation, the patient was encouraged to carry out tasks that he was not able to do. Thus, the patient never became fully aware of his deficits, nor did he find ways to adequately compensate for them. This resulted in the patient taking on employment that he eventually found overwhelming. He ultimately contemplated suicide in later years because he simply could not cope with the problems that his earlier cognitive remediation was supposed to reduce. This lesson emphasized the importance of teaching the patient and the therapist to be realistic about the deficits, the limits of compensation, and having the therapist educate the patient and family as to what will be realistic life choices concerning work, school, and so forth.

While a milieu or holistic neuropsychological rehabilitation program is typically the treatment of choice, a modified version has been attempted for some patients due to financial reasons. Keeping in mind the principles or guidelines suggested above, some practical things can be done for patients in this area.

An example is that of a young man who had an oligodendroglioma (a tumor) surgically removed from the right frontal area (see Figure 12.2 for Magnetic Resonance Imaging [MRI] findings and Table 12.3 for neuropsychological findings). This patient had many classic frontal lobe signs. There was an element of adynamia (i.e., loss of drive and initiative). He would frequently sit home and do very lttle. His wife, prior to retraining, thought that this was just laziness on his part. He frequently had difficulty organizing his day and initiating actions in the appropriate manner. There were also predictable problems in his memory for important daily events (despite a memory quotient of 101).

After the initial neuropsychological evaluation, the patient was referred to a psychiatrist because of the nature of his insurance coverage. The patient and his wife felt that that form of treatment was not helpful and eventually terminated treatment. They went to their church to get financial support to return for neuropsychological help. Given the limited funds, it was decided the patient would be seen for 20 sessions and that an individualized program would be attempted. This resulted in providing relatively few hours of direct intervention. Attempts were made, however, to work together with the patient and his spouse and focus on practical methods of coping with the higher cerebral deficits. An educational model was followed. The therapist worked with the patient 2 hours per week, in the presence of his wife, for 2 months. Then they were scheduled for once a week until 20 sessions had been reached. In the context of that work, the patient and wife were given material to read about frontal lobe damage and the behavioral consequences. The patient was also placed on a daily schedule that he, his wife, and the therapist collaboratively constructed. The patient was given instructions in using a notebook and did a number of paper-and-pencil cognitive retraining activities at home. The activities included speed of information processing, attention to detail, and so forth.

Within the context of this work, the patient showed modest improvement in his cognitive deficits, but now had a plan of action with which he could compensate for his problems. The wife also became much more knowledgeable of the patient's difficulties and focused on more realistic goals. Recognizing this information, they also decided that it would be best to thoroughly brief his union supervisor as to the nature of his deficits before taking a job that he thought he might be able to handle.

In this context, cognitive retraining activity included a series of individual training hours to improve basic higher cerebral functions. But, more

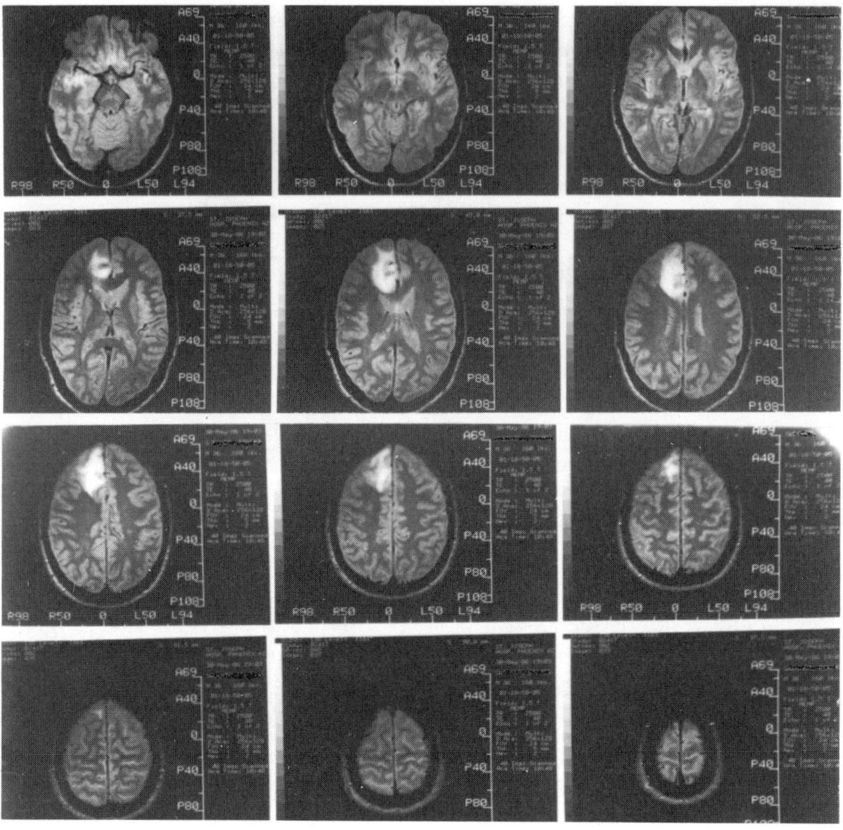

Figure 12.2. MRI scan of patient who had part of the right frontal region removed due to resection of oligodendroglioma. (Right side of brain is depicted on the left side of each scan.)

importantly, it was an educational experience for both the patient and spouse. A broad array of information was presented, explained, and gone over several times in order to ensure that the patient was more aware of the problems and understood the importance of compensation.

Also in this context, the therapist made a decided effort to establish a therapeutic alliance so that the patient would accept the various insights obtained through these interactions.[1]

[1] The author would like to recognize the efforts of Kevin O'Brien, PhD, a postdoctoral fellow at Barrow Neurological Institute, for his work with this patient and his wife.

THE HOLISTIC OR MILIEU ORIENTED NEUROLOGICAL REHABILITATION APPROACH

Ben-Yishay et al. (1985) and Prigatano and Others (1986) have written extensively about this approach. Basically, it incorporates cognitive retraining activities with psychotherapy activities within the context of a day treatment program. It is recognized that patients have both cognitive and personality difficulties that interact and that must be addressed in any educational experience or retraining. While some of the traumatic brain injured patients' problems look like learning disability problems, such patients also experience myriad cognitive and affective difficulties. This requires not only educational effort, but a therapeutic experience aimed at their psychiatric problems as well. Understanding patients' previous learning history, psychodynamics, and so forth, is necessary in order to effectively work with them. It requires, typically, psychologists, speech and language pathologists, occupational therapists, and physical therapists who are knowledgeable and sensitive to a variety of psychiatric as well as neurological factors. In most school settings, this is just not possible because of limitations of staff time and experience.

In working from a holistic model, it has become quite clear that a combination of cognitive retraining activities and psychotherapy activities must be utilized and that this eventually should include an actual vocational or work trial. Having patients working while they are undergoing rehabilitation provides the raw material by which they can now recognize how *generic cognitive and personality problems* impact on their ability to earn a living or go to school. With this type of information, patients can progressively be taught the nature of their problems and explore methods of compensating for them.

As recently described by Ben-Yishay and Prigatano (in press), there are at least six stages in this process. Figure 12.3 lists these stages. The holistic approach begins by encouraging the patient *to engage* in the rehabilitation activities. Many patients (and some learning disabled children) do not recognize the need to work on a problem. Once they are engaged in the activity, they begin to focus on progressive *awareness* of the problems. After that they are taught to *master* compensatory techniques for their cognitive deficits. As this is achieved they can learn to adequately *control* these compensatory activities in a more effective manner. From this emerges the possibility of *acceptance* of their deficits, which is never a purely cognitive act. From that finally emerges a new *identity*. Hopefully, the person can establish an identity characterized by dignity and enthusiasm for life. These six stages seem important in the overall restoration and adaptation to permanent traumatic brain injury.

TABLE 12.3
Case E.S.

Age:	36
Educ:	HS + 2 yrs college
Hand:	Right
D.O.I.	7/18/86
DX:	Partial right frontal lobectomy secondary to oligodendroglioma.
GCS:	N/A
MRI:	See Figure 12.2.

	TIME OF FOLLOW-UP
Aphasia Screening Test	**(4 mos)**
WAIS-R:	
FSIQ	111
VIQ	126
PIQ	92
Information	15
Digit Span	11 (7/6)
Vocabulary	13
Arithmetic	15
Similarities	15
Picture Completion	10
Picture Arrangement	7
Block Design	7
Digit Symbol	8
Wechsler Memory Scale:	
WMQ	101
Information	5/6
Orientation	5/5
Mental Control	8/9
Digits Total	13
Logical Mem.: Immed.	12+
Delayed	11
Visual Rep.: Immed.	8/14
Delayed	8/14
Assoc. Lrng.: Easy	5-6-6
Hard	4-4-4

TABLE 12.3 (cont.)

	Score	Impairment Rating
Halstead-Reitan Battery:		
Category Test	38 e-	1
Tactual Performance Test:		
Dominant Hand Time	7.1 min	1
Nondominant Hand Time	6.8 min	3
Both Hands Time	1.2 min	0
Memory (# correct)	7	1
Location (# correct)	4	2
Seashore Rhythm Test	2 e-	0
Speech Sounds Perception	0 e-	0
Finger Tapping:		
Dominant Hand	56	0
Nondominant Hand	50	0
Trails A	43 secs	2
Trails B	75 secs	1
Average Impairment Index		0.9
Wisconsin Card Sort	4 Categories	

Note. D.O.I. = date of injury; DX = diagnosis; GCS = Glasgow Coma Scale; MRI = Magnetic Resonance Imaging.

Present-day teaching methods are extremely important and useful in and of themselves. Ultimately, however, intervention directly into the nervous system will be necessary if brain damaged patients are to be helped in the most effective manner possible. Cotman and Nieto-Sampedro (1985) have recently summarized a series of interesting studies concerning the possible role of surgery for facilitating recovery after brain injury. They believe that the mature central nervous system may actually have some potential for recovery after injury if the temporal events in synaptogenesis (i.e., development of synapses) can be artificially induced, perhaps with neurotransplants. They suggest the following:

> Basic studies during the last quarter of the century on the response of the central nervous system (CNS) to injury have made it increasingly clear that, given the proper stimulus, most events necessary for the reconstruction of injured circuits in the CNS can take place in the mature adult. However, clinical evidence shows

IDENTITY

ACCEPTANCE

CONTROL

MASTERY

AWARENESS

ENGAGEMENT

Figure 12.3. Stages in neuropsychological rehabilitation. *Note.* From "Neuropsychologic Rehabilitation: Quest for a Holistic Approach" by Y. Ben-Yishay, J. Rattok, P. Lakin, E.B. Piasetsky, B. Ross, S. Silver, E. Zide, & O. Ezrachi, 1985, *Seminars in Neurology, 5*(3), 252–258. Reprinted by permission.

that most injuries to the mature CNS are not spontaneously repaired. Thus we are faced with a paradox of a CNS where individual molecular and cellular events leading to injury repair can take place, but where regeneration or repair of interrupted pathways nevertheless does not occur.

We believe that a key to this paradox is the lack of temporal organization of the events in adult synaptogenesis. Perhaps the most distinct feature of development is the strict temporal order of cellular and molecular events. The development of the nervous system depends on a complex series of steps, each of which must occur in the right place and at the right time. In our opinion, regeneration and reactive synaptogenesis, that is, synaptogenesis triggered by injury, could repair the damaged CNS in most cases if the various responses could take place in the proper ordered sequence, as they do in development. From this point of view, the role of the neurologist is to learn how to initiate and guide the steps of the repair process so as to allow each of them to occur at the appropriate moment. Interventive treatments need to be inserted into the natural repair

> process, completing it when natural repair is, as in the case of neuronal cell loss, clearly insufficient. (p. 83)

In addition to surgical intervention, the use of medications with brain injured patients is increasingly being considered to facilitate the activities associated with cognitive retraining.

PHARMACOLOGICAL INTERVENTION COUPLED WITH COGNITIVE RETRAINING

Before considering recent research on the use of physostigmine combined with memory retraining activities, it is important to reflect on the fact that recent studies have shown that some drugs may retard as well as potentially facilitate recovery phenomena. Porch, Wyckes, and Finney (1985) recently presented a stimulating paper suggesting that the administration of haloperidol may actually retard recovery from aphasia. The earlier work of Finney, Gonzalez, and Law (1982) emphasized that haloperidol slowed recovery from hemiplegia in the rat.

If medications can retard recovery, the opposite could well be true. Luria et al. (1969) suggested this concept, but until recently, no systematic studies have attempted to manipulate a pharmacological agent in conjunction with different forms of re-education or cognitive retraining to facilitate recovery of higher cerebral functions. A notable exception to this is the recent report by McLean, Stanton, Cardenas, and Bergerud (in press). McLean and his colleagues reported on the use of memory retraining combined with the use of oral physostigmine to aid memory in a young woman who had suffered carbon monoxide poisoning. While the problems of carbon monoxide poisoning are different from those of traumatic brain injury, there are nevertheless many areas of overlap, including significant memory problems. They used a double blind, single subject ABA design (A representing the baseline phase, B constituting the memory training combined with medication phase, and AA representing return to baseline condition). They reported, as others had, that immediate recall of a short story was only modestly affected by the combination of training and medication. However, medication substantially affected delayed recall in the positive direction. Their results will be published shortly and will highlight, perhaps for the first time, that *some* aspects of memory function can be substantially helped by the use of medications and memory retraining activities. As these types of findings begin to appear in the literature, hopefully group studies will clarify what aspects of training and medications produce the most notable positive effects. While the idea of combining cognitive retraining with medications has been around for many years (Luria suggested this as early as 1948, but his book was not published in English until

1963), McLean's study is perhaps one of the first to demonstrate how this can be done. The rationale for utilizing physostigmine to deal specifically with memory problems is based on the notion that this drug temporarily inhibits acetylcholinesterase, which is important for the establishment of memory traces.

Evans, Gualtieri, and Patterson (1987), utilizing only a psychostimulant (without cognitive retraining exercises), also reported improvement in attention and memory in a traumatic brain injured patient. This type of research should aid in expanding the utilization of various drugs with cognitive retraining activities to potentially increase their effectiveness.

SUMMARY AND CONCLUSIONS

The field of cognitive retraining is perhaps as variable and unpredictable as the behavioral recovery course following traumatic brain injury. While there have been no new scientific insights over the last few years that have substantially improved educational methods with brain injured patients, the fact that many of these young people survive and need to be reintegrated into as normal a life-style as possible has resulted in a proliferation of interest and techniques to retrain them. At the present time, the various techniques that are used under the label of cognitive retraining seem to have, at best, modest effects in improving cognitive functions (in some traumatic brain injured patients). As this article reviews, the most substantial improvement seems to take place when patients are able to use residual abilities to acquire new information. Frequently, patients require a combination of individual and group activities aimed at both cognitive and personality problems associated with traumatic brain injury. Within this context, a proportion of these individuals are able to improve their psychosocial adjustment. As described elsewhere (Ben-Yishay et al., 1985; Prigatano and Others, 1986), perhaps 50% of these individuals can substantially improve their quality of life given an intensive form of milieu or holistic oriented rehabilitation.

For the time being, however, researchers in the field must struggle with how the normal recovery process takes place and how various types of teaching and pharmacological agents can be applied to facilitate that process. In the long run, much of what is done in the name of treatment or rehabilitation is simply to facilitate the natural process of repair that the central nervous system may have within its potential. As John Hughlings Jackson suggested in 1878 and as Cotman and Nieto-Sampedro have stated in 1985, there may be a greater potential for recovery in higher brain functions after trauma than was previously recognized. It is hoped that within the next 10 years, methods of re-education or cognitive retraining will be substantially more effective than they have been in the last 10 years.

REFERENCES

Bach-y-Rita, P. (Ed). (1986). *Recovery of function: Theoretical considerations for brain injury rehabilitation*. Toronto: Hans Huber.

Basso, A., Capitani, E., & Vignolo, A. (1979). Influence of rehabilitation on language skills in aphasic patients. *Archives of Neurology, 36*, 190–196.

Ben-Yishay, Y., & Diller, L. (1983). Cognitive remediation. In E. Griffith & M. Rosenthal (Eds.), *Rehabilitation of the head injured adult*. Philadelphia: F.A. Davis.

Ben-Yishay, Y., Piasetsky, E.B., & Rattok, J. (1987). A systematic method for ameliorating disorders in basic attention. In M.J. Meier, A.L. Benton, & L. Diller (Eds.), *Neuropsychological rehabilitation* (pp. 165–181). London: Churchill Livingstone.

Ben-Yishay, Y., & Prigatano, G.P. (in press). Cognitive remediation. In E. Griffith & M. Rosenthal (Eds.), *Rehabilitation of the adult and child with traumatic brain injury*. Philadelphia: F.A. Davis.

Ben-Yishay, Y., Rattok, J., Lakin, P., Piasetsky, E.B., Ross, B., Silver, S., Zide, E., & Ezrachi, O. (1985). Neuropsychologic rehabilitation: Quest for a holistic approach. *Seminars in Neurology, 5*(3), 252–258.

Bond, M.R. (1975). Assessment of the psychosocial outcome after severe head injury. In Ciba Foundation Symposium, *Outcome of severe damage to the central nervous system* (pp. 141–157). New York: American Elsevier/Excerpta Medica/North-Holland.

Brooks, D.N. (1976). Wechsler memory scale performance and its relationship to brain damage after severe closed head injury. *Journal of Neurology, Neurosurgery, and Psychiatry, 39*, 593–601.

Brown, J.C. (1975). Late recovery from head injury: Case report and review. *Psychological Medicine, 5*, 239–248.

Chapman, L.F., & Wolff, H.G. (1959). The cerebral hemispheres and the highest integrative functions of man. *Archives of Neurology, 1*, 375–424.

Cotman, C.W.W., & Nieto-Sampedro, M. (1985). Progress in facilitating the recovery of function after central nervous system trauma. In F. Nottebohm (Ed.), *Hope for a new neurology. Annals of the New York Academy of Sciences*. New York: New York Academy of Sciences.

Diller, L., & Weinberg, J. (1986). Learning from failures in perceptual cognitive retraining in stroke. In. B.P. Uzzell & Y. Gross (Eds.), *Clinical neuropsychology of intervention* (pp. 283–293). Boston: Martinus Nijhoff.

Evans, R.W., Gualtieri, C.T., & Patterson, D. (1987). Treatment of chronic closed head injury with psychostimulant drugs: A controlled case study and appropriate evaluation procedure. *The Journal of Nervous and Mental Disease, 175*(2), 106–110.

Finney, D.M., Gonzalez, A., & Law, W.A. (1982). Amphetamine, haloperidol, and experience interact to affect rate of recovery after motor cortex injury. *Science, 217*, 855–857.

Goldstein, K. (1942). *Aftereffects of brain injury in war*. New York: Grune & Stratton.

Goldstein, F.C., & Levin, H.S. (1987). Disorders of reasoning and problem-solving ability. In M.J. Meier, A.L. Benton, & L. Diller (Eds.), *Neuropsychological rehabilitation* (pp. 327–354). New York: Churchill Livingstone.

Hagen, C. (1982). Language-cognitive disorganization following closed head injury: A conceptualization. In L.E. Trexler (Ed.), *Cognitive rehabilitation: Conceptualization and intervention* (pp. 131–172). New York: Plenum Press.

Jackson, J.H. (1898). Relation of different divisions of the central nervous system to one another and to parts of the body. *Lancet, 1*, 78–87.

Jennett, B., & Teasdale, G. (1981). *Management of head injuries*. Philadelphia: F.A. Davis.

Lashley, K.S. (1938). Factors limiting recovery after central nervous lesions. *The Journal of Nervous and Mental Diseases, 88*, 733–755.

Levin, H.S. (1985). Outcome after head injury: General considerations and neurobehavioral recovery, Part II: Neurobehavioral recovery. In D.P. Becker & J.T. Povlishock (Eds.), *Central nervous system trauma status report*, (17) (pp. 281–302). Washington, DC: National Institute of Health, National Institute of Neurological and Communicative Disorders and Stroke.

Levin, H.S., Benton, A.L., & Grossman, R.G. (1982). Neurobehavioral recovery. In D.P. Becker & J.T. Povlishock (Eds.), *Central nervous system trauma status report* (pp. 281–299). Washington, DC: Neurological and Communicative Disorders and Stroke.

Lezak, M.D. (1979). Recovery of memory and learning functions following traumatic brain injury. *Cortex, 15*, 63–72.

Lezak, M.D. (1983). *Neuropsychological assessment*. New York: Oxford University Press.

Luria, A.R. (1963). *Restoration of function after brain trauma*. London: Pergamon.

Luria, A.R., Naydin, V.L., Tsvetkova, L.W., & Vinarskava, E.N. (1969). Restoration of higher cortical function following local brain damage. In P.J. Vinken & G.W. Bruyn (Eds)., *Handbook of clinical neurology* (Vol. 3, pp. 368–433). New York: Elsevier-North Holland.

McLean, A., Stanton, K.M., Cardenas, D.D., & Bergerud, D.B. (in press). *Memory training combined with the use of oral physostigmine*.

Miller, E. (1984). *Recovery and management of neuropsychological impairments*. New York: Wiley.

Newcombe, F. (1985). Rehabilitation in clinical neurology: Neuropsychological aspects. In P.J. Vinken, G.W. Bruyn, H.L. Klawans, & J.A.M. Frederiks (Eds.), *Handbook of clinical neurology* (Vol. 46). New York: Elsevier-North Holland.

Porch, B., Wyckes, J., & Finney, D.M. (1985). *Haloperidol, thiazides and some antihypertensives slow recovery from aphasia*. Paper presented at Society for Neuroscience Meeting, Dallas.

Prigatano, G.P. (1986). Higher cerebral deficits: The history of methods and assessment and approaches to rehabilitation: Part 2. *BNI Quarterly, 2*(4), 9–17.

Prigatano, G.P. (1987). Neuropsychological deficits, personality variables and outcome. In M. Ylvisaker & M.R. Gobble (Eds.), *Community reentry for head injured adults*. San Diego: College-Hill.

Prigatano, G.P. (in press). Emotion and motivation in recovery and adaptation to brain damage. In S. Finger, T. LeVere, C.R. Almli, & E. Stein (Eds.), *Theoretical and controversial issues in recovery after brain damage*. New York: Plenum Press.

Prigatano, G.P., & Klonoff, P.S. (1988). Psychotherapy and neuropsychological assessment after brain injury. *Journal of Head Trauma Rehabilitation, 3*, 45–56.

Prigatano, G.P., Klonoff, P.S., & Bailey,

I. (1987). Psychosocial adjustment associated with traumatic brain injury: Statistics BNI neurorehabilitation must beat. *BNI Quarterly, 3*(1), 10–17.

Prigatano, G.P., & Others (1986). *Neuropsychological rehabilitation after brain injury.* Baltimore: Johns Hopkins University Press.

Schacter, D.L., & Crovitz, H.F. (1977). Memory function after closed head injury: A review of the quantitative research. *Cortex, 13,* 150–176.

Schacter, D.L., & Glisky, E.L. (1986). Memory remediation: Restoration, alleviation and the acquisition of domain-specific knowledge. In B.P. Uzzell & Y. Gross (Eds.), *Clinical neuropsychology of intervention* (pp. 257–282). Boston: Martinus Nijhoff.

Thomsen, I.V. (1984). Late outcome of very severe blunt head trauma: A 10–15 year second follow-up. *Journal of Neurology, Neurosurgery, and Psychiatry, 47*, 260–268.

Uzzell, B.P., Dolinskas, C.A., Wiser, R.F., & Langfitt, T.W. (1987). Influence of lesions detected by computed tomography on outcome and neuropsychological recovery after severe head injury. *Neurosurgery, 20*(3), 396–402.

Vignolo, L.A. (1964). Evolution of aphasia and language rehabilitation: A retrospective exploratory study. *Cortex, 1*, 344–367.

Von Zomeren, A.H., & Deelman, B.G. (1978). Long-term recovery of visual reaction time after closed head injury. *Journal of Neurology, Neurosurgery, and Psychiatry, 41*, 452–457.

Wilson, B. (1987). *Rehabilitation of memory.* New York: Guilford.

13

Effective Traumatic Brain Injury Rehabilitation: Team/Patient Interaction

GEORGE P. PRIGATANO

Rehabilitation, as a branch of medicine, focuses on the avoidance of physical complications (Stern, McDowell, Miller, et al., 1971) and *teaching* patients to understand and manage their disabilities in as normal an environment as possible (Diller, 1987). While neuropsychologically oriented rehabilitation may have a more direct impact on remediation of higher cerebral deficits in the future (Prigatano, 1986), at present it is confined to helping patients better understand their disabilities and enhancing psychosocial adjustment (Prigatano, 1987; Prigatano and Others, 1986; Prigatano & Klonoff, 1988). This is no small contribution in light of the fact that for many traumatic brain injured (TBI) patients, the "lack of understanding" may have an organic basis (Prigatano, in press), and if patients are not taught better psychosocial skills the long-term prognosis is indeed poor.

Teaching TBI patients about their disabilities and improving their psychosocial adjustment can be a demanding task that leaves many rehabilita-

---

This chapter is an expanded version of an article by Dr. Prigatano (1988) titled "Bringing It Up in Milieu: Toward Effective TBI Rehabilitation," originally published in the *Journal of Rehabilitation Psychology, 34*(2). Reprinted by permission.

tion therapists tired, frustrated, and eventually angry. Gans (1983) has written insightfully about this problem and has suggested one method for helping acute care rehabilitation team members improve their effectiveness with patients (Gans, 1987).

The purpose of this chapter is to describe another method to help rehabilitation team members improve their effectiveness in returning post-acute-TBI patients to work. The observations reported stem from the author's experience in developing two neuropsychologically oriented rehabilitation programs and consulting with five other programs over the last 8 years. During that time, it has become obvious that even technically competent therapists find it difficult to work with the psychosocial manifestations of cognitive and personality disorders in post-acute-TBI patients. Repeatedly, psychologists, physical therapists, speech and language therapists, occupational therapists, recreational therapists, nurses, social workers, and others become uncomfortable in dealing with these problems, which (if not managed) ultimately deprive the patient of a productive life-style.

Why is this? Like family members, therapists are often afraid that their attempts to confront brain injured patients with their inappropriate behavior will result only in the patient becoming more upset and in an erosion of an already tenuous working relationship. This belief is based on three major problems *within* the therapist:

1. At a conscious or unconscious level, the therapist "needs" the patient more than the patient perceives "needing" the therapist.
2. The therapist has not learned how to give negative feedback to patients in a supportive way that helps patients learn responsibility for their actions.
3. The therapist has not fully understood the nature of the cognitive and personality problems of a given patient. This can lead to an assumption that the patient could do better only if he or she "tried harder." This frequently leads to frustration in both the patient and the staff.

As a result of these three difficulties, many behavioral problems of TBI patients that typically alienate others are simply observed by the treatment team during the rehabilitation day with a feeling of frustration and ultimate despair. Often therapists will try to talk with patients privately, and this can help. Yet, if not corrected, the three problems listed above continue to exert their negative influence. With time, therapists can become defensive and even destructive in their reactions to patients. Cliques form between therapists, and they struggle to find emotional support from one another as patients' psychosocial manifestations of their cognitive and personality disorders remain unmanaged. "Turf" issues between disciplines and even within disciplines can be a manifestation of the anxiety and anger therapists feel when they are unable to deal effectively with these patients. Finally, the problem of professional "burnout" (see Maslach, 1982) emerges, and the inevitable consequences of depression, anger, and desire to leave the job setting take place.

To avoid these consequences, clinical directors of post-acute-rehabilitation programs for TBI patients need to educate staff members regarding cognitive and personality problems of these patients and teach staff to give feedback in a way that helps patients cope with the effects of brain injury. Choosing staff members who can do this work becomes especially important.

Elsewhere, the rationale of a milieu oriented neuropsychological rehabilitation program is described (Prigatano and Others, 1986). In the context of that program, at the end of the treatment day there is a milieu therapy time. This is officially a business meeting in which all therapists and all patients meet to discuss the day's events, provide positive feedback for successful accomplishments, and gently confront *any* behavior *of patient or staff* that interferes with the patient's progress toward independence and the capacity for work. Issues that arise in the daily staff meeting frequently deal with individual patient care. Yet, translation of these discussions into meaningful actions requires the staff to bring up issues in the milieu therapy time. This is not always an easy task because of the three major problems *within* the therapists that were pointed out earlier. To facilitate change, the education and psychological support of therapists becomes necessary. Table 13.1 lists the various treatment times, including milieu and staff meetings, that are a part of' the Work Re-entry Program at the Barrow Neurological Institute.

A BRIEF LOOK AT OUTCOME STATISTICS

To help therapists see the need to deviate from traditional forms of delivering rehabilitation services (in the multidisciplinary or even interdisciplinary treatment models), the sobering outcome statistics concerning TBI patients need to be reviewed. Two to 4 years postinjury, about one-third of severe traumatic brain injured patients return to work (Prigatano, Klonoff, & Bailey, 1987). The few long-term follow-up studies suggest that 10 to 15 years postinjury this figure may actually drop to less than 10% (Thomsen, 1984).

One major cause related to the inability to return to work may be that patients do not fully understand their higher cerebral deficits secondary to organic disturbances in self-awareness. The families also do not fully understand these difficulties and are frequently described as denying the patient's problems or at least minimizing their severity. Sadly, many therapists also do not fully understand the patient's problems and for various reasons allow patients and family to pursue courses of action that ultimately are not in the patient's best interest.

TABLE 13.1
Typical Weekly Work Re-entry Program

	Monday	Tuesday	Wednesday	Thursday	Friday
08:15–08:55	Cognitive retraining	Cognitive retraining	Cognitive retraining	Cognitive retraining	Work trial (optional)
09:00–09:40	Individual therapies	Individual therapies	Individual therapies	Individual therapies	
09:40–09:50	Break	Break	Break	Break	
09:50–10:25	Individual group	Individual group	Individual group	Individual group	
10:30–11:10	Cognitive group	Cognitive group	Cognitive group	Cognitive group	
11:15–11:45	Group psychotherapy	Group psychotherapy	Group psychotherapy	Group psychotherapy	
11:45–12:00	Milieu	Milieu	Milieu	Milieu	
12:00–01:00	Lunch	Lunch	Lunch	Lunch	
01:00–05:00	Work trial	Work trial	Work trial	Work trial	Work trial (optional)
01:45–02:45		Relatives' Group			
03:15–04:30	Staff meeting	Staff meeting	Staff meeting	Staff meeting	
05:00–06:00		Relatives' Group			

During the first week of the work trial, patients will work 2 hours per day, then move to 3 to 4 hours in Week Two, if they can handle it. By Week Three, the goal is to have the patients working 3 to 4 hours four days a week, depending on the needs of the work supervisor and needs of the patient.

(Generally, Months 3 through 6 will be designated for less supervised activities.)

Note. From "Rehabilitation Interventions After Traumatic Brain Injury" by G.P. Prigatano, 1988, *BNI Quarterly, 4* (2), pp. 30–37. Reprinted by permission of *BNI Quarterly*.

Patients can be extremely demanding, persistent, and unreasonable. Eventually they can wear down family members and staff. The end result is often that patients take jobs that they cannot handle. This results in failure and an eventual drop-out from the work environment. While cognitive problems seem to decrease with time, many personality problems do not (see Fordyce, Roueche, & Prigatano, 1983; Thomsen, 1984).

Oddy, Coughlan, Tyerman, and Jenkins's (1985) work in this regard is especially informative. They report that, 7 years post-TBI, 40% of family members say that the patient remains childish and refuses to admit to difficulties. Patients will not admit to difficulites without social pressure, neuropsychological intervention, and so forth. Consequently, the need for group and milieu oriented therapies is vital. A milieu treatment time is in essence a "mini" real life experience in the course of the treatment day. It helps the patient learn to deal with others in a socially appropriate manner. Therefore, it is a very important time in neuropsychological rehabilitation. An example is now given of how this treatment time should theoretically be used.

A CLINICAL VIGNETTE DESCRIBING THE USE OF MILIEU THERAPY TIME

A patient named Troy begins the treatment day with an explosive, angry outburst. He is upset with having to repeatedly start a treatment hour on time and is overwhelmed with his lack of improvement on a certain cognitive retraining task. The young, inexperienced therapist working with him is understandably frightened and embarrassed over Troy's outburst. How does he respond? One way is to say very little to him in an attempt to extinguish his rude and disruptive behavior. Another reaction is for the therapist to immediately stand up to him and become angry in return for Troy's inappropriate actions. The third option, which often occurs, is that the therapist may say very little but show a look of disdain and later complain to co-therapists about the patient's behavior. With this type of reaction, the therapist withdraws and may avoid talking to the patient at other times during the treatment day. During that same treatment day, the therapist may begin to fantasize about changing careers or at least changing jobs, hoping to find a less stressful set of patients and job responsibilities.

In the course of a milieu oriented neuropsychological rehabilitation program, this behavior would ideally be dealt with in the following manner. The therapist would briefly recognize Troy's being upset and would firmly but gently ask him to participate in the retraining task. If he cannot, he is asked to at least sit quietly while others work. The therapist would then say that whatever difficulties Troy is experiencing can be discussed more fully in group psychotherapy and milieu.

To simplify our case, let us assume that Troy argues that by the time group psychotherapy and milieu are held he will forget what he is angry about secondary to his memory difficulties. He therefore wants to discuss his problems now! The therapist assures Troy, in a nonthreatening manner, that he will remember to bring up the issue in milieu if he forgets. Assuming that Troy can then participate, the treatment day continues.

After the cognitive retraining hour, Troy is seen in other therapies including group psychotherapy. Troy may bring up what has happened during that time. Or, he may elect not to bring it up or even forget to bring it up as he had mentioned. In these latter cases, nothing is said during group psychotherapy on that particular day. However, following group psychotherapy the milieu time begins. Various nonemotionally threatened items are discussed among different therapists and patients in a businesslike manner. The moment of truth for Troy then arrives.

The scenario may begin something like this. The inexperienced therapist may start off with, "I know this is going to upset you, Troy, but..." and before he can finish Troy again explodes with an angry outburst, cursing at him, the rehabilitation program, and so forth. At this point, the clinical director intercedes. She says: "Troy, obviously you are upset by something. If you can find it within you to discuss this problem with us calmly today we will do so, but if not we can drop it and come back to it tomorrow." Assuming that Troy again explodes, the clinical director calmly but firmly takes control of the group, informing Troy that she understands that he is upset, and purposely states, "Let's leave the topic for today, but we will come back to it later." The clinical director then looks at others and asks, "Is there any other business?"

Assuming Troy is now quiet but the situation is tense, the milieu hour continues in an orderly and businesslike fashion. The clinical director shows by her behavior that someone is in control and the group can adequately function even though tension is high. The message is also quite clear that no one is going to force anyone to talk about painful issues before they are ready. It is further emphasized, however, that eventually the upsetting behavior will be discussed within the context of that treatment time. This conveys an extremely important message to the patient. Namely, eventually one will have to face the consequences of his or her behavior in a social way. The milieu treatment time ends and the remaining rehabilitation day continues.

The next day, during the milieu time, the clinical director comes back to Troy. This is usually done after other business is discussed. Troy may now be ready to discuss the topic, or he may again show that he is unwilling to do so. Again, the clinical director does not force the issue but reminds Troy that if it is not today it will be brought up again tomorrow or the next day, as the case may be. The lesson learned is that eventually Troy will have to be responsible for his actions, but the treatment team will not be punitive. The treatment team is there to teach Troy the impact of his actions on others and the ultimate responsibility he has for his actions. Eventually Troy will talk about his blow-up and the therapist will discuss his true reactions to him, but again in a therapeutic manner. For example, the therapist may eventually be able to discuss his feelings of embarrassment at being yelled at in the group. He may also be able to discuss his frustration at not seeing more improvement in Troy's cognitive functioning and his frank fear of him when he becomes upset and threatens violence.

If therapists can learn to do this, with a therapeutic (i.e., not punitive or permissive) attitude, then psychological growth occurs in both the patient and the therapist as they both begin to face reality. Getting therapists to do this, however, is difficult. Therapists (just like patients) may not be ready to face the realities of brain damage and their personal reactions to patients. However, by picking relatively stable therapists and educating them, progress can be made. The remainder of this chapter presents some of what post-acute-rehabilitation team members need to be taught about cognitive and personality problems of TBI patients. Also, ideas concerning choosing the staff for this work and discussing why certain staff "need" the patient more than the patient "needs" them are considered.

TEACHING STAFF ABOUT COGNITIVE AND PERSONALITY PROBLEMS

A common assumption by both experienced and inexperienced rehabilitation staff members is that they already know what the typical cognitive and behavioral problems of TBI patients are. What they want to learn is what to do about those problems. The first step in working with a TBI rehabilitation team is to show them, in a nonthreatening manner, that in fact little is known about the nature of such problems (see Prigatano, 1986; Prigatano and Others, 1986). However, it is clear that therapists working with TBI patients should have an understanding of three basic concepts: (a) the catastrophic reaction, (b) neuropsychological damage that may be worse than is apparent, and (c) disordered self-awareness by the patient.

The Catastrophic Reaction

One concept that is extremely important to teach the staff is that of the catastrophic reaction. Goldstein (1942, 1952) was the first to point out that when patients experience inability to solve a task that they could previously perform quite easily prior to brain injury, an intense state of anxiety can occur and patients may react in a "catastrophic" manner. Many angry outbursts are a form of the catastrophic reaction. When a patient becomes easily upset or difficult to manage, the staff must ask themselves: Are the tasks they are confronting a patient with too difficult for that patient at that time? Therapists frequently assume that a given task is relatively easy for the patient, but this may reflect a tendency to overestimate the patient's actual cognitive and personality resources. As the staff begins to understand the concept of the catastrophic reaction, they can modify their treatment interventions in a way that helps the patient find alternative routes to dealing with tasks that are overwhelming or too difficult. Even teaching patients the concept of the catastrophic reaction goes a long way in helping them with their behavioral reactions. But before this can be taught, the staff must fully understand it.

Going back to the example of Troy, if the therapist can understand that Troy's outburst may reflect his catastrophic reaction over lack of improvement on a cognitive task, the therapist does not take it personally. The therapist can now teach Troy something about his behavior in a truly therapeutic manner.

Extent of Neuropsychological Impairment

A second point that must be emphasized to rehabilitation team members is that the higher cerebral deficits of TBI patients may be more severe than what is frequently thought and are often worse than what the formal neuropsychological tests show (Prigatano, Pepping, & Klonoff, 1986). There are numerous instances in which well-trained therapists will expect patients to follow a home exercise program or to self-initiate therapeutic activities in the course of a treatment day, when in fact the patients' memory problems and disorders of planning and organization are too severe for them to do this. The unsophisticated therapist will often assume at this point that a patient is just unmotivated and thoughts of discharging the patient emerge. Recognition by the therapists that patients do not fully understand the nature of their difficulties and cannot pick and choose therapies because of that becomes extremely important. This is why these individuals are referred to as patients rather than clients: They have disturbances in higher cerebral functioning that require guidance from experienced individuals.

Disordered Self-Awareness

Related to this problem of underestimation of the severity of difficulties by therapists is the associated problem of disordered self-awareness by patients after brain injury. While the classic neurological literature describes phenomena such as anosognosia (see Weinstein & Kahn, 1955), more recently there has been an appreciation that after significant brain injury prolonged and even permanent alteration in the capacity of individuals to perceive themselves in an objective manner can exist. As a consequence, many therapists do not fully understand disorders of self-awareness and oftentimes take a patient's behavior at face value. As we learn more about disorders of self-awareness (see Prigatano, in press), it becomes clear that these problems must actively be addressed in the context of neuropsychologically oriented rehabilitation. In fact, one of the most important contributions of this type of rehabilitation is to progressively help patients become aware of their residual strengths and weaknesses and help them learn to adjust to those realities as best as possible. As illustrated in Figure 12.3, once patients are engaged in a treatment program, the next major step is to help them become more aware of what their higher cerebral strengths and limitations are. From this, they are taught mastery and control of residual capacities. It is hoped that individuals can then learn to accept these realities and to form a new identity as brain injured patients who still have dignity and something to contribute to society (see Ben-Yishay and Prigatano, in press).

Besides helping therapists understand these three basic points (the concept of the catastrophic reaction, the notion that the degree of neuropsychological impairment may be worse than is obvious, and the importance of disordered self-awareness for rehabilitation), the treatment team must actually be taught a model that helps the staff give feedback to patients in a therapeutic manner. What specific techniques or guidelines can be used to help therapists provide positive and negative feedback in the milieu treatment time?

TEACHING STAFF TO GIVE FEEDBACK IN MILIEU

Five points have proven to be helpful in regard to teaching staff to give feedback in the milieu therapy situation. The first is to help the staff release intense negative feelings during the staff meeting before giving feedback to patients. Staff can become quite upset with a given patient. If they are to give useful feedback, they often need to first have a cathartic experience with fellow staff members. This is one major advantage to daily staff meetings. Second, staff need to listen to the intensity of a given therapist's reaction and provide support and guidance as to how feedback might be given. In the case of Troy, the staff can listen to a given therapist's personal reaction to Troy's apparently insulting comments and support the therapist with the notion that they too would be insulted given what Troy had said. After discussing Troy's premorbid personality characteristics, his reactions to brain injury, and his present neuropsychological deficits, the staff can help the therapist decide on how to therapeutically confront Troy. The use of the so-called "sandwich" technique is very helpful in this regard (point number three) (the author wants to recognize Yeduha Ben-Yishay for teaching him this method). With the "sandwich technique," the therapist begins by making a complimentary statement to the patient, then states whatever negative feedback has to be given, and ends up with thanking the patient for listening to such information.

For example, in the case of Troy, instead of starting off with the statement that the feedback that is about to be delivered is going to be upsetting to him, the therapist might take this approach. The therapist states that he would like to give some feedback to the patient. But before doing so, he emphasizes how much he appreciates Troy's attempt to work at "difficult and at times boring tasks." The therapist states that the feedback may be a little painful to hear, and it is not intended to hurt but rather to help. The therapist then states in a calm, nonthreatening way that Troy had a difficult time in the morning and became angry when it was pointed out to him that he was late for a given treatment hour. The therapist inquires as to Troy's perspective as well as other community members' perceptions. After the discussion, the therapist states appreciation for Troy's willingness to listen to this feedback and compliments Troy for having the courage to listen to negative feedback in the group setting. During this time, the community of patients and staff may suggest a plan for helping Troy, or a plan will be developed in other treatment times. This is the fourth point—not letting issues drop but seeking, when necessary, a community-based plan to help the patient.

The sandwich technique comes in many different forms, as do regular sandwiches, but its basic concept is extremely important for staff to learn. If the bread is too sweet or sour, the patient will spit it out. It has to be of such a flavor that the negative message can be heard, and this is the key that therapists must continually search for.

Learning the sandwich technique requires support from senior clinicians, and many times inexperienced therapists can simply learn to model what experienced clinicians say in the milieu therapy time. In this regard, a fifth and final point is important. The staff must make a conscious effort to ensure the accuracy of their feedback to patients and take a hard look at when they are trying to be punitive versus therapeutic. The capacity to do this relates directly to the staff understanding themselves and understanding what pressures might lead them to need the patient more than the patient needs them.

WHY DOES THE STAFF NEED THE PATIENT MORE THAN THE PATIENT NEEDS THE STAFF?

As indicated above, after severe TBI patients often do not fully understand the extent or the severity of their higher cerebral deficits. Consequently, they may not see the need for therapy and be very blunt about that. Therapists can become disarmed by this, because many of their therapies are predicated on the notion that the patient wants to learn and they do not know how to motivate a patient given this stance. An approach to this problem is considered elsewhere (see Prigatano and Others, 1986). It would be beyond the scope of this paper to describe this approach in detail, but suffice it to say that there are ways of getting patients involved in rehabilitation activities provided the therapist is willing to take a novel approach. Beyond teaching techniques for working with unaware or unmotivated patients, important influences can result in the staff "needing" the patient.

The first and the most obvious influences are the financial pressures placed on therapists to generate income. If therapists are in private practice, it is obvious that they need to keep their caseload up in order to meet the economic realities of life. If they are salaried by an institution, they are frequently reminded of the need to spend a predetermined number of hours in direct patient contact to justify their position. In this regard, it is extremely important that therapists in private practice as well as institutions set realistic economic goals if they are going to work with this population. If the overhead is too high or if the profits expected are too great, there will be an inordinate amount of pressure to force the patient to enter therapy and even stay in therapy without adequate sensitivity to what the patient's actual needs are.

Beyond these financial pressures, there are internal, personal pressures on therapists. One pressure has to do with therapists' need to prove their professional competency and their place on a treatment team. Be they psychologists, speech and language therapists, occupational therapists, and so forth, individual therapists are often aware that their professional services only partially meet the patient's needs. Yet, they charge a fair amount of money for their services and they want to feel that they are not exploiting the patient. Consequently, there is a strong desire to convince the patient that the services rendered are needed and will be helpful if the patient is motivated to learn. As therapists develop in their sophistication, they recognize that their services are indeed valuable but limited. To coerce the patient to behave in a certain way in order to feel professionally competent is always a mistake. Many competent therapists continually re-evaluate traditional ways of treating patients and alter therapy if their services are in fact going to be useful to a given patient. Clinical research to measure the efficacy of all forms of therapy (psychotherapy, cognitive retraining, physical therapy, speech and language therapy, etc.) is quite important and necessary for *staff* development (see

Prigatano and Others, 1986). Without such research, therapists will always have a "professional inferiority complex" and, in fact, may deserve it if they cannot demonstrate that their therapies are helping patients adapt and are cost effective.

A third point that can be painful to discuss is that many therapists who enter this field have a very strong need for admiration and love. Part of their desire to become clinicians is to treat and cure. Why does one get involved in needing to treat and cure? In our society, doctors, therapists, and various clinicians often receive the same admiration, love, and respect that the early priests and witch doctors had in primitive tribes. Therapists may choose this type of work, therefore, in hopes that they too will have a special place in society. If they feel that their work is ineffective, they often will move to other positions or blame the patient for failing to get better.

Related to this need for admiration and love are other psychological difficulties that therapists experience. Certain "patient problems" may reflect to some degree unresolved psychological problems within a given staff member. For example, some TBI patients are sociopathic and manipulative. Staff members can have milder versions of these same problems and consequently be attracted or repulsed by certain patients. Often, there is the unconscious hope that if the patient is "cured," therapists may cure the same problems in themselves. Other staff members may feel depressed or angry and hope that they can teach patients to cope better with these problems. The list goes on and on, but the basic point is that therapists bring to the treatment setting a host of psychological strengths and weaknesses that are going to be mirrored to some degree in the patient's behavior. If they can understand their own strengths and weaknesses, then they do not get into situations of having to force patients to get better in areas that the staff themselves have trouble with.

SELECTING THE TREATMENT STAFF

Given what has been said above, one might erroneously assume that the only effective rehabilitation staff for post-acute-TBI patients are fully trained, totally psychologically intact or developed individuals who are close to being independently wealthy or have a benevolent organization that is not going to put pressure on them to make a profit. If that were the case, we would have no rehabilitation programs in the United States or other countries for that matter. What has been described are issues or themes that need to be understood in order for the staff to effectively improve their working relationships with TBI patients. What ingredients should be attended to when choosing staff to do this work?

It may be obvious, but the first variable is intelligence. The staff has to be reasonably bright for them to learn how to work with these patients. However, intelligence in and of itself is not enough. The staff must be energetic over their efforts and truly have a desire to help the patient without it reaching pathological proportions. That is, they must have an energy and a creativity without feeling overwhelmed if the patient does not get better in all the ways they would like to see. The degree of professional competency that individual therapists have obtained as well as the degree of interpersonal stability in their lives are important to observe. While some very competent people have not achieved professional credentials (and our treatment team has one), it is important to look closely at the professional credentials of the various team members. Often, people with limited training are picked for positions because their salary level will be lower than individuals who have more extensive training. This is clearly a mistake.

Interpersonal stability in the therapist's life is also necessary. Looking at whether or not individuals have been able to make commitments in their own interpersonal lives to a spouse, children, and so forth, is quite important. If a therapist is not able to sustain interpersonal relationships and resolve conflicts in those relationships, the odds of them doing that in a treatment environment are very small indeed. Therapists who have multiple marriages, who have trouble dealing with children, or who hop from one job to the next within a very short period of time most likely are not the appropriate people for doing this work.

Finally, a fourth criterion is considered when selecting staff. Staff who are interested in broader rehabilitation issues than what their own discipline addresses are the best therapists for this type of work. For example, it is quite important to have a physical therapist who is interested in the problems of spasticity, balance, ambulation, and so on. Yet, that therapist must also be interested in the broader question of how his or her contribution to the patient ultimately impacts on the patient's capacity to be independent in the home, return to a productive life-style, and not require extensive further rehabilitative treatment (see Prigatano, 1988).

If therapists can take this stance, they often can participate very well in a treatment team approach and take an honest look at what they have to offer a given patient and a given team. Once such a team is established, it is truly a delight and one of the major reinforcers for continuing to work in this difficult area.

SUMMARY AND CONCLUSIONS

A psychologically healthy (but not perfect) rehabilitation staff can face adversity among themselves and with the patients they treat in interpersonal settings. The treatment team needs to consist of intelligent individuals who are capable of discussing their own feelings, particularly anxiety and depression as it relates to patient issues. If they can do this, the milieu treatment hour becomes a very useful vehicle for helping patients learn to cope with their behavioral problems in the real world. As therapists better conceptualize the cognitive and personality problems of these patients, they can learn to confront the patients in a therapeutic way, not in a permissive or punitive manner. Within this context, patients and staff learn to interact in a more harmonious manner like any effective social group unit.

As administrators and medical and clinical directors understand these principles, realistic rehabilitation goals are set for patients, and both the patient and institution substantially benefit. The old model of multidisciplinary versus interdisciplinary treatment approaches was simply the precursor for what might broadly be called the milieu approach to neurological rehabilitation. The therapeutic milieu allows the patient to again be a part of a group that has both brain-injured and non-brain-injured members. The degree to which patients can utilize the milieu treatment time is often the best predictor of their ability to find productivity and meaning when eventually discharged.

REFERENCES

Ben-Yishay, Y., & Prigatano, G.P. (in press). Cognitive remediation. In E. Griffith & M. Rosenthal (Eds.), *Rehabilitation of the adult and child with traumatic brain injury.* Philadelphia: F.A. Davis.

Diller, L. (1987). Neuropsychological rehabilitation. In M.J. Meier, A.L. Benton, & L. Diller (Eds.), *Neuropsychological rehabilitation* (pp. 3–17). New York: Guilford.

Fordyce, D.J., Roueche, J.R., & Prigatano, G.P. (1983). Enhanced emotional reactions in chronic head trauma patients. *Journal of Neurology, Neurosurgery, and Psychiatry, 46*, 620–624.

Gans, J.S. (1983). Hate in the rehabilitation setting. *Archives of Physical Medicine and Rehabilitation, 64*, 176–179.

Gans, J.S. (1987). Facilitation staff/patient interaction in rehabilitation. In B. Caplan (Ed.), *Rehabilitation psychology desk reference* (pp. 185–218). Aspen.

Goldstein, K. (1942). *Aftereffects of brain injury in war.* New York: Grune & Stratton.

Goldstein, K. (1952). The effect of brain damage on the personality. *Psychiatry, 15*, 245–260.

Maslach, C. (1982). *Burnout—The cost of caring.* New York: Prentice-Hall.

Oddy, M., Coughlan, T., Tyerman, A., & Jenkins, D. (1985). Social adjustment after closed head injury: A further follow-up seven years after injury. *Journal of Neurology, Neurosurgery, and Psychiatry, 48*, 564–568.

Prigatano, G.P. (1986). Higher cerebral deficits: History of methods of assessment and approaches to rehabilitation: Part II. *BNI Quarterly, 2(4)*, 9–17.

Prigatano, G.P. (1987). Recovery and

cognitive retraining after craniocerebral trauma. *Journal of Learning Disabilities, 20(10)*, 603–613.

Prigatano, G.P. (1988). Rehabilitation interventions after traumatic brain injury. *BNI Quarterly, 4(2)*, 30–37.

Prigatano, G.P. (in press). Anosognosia, delusions, and altered self awareness after brain injury. *BNI Quarterly.*

Prigatano, G.P., and Others. (1986). *Neuropsychological rehabilitation after brain injury.* Baltimore: Johns Hopkins University Press.

Prigatano, G.P., & Klonoff, P.S. (1988). Psychotherapy and neuropsychological assessment after brain injury. *Journal of Head Trauma Rehabilitation, 3(1)*, 45–56.

Prigatano, G.P., Klonoff, P.S., & Bailey, I. (1987). Psychosocial adjustment associated with traumatic brain injury: Statistics BNI neurorehabilitation must beat. *BNI Quarterly, 3(1)*, 10–21.

Prigatano, G.P., Pepping, M., & Klonoff, P. (1986). Cognitive, personality, and psychosocial factors in the neuropsychological assessment of brain-injured patients. In B.P. Uzzell & Y. Gross (Eds.), *Clinical neuropsychology of intervention* (pp. 135–166). Boston: Martinus Nijhoff.

Stern, P.H., McDowell, F., Miller, J.M., et al. (1971). Factors influencing stroke rehabilitation. *Stroke, 2*, 213–218.

Thomsen, I.V. (1984). Late outcome of very severe blunt head trauma: A 10–15 year second follow-up. *Journal of Neurology, Neurosurgery, and Psychiatry, 47*, 260–268.

Weinstein, E.A., & Kahn, R.L. (1955). *Denial of illness.* Springfield, IL: Charles C. Thomas.

14

Psychotherapy and Neuropsychological Assessment After Brain Injury

GEORGE P. PRIGATANO

PAMELA S. KLONOFF

The assessment of brain-behavior relationships is, of course, the core of both experimental and clinical neuropsychology. The use of this information for diagnostic purposes, medicolegal reasons, patient management, and research has been the traditional focus. Progressively, however, the application of neuropsychological test findings to a broader array of problems has occurred. Is the patient capable of returning to work? What school placement should be attempted? Can the patient safely operate a motor vehicle? Can he or she be left alone in the home, or is supervisory care required? These are the real-life questions clinical neuropsychologists are being asked daily, particularly in rehabilitation settings. To this list can be added still another question: Can anything be done to help the patient and family understand the effects of brain damage and to adjust better to these problems? The role of neuropsychological assessment is clearly expanding, and the use of the

---

Adapted from the *Journal of Head Trauma Rehabilitation*, Vol. 3, No. 1, pp. 45–56, with permission of Aspen Publishers, Inc., ©March 1988.

information it obtains is being applied more and more to patient management and care issues. This chapter focuses on neuropsychological assessment as it relates to psychotherapeutic activities with brain damaged patients.

NEUROPSYCHOLOGICAL ASSESSMENT

Disorders of brain function are known to produce fairly predictable neuropsychological symptoms and syndromes (Frederiks, 1985; Heilman & Valenstein, 1979; Luria, 1966). Methods of assessing disorders of higher cerebral functioning are expanding (Lezak, 1983), and the effects of various neurological and nonneurological factors on the total clinical picture (Lishman, 1978) and neuropsychological test findings in particular (Parsons & Prigatano, 1978) are becoming better appreciated. While the primary focus of the neuropsychological examination has traditionally (and rightfully) been the assessment of the nature and severity of higher cerebral dysfunctions (Prigatano, 1986), more is needed in a contemporary neuropsychological examination.

Three interrelated diagnostic questions face the clinical neuropsychologist who is asked to evaluate traumatically brain injured adults (Prigatano, Pepping, & Klonoff, 1986):

1. What is the nature and severity of higher cerebral dysfunction?
2. What is the patient's personal reaction to these deficits?
3. What is the the cumulative effect of these two dimensions on interpersonal or psychosocial adjustment?

These questions require that the clinical neuropsychologist not only consider how specific cognitive, motor, linguistic, or affective deficits emerge following a brain injury but also how these deficits impact the patient's retained cognitive and personality resources. The questions also require that clinicians concern themselves with how neuropsychological test findings (quantitative and qualitative features) relate to practical adjustment issues as they emerge in the hospital, at home, and in the work setting. Traditionally, neuropsychological assessment was done essentially to expand the neurological examination findings (Prigatano, 1986). As neuropsychology has been applied increasingly to the rehabilitation phase of medicine, as opposed to its diagnostic role, the need to expand the scope of the questions that the neuropsychological examination addresses has become obvious.

Some may argue that neuropsychological test findings are not intended for this latter purpose and that is unfair and professionally dangerous to extrapolate as to the psychosocial and psychiatric consequences of disorders of higher cerebral functioning. It is true that many of the tests that are used by neuropsychologists were not developed for the purpose of assessing overall psychosocial adjustment or personal reaction to deficits. However, as more neurological patients survive the life-threatening aspects of their illness, the impact of their brain-behavior disorders on practical aspects of life require and deserve extensive attention. Such attention is no less important *for the neuropsychologist* than is a careful neurolinguistic analysis of the impact of a lesion in the left inferior gyrus of the frontal lobe. Moreover, it is the authors' position that it is precisely the responsibility of the clinical neuropsychologist to attempt this evaluation and to meaningfully contribute to rehabilitation efforts of brain dysfunctional patients.

Neuropsychologically oriented rehabilitation after brain injury includes efforts at cognitive retraining and psychotherapy (Prigatano and Others, 1986). Currently, formal neuropsychological test findings only moderately contribute to these two ventures because the extent and nature of neuropsychological consequences of brain injury need to be assessed not only in a standardized testing situation but also as they emerge in unstandardized, unstructured events of life. Psychological tests often underestimate the impact of a neuropsychologic deficit on day-to-day functioning (Prigatano and Others, 1986). It is primarily in the unstructured, unpredictable events of life that the effects of brain injury reveal themselves in their most florid, albeit less controlled, manner. To effectively use information concerning neuropsychological deficits and strengths to guide cognitive remediation and psychotherapy, it is necessary to appreciate a patient's behavior on formal testing and as it emerges in various life situations. While careful psychometric assessment of brain injured patients is always necessary, it may not be sufficient when attempting to plan rehabilitation activities. Recently Diller (1987) has compared the philosophies of neuropsychology and rehabilitation and has pointed out that the language of neuropsychology has primarily been based on the neurosciences and has focused on deficits of brain function. The language of rehabilitation, however, has emphasized an educational model and the need to manage the patient given diverse sets of information.

The works of Luria (1966) and Luria, Naydin, Tsvetkova, et al. (1969) often are cited as the models by which neuropsychological test findings are directly applied to the re-educational process of brain dysfunctional patients. While Luria has certainly described many important ingredients in approaching higher cerebral deficits from a rehabilitation point of view, his principles of restoration of higher cerebral functioning require a great deal of experience on the part of the clinician to be put into practice. His concept that one should have a thorough psychological analysis of cognitive, perceptual, motor, and linguistic deficits before planning remediation activities is the ideal example. Accomplishing such an analysis in everyday life is often quite difficult because how the brain codes information and how higher cerebral deficits actually emerge are still not well understood. To date, the best that can be done is to use models of cognitive structures to guide testing and to "patch together" some rudimentary ideas concerning the nature of the deficit and the point at which the rehabilitation process might be initiated. Frequently it is said, for example, that there is a deficit in verbal memory versus nonverbal memory. Often the severity of the deficit is rated as mild, moderate, or severe. Yet what does a mild or even moderate verbal learning and memory problem mean for a given patient? It certainly could be quite varied depending on the patient's life circumstances, premorbid characteristics, and tasks that are presented to him or her. For some patients a "mild" memory deficit may be devastating in light of their chosen work.

These statements are made, not to discourage the notion that careful neuropsychological assessment should be attempted in every patient, but only to emphasize the reality that even with the most careful assessment clinicians still do not know how to proceed in remediation activities (be it under the rubric of cognitive retraining or psychotherapy). Given this, what neuropsychological test findings seem to be helpful to the clinician who attempts psychotherapy with brain injured people?

DEFINING PSYCHOTHERAPY BEFORE AND AFTER BRAIN DAMAGE

There is nothing magical about psychotherapy, and the more it is mystified or made to seem mysterious the less likely it will help anyone—brain injured or not. For people who typically have a medical diagnosis, psychotherapy is an educational process. The educational process is geared to teaching the patient (brain injured or not) as much as possible about the nature of his or her behavioral or personality disorder. It is hoped that this educational process allows the patient to cope with life's problems better than he or she would have been able to without this process. It is obvious from this definition that assessing the efficacy of psychotherapy has many inherent methodological problems. Nevertheless people have a variety of difficulties in coping with life's frustrations, and they seek helpers to aid them in this process.

While the ingredients and elements of psychotherapy after brain injury are discussed in more detail elsewhere (Prigatano and Others, 1986), a few comments will be made concerning the psychotherapeutic process and what it attempts to address.

Psychotherapy is really a process by which an individual learns to behave in his or her own best self-interest. This clearly does not mean selfish interest. It means teaching the patient to better understand who he or she is, what his or her basic needs are in life, and how best to get those needs met. The understanding of the nature of the needs will change as the patient and therapist get to know themselves and one another better. Helping the patient to address practically areas of conflict or maladjustment is the goal. In this process the clinician frequently has to define the major life problems that patients experience, particularly those after brain injury.

In this regard Freud has clearly led the way. On stepping off a train in London, Freud purportedly was asked, "What does it mean to be psychologically healthy?" Despite his numerous technical papers, Freud supplied an answer that seems to have withstood the test of time. In very simple terms he stated that there are two major ingredients to psychological health: the capacity to work and to love. If one can do both of these things, one in essence has achieved about as much psychological normality as his or her fellow human. But what are the ingredients of working and loving? Certainly they are complicated phenomena, and there are no simple answers. From clinical interaction with brain injured patients, the authors have developed certain ideas concerning the nature of work that can be indirectly addressed by the neuropsychological examination. Also recent theoretical ideas by Sternberg (1986) on the nature of love add a great deal to our understanding of what practical things to look for in the neuropsychological assessment of brain injured patients that bear on the dimension of love.

IF LOVE IS A TRIANGLE, WORK IS A SQUARE

In the clinical neuropsychological rehabilitation of young adult, traumatically brain injured patients, four dimensions seem important for work (Figure 14.1a). In describing the ingredients of "love," Sternberg (1986) has suggested three dimensions, or a so-called triangular theory of love (Figure 14.1b).

Work involves, at a minimum, an attitude of cooperation, a capacity to be reliable or responsible, and a capacity to do the job efficiently and effectively. In neuropsychological assessment the degree of cooperation is assessed by *how* the patient engages easy and demanding tasks. Does the patient get overwhelmed and give up? Does the patient show an honest effort while working on psychometric tasks? Does the patient become easily irritated or angry if asked to do something that he or she does not wish to do? Moreover, does the patient's history suggest an individual who has been able to get along with others and to work in a reasonably calm manner despite differences of opinion with coworkers? Based on the history, observations of the patient during testing, and rehabilitation activities, what seem to be the relevant reinforcers for achieving a cooperative attitude in a given patient?

Reliability is assessed by the history and neuropsychological assessment of memory and judgment. Patients who have never been reliable (i.e., who were unable to commit to doing what they had said or promised prior to their accident) typically have major problems with reliability after brain injury.

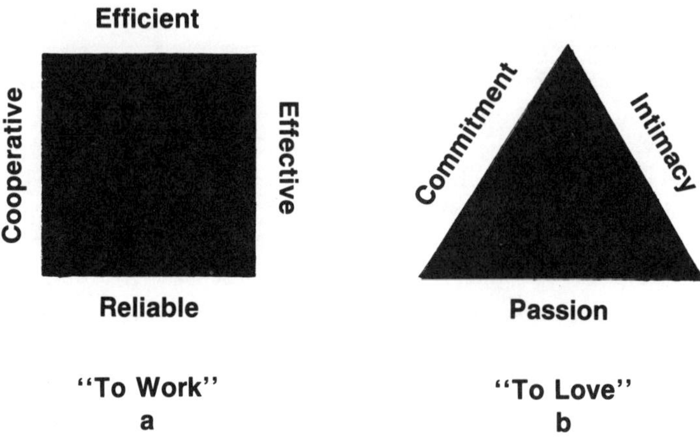

Figure 14.1. The "ingredients" of work for brain-injured patients **(a)**, and the "ingredients" of love according to Sternberg (1986) **(b).** Both dimensions need to be indirectly or directly evaluated by neuropsychological observation and testing.

Patients who have severe memory or amnesic problems will simply be unable to follow through on obligations despite their best intentions. Patients who do not understand the complexity of what they agree to do will also prove to be unreliable in certain jobs. In the authors' own clinical work a Wechsler Memory Quotient below 80 seriously raises the question of whether or not the individual is going to be reliable without a great deal of environmental structure and support. If the patients do poorly on such tests as the Picture Arrangement subtest of the Wechsler Adult Intelligence Scale–Revised (WAIS-R) (e.g., scale score of 6 or below) or the Wisconson Card-Sorting Test (e.g., do not achieve 6 categories), concerns are raised about their judgment, their ability to learn from mistakes, and their capacity to be reliable.

Efficiency and effectiveness are greatly influenced by the structure of intellect, the capacity to remember, the speed of information processing, and the presence of significant motor, psychomotor, and linguistic difficulties. It would be difficult, if not impossible, to list every type of deficit that impinges on these two dimensions. Nevertheless, in the clinical assessment it is necessary to figure out the important dimensions for predicting effectiveness and efficiency for a given patient looking at a given job.

In this regard it may be useful to point out some clinically helpful general guidelines. The Digit Symbol Subtest of the WAIS-R is a useful measure of the speed of information processing and often predicts the basic ability of the patient to be efficient. Patients who are extremely slow on this test (e.g., who have a Digit Symbol Subtest score of 5 or below) are frequently not in a position to return to full-time competitive, gainful employment. Knowledge of this information can be helpful in guiding the patient to consider other alternatives (e.g., voluntary work). Helping the patient recognize and accept this is an important goal of psychotherapy after brain injury. One such patient, for example, 2 years following traumatic brain injury had a Digit Symbol Subtest score of 3. Despite repeated efforts this basic ability could not be substantially improved. It became very important, therefore, for the patient to recognize that the likelihood of gainful employment was, in essence, nil. Helping the patient face and accept this reality resulted in allowing him to work on a voluntary work trial. This is a typical example of how neuropsychological test findings (which we know are sensitive to brain damage; Chapman & Wolff, 1959) can guide what is done with a patient in the psychotherapeutic process. This information helped the clinician talk with the patient about a painful reality (i.e., being too "slow" to return to work). Without knowing that reality the clinician may inadvertently encourage the patient to pursue unrealistic work goals.

Certainly level of performance on such tests as the Logical Memory, Visual Reproduction, and Paired-Associate Learning of the Wechsler Memory Scale is important for psychotherapeutic management. Very poor scores require the patient to review daily (and sometimes several times daily) salient ideas concerning his or her condition and the issues confronting him or her. When solutions are arrived at they too must be repeatedly reviewed. The Block Design, Vocabulary, and Similarities subtests of the WAIS-R provide very important guidelines for talking to a patient. The ideas presented and the actual words used must match the patient's knowledge of words and abstract reasoning capacity. This necessity to match is often forgotten when the psychologist is verbal and accustomed to concepts and ideas not readily available to some patients.

Heaton and Pendleton (1981) have specifically evaluated how the neuropsychological test scores predict capacity to work. Their findings emphasize that the performance IQ has perhaps more to do with successful vocational adjustment than does Verbal IQ. They and others (Klonoff & Prigatano, 1987) have also noted that basic speed of motor functioning, as reflected by the finger tapping test, seems to be an important predictor of work.

The constellation of neuropsychological strengths and limitations that predict work depends on the level of work that the individual wants. Speed of motor movement may well be an important dimension for gainful employment. Interestingly, the self-reported degree of depression does not tend to identify patients who go back to work (Heaton, Chelune, & Lehman, 1978). When asked to evaluate effectiveness for a given patient, the Performance IQ, the average impairment rating, and the patient's activities in various social settings are considered. Currently the authors are expanding the evaluation by considering how specific cognitive retraining activities may be predictors of activities at work. A work skill competency questionnaire has been developed that evaluates a patient's performance in a variety of areas including attendance, personal hygiene, productivity, work attitude, and interpersonal work behaviors with coworkers and supervisors. This questionnaire is completed by the patient and the program therapist involved in the work trial as well as by the job supervisor. Work questionnaire responses are compared and related to performance during cognitive retraining. Similar patterns of behavior and performance will likely be seen in both the cognitive retraining activities and work environments. This research should help demonstrate that observation during rehabilitation activities expands upon neuropsychological test findings and provides relevant information regarding a patient's real-world functioning.

Neuropsychological clinicians, therefore, must attempt to determine the basic ingredients of work and look upon the neuropsychological examination as providing information that they must interpret for a given patient. The accuracy of the interpretation must then be evaluated by ongoing research.

As noted above, Sternberg (1986) has suggested that the three ingredients of love are passion, intimacy, and commitment. How does the neuropsychological assessment relate to these ingredients? The ability to have passion may be obvious from the clinical examination and history as well as from talking to the spouse or "significant other." If the patient is obtunded, apathetic, or demonstrates a clear state of adynamia, he or she most likely will not have the necessary drive level or libidinal interest to engage others and thereby to establish a love relationship. However, most young adult traumatically brain injured patients have this capacity, and usually it is unchecked, that is, passion may be expressed in a disinhibited, inappropriate manner, which makes the second ingredient, intimacy, a much more demanding and difficult task. Clinically it appears that the major factors that interfere with intimacy have to do with childishness, impairment in abstract reasoning, paranoia, and deceitfulness.

Prefrontal injuries often result in more childish behavior (Stuss & Benson, 1986). It is difficult for a healthy spouse to have a sense of intimacy with a partner who behaves more like a child than an adult. This component is not easily assessed by formal aspects of testing but is revealed in the clinical interview and in how the patient interacts with others. Also ratings by family members as to whether or not the patient is childish are very useful (Oddy, Coughlan, Tyerman, et al., 1985). A second factor is whether the patient can "see the big picture of things" or whether he or she simply appreciates small aspects of a given situation (i.e., loss of abstract attitude). For example, if the patient overreacts to very small details and does not understand the complexity of life issues, establishing an adult relationship is difficult. Many spouses say that they have "three children," as opposed to their actual two, when this problem emerges. Establishing intimacy is difficult if one adult is childish and does not see the complexities of life. Helping the individual improve in abstract reasoning and reduce childlike behavior, therefore, is an important goal of neuropsychological rehabilitation. Paranoia and deceitfulness undercut any willingness to be "open" because both run directly counter to open, honest, and fair dialogue.

Commitment may be best assessed by the individual's previous level of functioning. However, it is perhaps a little easier for an individual to be committed after brain injury because the patient does not readily see various options. If placed in a setting that is protected and committed to the patient, that individual will often "latch on" and become committed in return. The same dynamics are seen in people with advancing age.

Psychotherapy, therefore, is guided by the neuropsychological examination findings insofar as the examination provides information relevant for the capacity to work and to love. While certainly the classic neuropsychological examination does not directly address these questions, examination findings have to be analyzed in light of the seven dimensions described in Figure 14.1. How the clinician goes about doing this is, of course, a function of clinical experience and skill. However, these components can be taught and have relevance to beginning clinicians as well as to seasoned ones. Before considering actual techniques of psychotherapy after brain damage, the impact of financial factors and family issues in the psychotherapeutic process are addressed briefly.

WORKERS' COMPENSATION, LAWSUITS, AND DECOMPENSATION

From Freud to present-day theorists there has been a recognition that for patient behavior to change the patient must be motivated to change. Motivation is difficult to define. Neuropsychologically oriented definitions describe it as including the arousal component that parallels an ongoing goal-seeking behavior (Prigatano and Others, 1986). Behavior therapists define the concept typically in terms of the environmental response (or reinforcement) to a given behavior. After brain injury motivation is no less important in behavior change and adaptation to the effects of a brain lesion.

Patients are often motivated to deal with their feelings of self-inadequacy, depression, and so on, if the reward for doing this is clear and appropriate. If patients recognize a real economic threat to being unemployed after brain injury, this mobilizes the energy component to work. One young man, who was covered by workers' compensation insurance, desperately wanted to return to work to regain his sense of self-respect and to assist his wife economically so she could return to graduate school. He recognized the need to lower his job ambitions to accomplish these goals. His workers' compensation insurance was vital to their economic security and provided the financial basis for getting rehabilitative services that led to his employment. To date he is working as a postman and has done quite well over the last four years.

In contrast, some patients can actually deteriorate when the financial rewards associated with their disability are too inviting and stimulate underlying issues of greed. For example, another patient who had workers' compensation and an ongoing lawsuit began to fantasize (partly fueled by his attorney) that he could become independently wealthy because of his residual neurological and neuropsychological deficits. His situation was complicated because his abstract reasoning skills were impaired and his premorbid personality style was psychopathic. These factors made it impossible for him to embrace a true psychotherapeutic relationship. Despite his need to face the truth about his brain injury, both he and his wife were so tied into his lawsuit that facing the truth was impossible. In this case, workers' compensation insurance and the lawsuit actually resulted in "decompensation" rather than a "compensation" for the patient's psychosocial difficulties.

WORKING WITH THE FAMILIES

It is not uncommon to see family members who need psychological help in coping with a brain injured relative. As the families become better educated about the complexity of the problems of a brain injured relative, they become more realistic and hopefully manage the patient more effectively. Perhaps effective psychotherapy cures very little but does manage problems much better.

Elsewhere (Klonoff, Costa, & Snow, 1986), the authors have tried to describe some of the typical reactions that family members go through and how to approach family members in the context of a neuropsychological rehabilitation model. Basically there are three avenues for working effectively with family members. The first is to share with family members, in detail, the neuropsychological test findings. No secrets are kept. The psychotherapist tries to help the family members understand how the person has been affected. Initially family members may think the psychotherapist is overstating the problems and will simply not trust his or her judgment. As the problems become more real to them, family members then think back on what they have been told, and often this helps establish a substantially better working relationship.

Next, working with groups of relatives is very useful. In this context the relatives of a patient meet with the psychotherapist once a week in a round-robin technique (e.g., each family member describes what he or she is experiencing with a given patient during the week). Information about a patient when away from the institution is especially useful. The psychotherapist then conveys what he or she sees in a given patient. This sets the tone for open dialogue and encourages families to listen to others about how they cope with the majority of problems these patients present.

The third avenue is, of course, individual family therapy, with or without the patient present. During these hours the specific needs of a given family are addressed. These three activities are extremely important, since psychotherapy with brain injured patients would be ineffective if there is not an equally ongoing work relationship with family members.

TECHNIQUES OF PSYCHOTHERAPY AFTER BRAIN INJURY

While there are no specific techniques of psychotherapy after brain damage, the authors have found several approaches useful. First, patients are worked with individually and also in groups. Group feedback to patients can be invaluable, as patients may accept suggestions and criticisms from peers more readily than from therapists. Group therapy can also be valuable in helping less aware patients become more sensitive to their negative social impact on others.

The authors rely heavily on a psychoeducational model that presents and explains patients' behavior in, it is hoped, concise, digestible units. This is particularly important after significant brain injury, when patients may have difficulty with auditory comprehension, memory, and abstract reasoning. One example of a model of behavior that commonly emerges is the "catastrophic reaction" (Goldstein, 1942). Often after brain injury patients' difficulties with interpersonal functioning can be related to their becoming overwhelmed with tasks that are too difficult for them. This may result in feelings of anger, depression, or frustration, which in turn may be projected onto people in the environment, including family members, coworkers, and supervisors. When this model is explained to patients (and their families), patients often respond with a sense of relief, as they then have a framework in which to interpret their behavior.

Providing simple models in diagrammatic or symbolic form is also helpful. Often patients will "hook onto" a simple diagram of a particular behavioral characteristic they are experiencing and will be able to critically evaluate their own subsequent behaviors in light of it. For example, consider a patient who had substantial difficulty seeing the big picture and who would often focus on small details, lose perspective, and get into many interpersonal conflicts. By diagrammatically explaining this with a simple picture (Figure 14.2), the patient was able to understand better this problem and to recognize his tendency to do this in other situations. Diagrams such as this can be especially helpful for patients who have trouble processing abstract or verbal information.

Related to this, psychotherapists may take a more direct, gently confrontative approach to issues. This is not to say that they are didactic or intolerant of patients' attitudes or beliefs; instead therapists try to be instructive in their style, providing options and guidance where necessary. For patients with significant problems with judgment, reasoning, or reality testing, the therapist may act as the "auxiliary ego" (Werman, 1984) and help patients with decisions that they are genuinely unable to make independently. A common example of this type of guiding approach might occur when patients are unrealistic about work aspirations.

Other techniques that are often helpful include the use of examples of other patients' attempts to struggle with similar problems. Again, this technique is particularly useful in helping patients accept positions with lower work status or face the consequences of unawareness or unacceptance of their

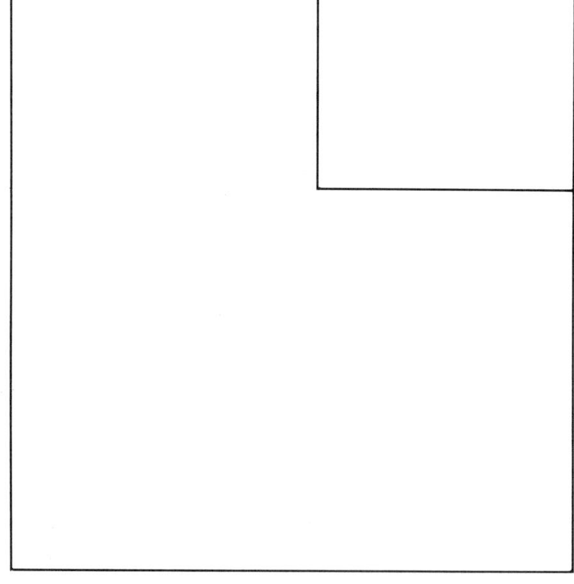

Figure 14.2. An example of an analogy used in psychotherapy with brain injured patients. Patients are shown this drawing and are told that they think that they are looking at the larger square when in fact they are looking at the smaller one. This analogy helps patients to recognize that they have trouble seeing the big picture and, consequently, are reacting to only part of a complex situation.

brain injury. Helping patients forgive themselves and others for the accident and re-establish a purpose in life is also done with other patient examples.

The authors also incorporate the use of analogies when it is feasible. For example, a group of psychotherapists worked with a patient who sustained a very severe brain injury as a result of a bicycle accident. He was severely depressed over his memory difficulties. Prior to the accident he was an avid hiker, camper, and outdoorsman. As his depression deepened he would experience catastrophic reactions when he became overwhelmed by his memory difficulties. The authors developed an analogy of this behavior and referred to it as the patient "packing up his tent." Whenever therapists observed this behavior in the program or at work, they would use this analogy to cue him regarding his behavior. He was able to relate to this analogy and to better appreciate the impact of this behavior on his environment. This proved to be a useful therapeutic tool to help him adapt his behavioral response to this injury. Humor can also be an invaluable tool, especially when patients so often confront the devastating effects of their injury. No matter what the problems and style of communication used, therapists should repetitively review this material to help ameliorate the effects of memory difficulties.

SUMMARY AND CONCLUSIONS

In this chapter we have tried to emphasize, first of all, that it is extremely important to provide a model the patient understands and can use in coping with his or her problems. Second, it is extremely important to help the patient to understand the meaning of brain injury in his or her life. Third, the patient must be helped to achieve a sense of self-acceptance and ultimately to forgive himself or herself and those who caused the accident. Without these accomplishments, the patient continues to spend a great deal of energy on these problems. Next, the patient needs to make realistic commitments to work and to interpersonal relationships. Fifth, the patient must be taught how to behave in different social situations to improve interpersonal competence. Behavioral techniques are extremely useful here. Also the patient needs to be taught specific behavioral strategies when compensating for neuropsychological deficits. Finally, fostering a sense of realistic hope is extremely important if patients are going to be worked with effectively (Prigatano and Others, 1986).

To achieve these goals the use of symbolism is often quite important. The last two figures presented are drawings by patients. These types of drawings have been found to be extremely important in helping patients understand how their neuropsychological functioning has affected them and their life. In Figure 14.3 are caricatures the patient drew of himself preinjury and post-

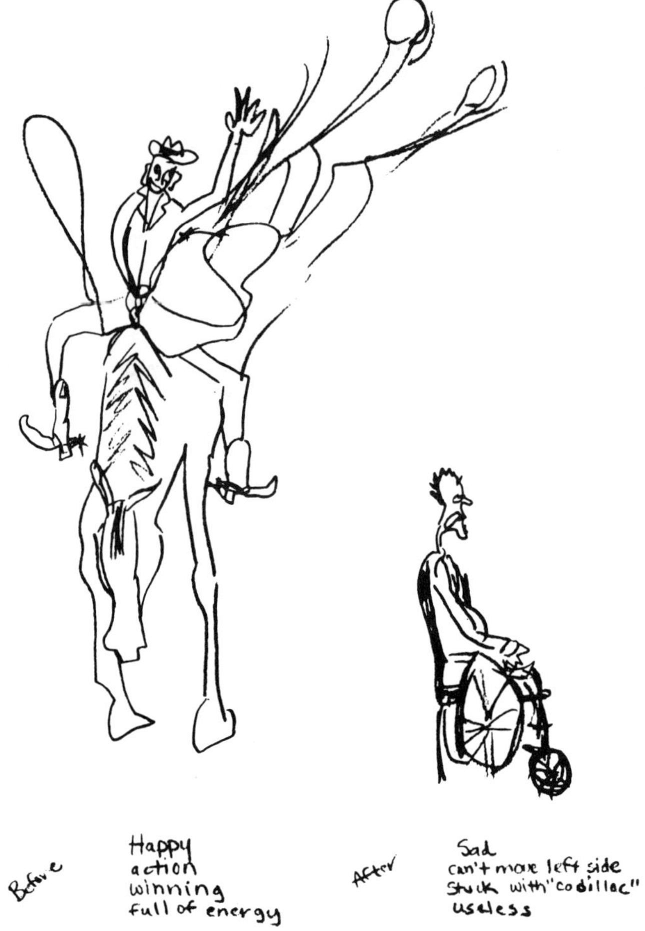

Figure 14.3. A drawing by a traumatically brain injured patient depicting himself pretrauma and posttrauma. (The authors thank the spouse of this individual for permission to print these drawings.)

injury. While the psychotherapy of this patient was ineffective, the issues his drawings presented are crucial for the psychotherapist attempting to work with brain injured patients. In a sense a patient's drawings are as diagnostic and useful for psychotherapy as are formal neuropsychologic assessment procedures. Each drawing in Figure 14.3 reflects what the patient has experienced and how he thinks after brain injury.

The final figure (Figure 14.4) was provided to the authors by a speech and language pathologist who is working with a brain dysfunctional patient. It illustrates how the patient experiences herself as being "normal" after a very severe injury. "Only part of her head" has been affected. She wonders if she is in a "never, never land." How can one lose part of her head and be normal? The picture reflects the eternal struggle of brain injured patients to establish a sense of wholeness and meaningfulness after brain damage. The degree to which psychotherapists can help patients understand these symbolic representations and re-establish purpose and meaning in life is the measure of the effectiveness of psychotherapy and ultimately the usefulness of the neuropsychological assessment of those patients.

I am a normal
person with part
of my head off in
Never Never
land. (Will I ever
retrieve it?)

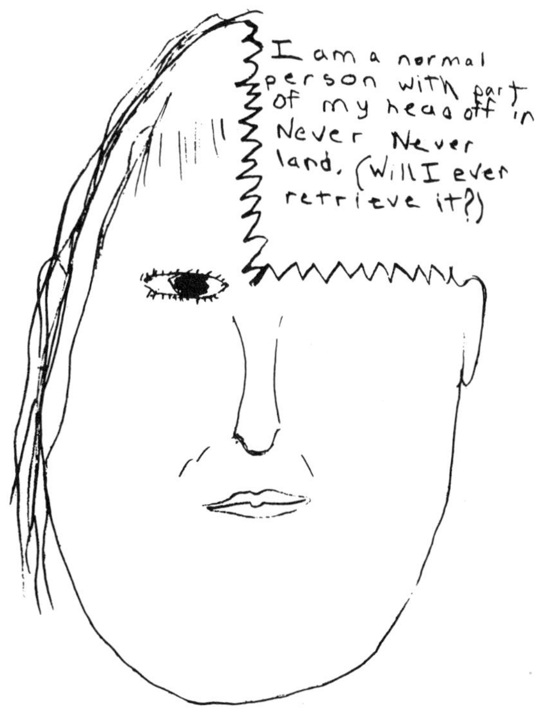

Figure 14.4. A drawing by a traumatically brain injured patient illustrating the self-perception of normality and yet questioning her ultimate recovery. (The authors thank Karen Tripp, speech and language pathologist, for providing this picture.)

REFERENCES

Chapman, L.F., & Wolff, H.G. (1959). The cerebral hemispheres and the highest integrative functions of man. *Archives of Neurology, 1*, 357–424.

Diller, L. (1987). Neuropsychological rehabilitation. In M.J. Meier, A.L. Benton, & L. Diller (Eds.), *Neuropsychological rehabilitation* (pp. 3–17). New York: Guilford.

Frederiks, J.A.M. (1985). Clinical neuropsychology: The neuropsychological symptom. In P.J. Vinken, G.W. Bruyn, H.L. Klawans, et al. (Eds.), *Handbook of clinical neurology: Clinical neuropsychology* (vol. 45, pp. 1–6). New York: Elsevier Science.

Goldstein, K. (1942). *Aftereffects of brain injuries in war.* New York: Grune & Stratton.

Heaton, R.K., Chelune, G.J., & Lehman, R.A.W. (1978). Using neuropsychological and personality tests to assess the likelihood of patient employment. *Journal of Nervous and Mental Disorders, 166*, 408–416.

Heaton, R.K., & Pendleton, N.T. (1981). Use of neuropsychological tests to predict adult patients' every day functioning. *Journal of Consulting Clinical Psychology, 49*, 807–821.

Heilman, K.M., & Valenstein, E. (Eds.). (1979). *Clinical neuropsychology.* New York: Oxford University Press.

Klonoff, P.S., Costa, L.D., & Snow, W.G. (1986). Predictors and indicators of quality of life in patients with closed head injury. *Journal of Clinical and Experimental Neuropsychology, 8*, 469–485.

Klonoff, P.S., & Prigatano, G.P. (1987). Family and staff's reactions in the rehabilitation of brain injured patients: Clinical and research findings. In M. Ylvisaker (Ed.), *Adult head injury rehabilitation: Community re-entry.* San Diego: College-Hill.

Lezak, M.T. (1983). *Neuropsychological assessment* (2nd ed.). New York: Oxford University Press.

Lishman, W.A. (1978). *Organic psychiatry.* Boston: Blackwell Scientific.

Luria, A.R. (1966). *Higher cortical functions in man.* New York: Basic Books.

Luria, A.R., Naydin, V.L., Tsvetkova, L.W., et al. (1969). Restoration of higher cortical functions following local brain damage. In P.J. Vinken & G.W. Bruyn (Eds.) *Handbook of clinical neurology* (vol. 3). New York: Elsevier-North Holland.

Oddy, M., Coughlan, T., Tyerman, A., et al. (1985). Social adjustment after closed head injury: A further follow-up seven years after injury. *Journal of Neurology, Neurosurgery, and Psychiatry, 48*, 564–565.

Parsons, O.A., & Prigatano, G.P. (1978). Methodological considerations in clinical neuropsychological research. *Journal of Consulting Clinical Psychology, 46*, 608–619.

Prigatano, G.P. (1986). Higher cerebral deficits: The history of methods of assessment and approaches to rehabilitation: Part I. *BNI Quarterly*, 2(3), 15–26.

Prigatano, G.P., and Others. (1986). *Neuropsychological rehabilitation after brain injury.* Baltimore: Johns Hopkins University Press.

Prigatano, G.P., Pepping, M., & Klonoff, P. (1986). Cognitive, personality, and psychological factors in the neuropsychological assessment of brain injured patients. In B.P. Uzzell & Y. Gross (Eds.), *Clinical neuropsychology of intervention* (pp. 135–166). Boston: Martinus-Nijhoff.

Sternberg, R.J. (1986). A triangular theory of love. *Psychological Review,*

93, 119–135.

Stuss, D.T., & Benson, D.F. (1986). *The frontal lobes.* New York: Raven.

Werman, D.S. (1984). *The practice of supportive psychotherapy.* New York: Brunner/Mazel.

15

Disorders of Attention and Their Treatment in Traumatic Brain Injury Rehabilitation

RODGER LI. WOOD

Abnormalities of attention in association with brain injury have been described in the psychological literature since 1904 (see Wood, 1987, for a review). In the majority of studies, abnormalities of attention have been described in terms of how attention interacts with a person's performance on psychological tests. Only quite recently has the attention process been used to explain some of the problems of behavior and new learning that a therapist might encounter during the rehabilitation of a head injured patient (Mack, 1986; Nissen, 1986; Webster & Scott, 1983; Whyte, 1986; Wood, 1986, 1987).

Wood (1987) discusses the mechanisms by which brain injury interferes with attention and deregulates the mechanisms of information processing. Geschwind (1982) has described attention disorders as one of the most common deficits of higher mental function encountered by neurologists, while Newcombe (1985) points to the way attention disorders can produce incoherent thinking and a failure to recognize or respond to cues that are present in the individual's immediate environment. The probable reason for this is that attention is a *control process* that allows us to select from a complex stimulus array those factors that are important to behavior, thereby influencing the process of decision making and the cognitive strategies that are necessary for day-to-day living.

Some attempts at rehabilitation therapy are unsuccessful because the therapist has not considered how a brain injury can impose limitations upon the attentional capacity of an individual or prevent a person from focusing or sustaining attention for a long enough period of time to allow learning to take place (see Wood, 1986). Wood (1987) showed how attention was more important than intelligence (measured by IQ) during the learning of a simple discrimination task.

The purpose of this chapter, therefore, is to try to describe how the attentional process permeates all aspects of behavior, making it a fundamental neuropsychological thread in the fabric of rehabilitation therapy. In order for rehabilitation staff to have a reasonable clinical frame of reference for understanding attentional disorders in the context of brain injury, it is necessary to appreciate the theoretical basis of attention as an operational process mediating many aspects of behavior and cognitive function. Such a framework has been evolving for some time, and the recent description given by Posner and Rafal (1987) provides an excellent foundation from which the rehabilitation therapist can apply clinical observations and treatment (or training) strategies. In order to do this successfully, however, it is important to have a clear understanding of the diversity of attention and its status following head injury.

WHAT IS ATTENTION?

Stuss and Benson (1986) point to a continuing confusion in the way *attention* is defined. They suggest that this lack of clarity is one factor that prevents the attentional process from having universal acceptance by clinicians as a fundamental process regulating many aspects of intelligent behavior.

At the phenomenological level, no attempt to define attention can ignore the original description of attention presented by James (1890), which states that attention "is the taking possession by the mind, in a clear and vivid form, one out of what seems several simultaneously possible objects or trains of thought" (p. 403). This statement combines virtually all the components that exist as part of the attentional process. The description "taking possession by the mind" can explain the conscious *effort* that we must sometimes make to regulate our attention and maintain concentration. The phrase "one out of what seems several simultaneously possible objects or trains of thought" implies a withdrawal of attention from some things in order to deal more effectively with others — the process of *selective attention*. The combination of selectivity and effort requires a level of arousal in the brain that will allow these components of attention to operate at an optimal level and produce a speedy response to some stimulus configuration.

The diversity of the attention process, incorporating arousal, selectivity, and effort (or vigilance), was originally described by Posner and Boies (1971) and recently reviewed by Posner and Rafal (1987). These different attentional categories relate very well to the cognitive problems that influence the behavior, social learning, and functional skill training in those individuals who have sustained head injuries of all degrees of severity. As Ben-Yishay, Piasetsky, and Rattok (1987) comment, "the clinical manifestations of disturbed attention in patients with traumatic head injury in remedial rehabilitation, conform well to Posner and Rafal's layered partitioning of the attentional processes" (p. 165). This review of attention and attentional deficits is of particular interest to neuropsychologists and rehabilitation professionals because it relates many of the phenomenological aspects of attention to underlying neural mechanisms and, where possible, specific neurological disorders. If the Posner and Rafal chapter has a weakness, it relates to not describing attention in the context of head injury per se. This is probably due to the diffuse nature of such injuries and the fact that so many attentional variables are involved, making it difficult to separate out the contributions made by arousal, selectivity, and effort to a person's attentional capabilities and cognitive performance. For this reason there is probably some merit in restricting a description of attention in the context of head injury to its behavioral manifestations in order that rehabilitation professionals will recognize how attention plays a part in some of the clinical problems that confront them as a routine part of their work.

In order to understand the phenomenon of attention as it relates to brain injury rehabilitation, it is probably best to try and separate attention as a *cognitive process*, from attention as a *neuropsychological system*. The former relates to, and is part of, the behavior we *observe*, while the latter represents the substrate of cognition that we *infer*. Using this distinction as an argument for presenting problems of attention in a cognitive mode, the information processing model proposed by Shiffrin and Schneider (1977) seems to offer a good framework for understanding how attention is involved in learning many of the skills contained in a comprehensive program of rehabilitation therapy.

The application of this cognitive model to brain injury rehabilitation has been discussed by Wood (1987), who emphasized the dual nature of attention, which can operate in a *conscious mode* during the *acquisition* of a skill or the solving of a conceptual problem, or in an *automatic mode* during the *performance* of a skill (motor or verbal), once that skill has been acquired and refined through practice. The essential difference between these two modes of operation is that the conscious mode is a slow form of information processing that emphasizes the *effort component* of attention. In this mode an individual has to maintain a level of concentration and a focus of attention on the relevant task parameters. As such, there is a limit to the amount of information that one can deal with at any given time, indicating the restrictions on attentional capacity that can influence all aspects of our behavior and learning ability. The conscious mode operates on the basis of serial processing; if there are 10 facts or units of behavior involved in the acquisition of a particular skill, then one has to attend to each of these facts in turn because the learning process would be inefficient if one had to try to learn 10 different, but related, facts, at more or less the same time. Attention in the *automatic mode* does not require the same degree of conscious effort because skills that are learned seem, in many respects, to be performed more or less automatically, without us necessarily being aware of them. This is assumed to indicate a fast form of information processing, one in which information is processed in *parallel* rather than in *series*.

An obvious example that compares and contrasts the two modes of information processing is learning to drive a car. At first, we have to give conscious attention to the position of the steering wheel, pressing the accelerator and clutch pedal, moving the gear stick, plus a host of other driving-related motor actions. The process is tiring, the movements are effortful and sometimes clumsy, and there is a hesitant quality with respect to the performance of the driving task. We feel that we can attend to only one thing at a time. With practice, however, we become less aware of the individual or discrete units of activity that combine to make up the sequence of movement involved in driving. Instead of performing one action at a time, the whole process becomes more fluent and we pay less attention to its individual components, allowing us to drive, listen to the radio, talk to a passenger, or admire the scenery, while still (hopefully) maintaining an awareness of traffic conditions and a safe driving style. This would represent a change from the laborious conscious mode of information processing to an almost effortless automatic mode of processing.

HABIT AND ATTENTION

The difference between automatic and conscious modes of behavior is central to the process of learning new skills or strategies that compensate for residual disability following brain injury. The reason for this is that much of adult behavior operates at a more or less automatic level in the form of a habit sequence. Habit is a process that is central to many forms of behavior; therefore, one of the aims of rehabilitation must be to re-establish those complex habit sequences that constitute social and functional skills. These habit sequences represent automatic forms of behavior that become disrupted by brain injury. The cognitive processes, which normally regulate these behaviors, fail to operate properly; subsequently, a person has to revert to a more conscious mode of behavior regulation.

As a result of brain injury, many habit sequences are lost, either because the motor action producing them is impaired or the cognitive process coordinating or organizing the action has been damaged. Luria (1961) emphasized the importance of interpreting these sequences of behavior in terms that describe some "common mental action." This "common mental action" is described by Luria as the process of "inner speech," which he believed played a critical role in the cognitive mediation of complex forms of behavior (Luria, 1961). He believed that disorders of attention were themselves a product of the disruption in covert aspects of speech (Luria, 1982). The question of whether covert speech mediates attention, or is itself mediated by attention, is analogous to the chicken and the egg conundrum! From a clinical or therapeutic point of view, it is not necessary to get embroiled in the argument, but it is necessary to understand how one process is involved in the other for the purpose of cognitive remediation (see below).

The involvement of habit in behavior and attention was not overlooked by William James. In his original presentation of the interaction between cognition and behavior he stated that "habit diminishes the concentration with which our acts are performed" (James, 1890, p. 114). Reason (1984), when describing the impact of James's work on our present understanding of lapses of attention in everyday life, suggests that a diminishing effect of habit on conscious attention is "a self-evident truth [which] does not alter the fact that understanding how automisation comes about still remains one of the central problems in psychology" (p. 515). He describes how both habit and attention have prominent roles in the guidance of behavior, but it is still not clear how much attention is needed (even at an automatic level of processing) to regulate a habit sequence of behavior.

DIVIDED ATTENTION AND ATTENTIONAL CAPACITY

Much research in attention assumes that there is a limited pool of attentional resources that can be distributed across tasks (Kahneman, 1973). This is generally referred to as attentional capacity. Schneider, Dumais, and Shiffrin (1984) try to explain this by suggesting that "simple capacity models" would predict that if a person has 100 units of attentional capacity but is required to perform two tasks, each requiring 75 units, then performance on these tasks will decline if the behavioral response demands that instead of performing the tasks individually they should be performed simultaneously. The automatic versus conscious control processing theories assume that attentional capacity is limited as a result of the competition between different activities that require conscious attention. If one combines tasks in which conscious control is needed, then the demands of the tasks will overload the information processing system and this will result in reduced or impaired performance.

When one considers the richness and complexity of the information that is presented to our senses at any one time, it is not difficult to appreciate the risk of confusion produced by attentional overload. In response to this, we are expected to produce diverse and often incompatible responses, and, depending upon the type or combination of response required to any set of complex stimuli, there may be a risk of what Kahneman and Treisman (1984) describe as "cognitive paralysis and incoherence." The attention mechanism tries to provide order to this complex cascade of sensory stimuli by, on the one hand, a process of selective information processing and, on the other hand, the adoption of an appropriate perceptual (or attentional) set. The success of attention in dealing with this complex stimulus array depends upon the extent to which attention can be divided across such information, which, in turn, depends very much on the operating capacity of the information processing system and the similarity (or disparity) between the"messages" that system has to act upon.

It is inevitable that, following brain injury, the information processing system of the brain will be impaired. This imposes limitations on attentional capacity and reduces the extent to which attention can be divided across different stimulus configurations. The more alternatives a head injured patient has to respond to, the slower and more unreliable his or her response to a stimulus will be. Van Zomeren and Deelman (1978), using a choice reaction time task, found that the amount by which the rate of information processing in the head injured would slow down was proportional to the duration of coma after injury.

The problem with understanding divided attention is that one is not simply referring to attentional *capacity* (i.e., the degree to which one is able to spread one's attention over a number of things at any given time). It also refers to the ability to focus attention, in order to recognize which, out of a number of diverse stimuli that are present at any given time, are the important cues that guide or regulate behavior in any particular situation. In the case of head injury, clinical observations suggest that the attentional capacity of patients is limited, meaning that they cannot divide their attention equally over the same number of stimuli, as a non-brain-injured person can. This means that the quality of attention or recognition that they can give to any individual stimulus is inevitably reduced. As the studies by Van Zomeren and Deelman have shown, when an individual's attentional capacity is stretched beyond a certain level it is not only the extra stimuli that fail to be properly attended to. Rather, all stimuli within that chunk of information are affected and responded to poorly, slowly, or unreliably.

ATTENTION TRAINING

Although there would appear to be general agreement that attention is an important element of cognition, studies that have attempted to show the value of cognitive rehabilitation techniques have largely neglected attention in favor of memory or perceptual training. Inevitably, these cognitive processes incorporate attention, but the attentional variable is never isolated as a relevant parameter in order to measure the outcome of a training procedure. Apart from the author's own work (Wood, 1986, 1987), the only other study specifically devoted to attention training is that of Ponsford and Kinsella (1988), although Diller and Weinberg (1977) also recognized the importance of attention in the training of patients with visual neglect.

The concept of attention, as it affects rehabilitation, can be divided into two broad areas. The first involves a behavioral component of attention (attentiveness), the second, a cognitive component, roughly equivalent to information processing. Methods that have attempted to improve attention in both these areas have been described in the literature and are discussed in the following sections.

Attention Span

The literature on attention has suggested that the concept of attention span refers to the number of distinct objects that can be perceived in a single momentary representation or, more simply, how many things can we attend to in a single instant of time? There is, however, a second definition that refers to the *length of time* a person can attend to one thing. In rehabilitation, therefore, *attention span* has been extended as a concept to incorporate sustained attention, which is of greater interest to rehabilitation therapists because it incorporates many other aspects of the attentional process, namely, selectivity, resistance to distracting influences, attentional capacity, and scanning ability.

The length of time a person can attend to one thing was initially referred to as voluntary attention (James, 1890). As such, it also incorporates factors such as effort and motivation. We therefore have a certain form of behavior that has been described by different neuropsychological terms. As Parasurman (1984) states, sustained attention and vigilance are used interchangeably to describe *span* of attention. The word *vigilance* has been preferred by neurologists and physiologists as a term to describe arousal, the degree of cortical tone that is necessary for a number of brain functions to operate. In 1926, Sir Henry Head defined vigilance as "a state of high grade efficiency of the nervous system" (p. 128). Parasurman prefers to regard the concept of vigilance as an aspect of attention rather than arousal because arousal is a general state of the organism that affects the ability to carry out various functions of attention, including remaining vigilant.

Problems of short attention span were recognized as early as 1904, when Kuhlman proposed that it could explain the learning difficulty experienced by mentally handicapped people. Strauss and Kephart (1947), in *Psychopathology and Education of the Brain Injured,* considered short attention span to be the main problem underlying the difficulty that brain injured children displayed in attending to task for any length of time and learning new skills.

Operant conditioning procedures offer a powerful tool to manipulate the length of time individuals can attend to a particular task. The most important single principle in changing behavior is the application of reward for attentive behavior. The work of Wood (1986, 1987) has shown how the application of systematic reinforcement for attentive behavior significantly improves the amount of time individuals attend to task and ignore distracting stimuli in a therapy setting, thereby increasing the amount of therapy that they receive and improving potential for recovery through the process of rehabilitation.

A behavioral method also formed the basis of a training procedure to improve hemi-inattention (Diller & Weinberg, 1977). Diller and Weinberg construed hemi-inattentiveness and visual neglect as a failure to systematically scan one's visual environment. This scanning could be improved by increasing the salience of a stimulus (making it more noticeable) while at the same time providing cues as to the direction that scanning should take, followed by feedback of the patient's performance. A *shaping* procedure was employed because, as scanning ability increased, the cues and salience factors were gradually removed. Diller and Weinberg found that this process could help patients compensate for a visual field deficit, and the improved visual performance was evident in real-life situations outside the clinic.

Content of Attention

Content of attention refers to the *cognitive component* of attention, not just "attentiveness," which simply refers to a behavioral readiness to receive information. As such, "content" is closely related to memory, and there is now a fairly general agreement as to the relationship between attention and memory, and the dependence of the latter upon the former. Nissen (1986) stated that "information that is not attended to is poorly remembered" (p. 17). She clearly felt that new learning was also dependent upon attending, commenting that "the acquisition of new information is strongly dependent upon attention processing" (p. 18). Craik and Lockhart (1972) proposed that an event was more likely to be remembered if it achieved a deeper "level" of processing than an event that was only processed briefly or superficially. The act of processing, in their sense of the word, implies that one gives attention to an event, making it more meaningful and more memorable.

So far, however, there is not a great deal of evidence to show that we can influence the *content* of attention. Nissen (1986) refers to a number of studies that describe the importance of attention to memory, but there is little documented evidence to support the idea that by improving attentional processing we can increase aspects of memory. Wood (1986) found that for patients who made significant progress on attention training tasks, improving aspects of (a) attention span, (b) discriminated visual processing, and (c) speed of response failed to generalize that ability to memory tasks, even though the measures of recall, recognition, and new learning ability, used as independent outcome criteria, all rely on the efficient processing of information.

This observation has been repeated in a more recent study (Wood & Fussey, 1987) that employed a control group design composed of a normal control group plus two matched patient groups, each containing 10 severely brain injured patients, with an average posttraumatic amnesia of 2 months. All the patients were more than 2 years postinjury. An attempt was made to evaluate the success of a computer-based attention training procedure and assess its generalization to tasks that required visual-motor skills, but not those used during the computer training task itself. The results of this study supported the earlier observation. The computer task, which trained sequential aspects of information processing, speed of processing, visual discrimination, and decision and motor reaction time, did show a difference between the patient group that received 1 hour of training each day for 28 days, and the two control groups that were exposed to the computer task only on Day 1 and Day 28 of the training procedure. There was no evidence, however, that the improved performance of the patients trained on the computer task generalized to a number of independent outcome measures that were tested for all three groups at Days 1 and 28 of training. It appears that the apparent improvement in the content of attention, as far as performance on the computer is concerned, may be task specific!

The recent study by Ponsford and Kinsella (1988) concentrated on speed and selectivity of information processing as the relevant attentional variables in 15 patients who had sustained severe closed head injury. This study used patients who were less than 12 months postinjury and had a posttraumatic amnesia in excess of 24 hours. Generally speaking, therefore, they were a far less severely injured group than those subjects that constituted the Wood and Fussey (1987) study. The results were largely consistent with the previous studies described. Subjects showed a gradual improvement on the computer training task but there was no evidence that this specific skill generalized to any other aspect of cognitive ability. Neither could the authors confirm that the improvement on the training task itself was anything more than might be expected from a process of spontaneous recovery.

The findings of Ponsford and Kinsella (1988) are important because of the rigorous experimental methods employed during this clinical study. They not only employed a controlled group design but also subjected the performance of individual subjects to analysis using single case study methods based on a multiple baseline design. This suggests that we must view with caution other computer training procedures that have not employed such carefully controlled methods of evaluation, yet claim success in cognitive training procedures that have a major attentional emphasis.

Bracy (1983) provided evidence on two patients who received computer training 3 years postinjury. This training was not specifically oriented toward the attention process but did demand good information capabilities and aspects of selective attention. Bracy showed that an improvement could be obtained on the training task and that this improvement was associated with an improvement in IQ because the scores of the two patients on the Wechsler Adult Intelligence Test increased by 23 and 28 points, respectively.

The significance of this finding is somewhat undermined by the general agreement that IQ is notoriously poor as an index of progress of recovery in rehabilitation because it does not correspond to observations of functional ability or social independence. It may be, therefore, that a useful method for retraining attentional capabilities is not being properly utilized because of the use of inappropriate outcome measures.

Trexler (1987) also describes a computer-based training procedure that has a number of attentional components, namely, visual scanning, perception, and the processing of these percepts into memory for later recall and recognition. Unfortunately, no data are given to show the efficacy of such a procedure, but Trexler does comment on the difficulty of performing "empirical research" because patients tend to receive treatment that has been individually designed, thereby preventing an analysis of group data. This is an understandable but not a sufficient argument for failing to evaluate the process of attention training. Single case design methods are available to evaluate clinical procedures that, by their nature, have to be applied according to variable criteria. In order to have these computer methods accepted as being clinically credible, a greater effort must be spent in devising appropriate (functional) ways of evaluating the training process.

It would be wrong to consider attention training as relying entirely on computer technolgy. Some success has been reported in aspects of information processing ability and attention when other forms of cognitive training have been used. Webster and Scott (1983) used a cognitive-behavioral procedure based on a verbal mediation strategy (Meichenbaum, 1974) to increase attentional capacity and improve memory in a single case study of a head injured patient, 2 years postinjury. They trained the patient to verbally regulate aspects of his behavior and found that focused attention improved and the patient showed better ability for retaining memories of his behavior and other aspects of information.

The procedure used by Webster and Scott (1983) combined principles of behavioral learning and neuropsychology, the latter based on the concept of "inner speech" in the organization of behavior (Luria, 1982). By utilizing, in an overt way, cognitive controls that normally operate without conscious awareness, they have shown that aspects of behavior can be regulated in a way that helps the individual focus attention upon them, elevating their significance and, therefore, the person's awareness of them. This might assist the process of memory, comprehension, and the organization of behavior.

This has been demonstrated by Wood (1987) in a severely head injured female, 4 years postinjury. She was not able to regulate the content of her conversation, and therefore produced a number of stereotyped themes that were very boring to those who had to spend long periods of time in her company (e.g., family and attendant-companions). A purely behavioral approach failed to change her style of conversation, but a cognitively oriented approach that drew her attention to these stereotyped phrases resulted in a significant reduction in these phrases and a greater level of awareness for the need to produce socially appropriate speech.

DISCUSSION

There is little evidence of the versatility or clinical reliability of attention training procedures. This is surprising given the apparent consensus of opinion regarding the importance of attention as a cognitive variable.

The use of the computer as the primary means of training aspects of attention remains quite prominent, but because of the lack of observable clinical change in many of these patients, more therapists are giving consideration to other methods that help focus and sustain attention. Behavioral methods are emerging as a reliable way of improving attentiveness and thereby increasing cooperation, effort, and learning ability in all aspects of rehabilitation therapy. Similarly, the use of cognitive mediators, such as language regulation or visual imagery (Wilson, 1984), will assist in giving greater attention to aspects of our environment or other forms of information that are important to ongoing behavior.

Whatever the method of training, it is clear that more consideration needs to be given to evaluating, objectively and functionally, the whole concept of cognitive rehabilitation, and attention training in particular. Without this, the fund of knowledge needed to develop procedures that are likely to facilitate the efficient processing of information and help establish a reliable memory system, will not become available and the potential of many individuals to reach a level of independence in their social behavior will not be realized.

REFERENCES

Ben-Yishay, Y., Piasetsky, V., & Rattok, J. (1987). A systematic method for ameliorating disorders in basic attention. In M. Meier, A. Benton, & L. Diller (Eds.), *Neuropsychological rehabilitation* (pp. 165–182). New York: Churchill Livingstone.

Bracy, O. (1983). Computer-based cognitive rehabilitation. *Cognitive Rehabilitation, 1*(1), 7–9.

Craik, F.I.M., & Lockhart, R.S. (1972) Levels of processing: A framework for memory research. *Journal of Verbal Learning and Verbal Behavior, 11*, 671–684.

Diller, L., & Weinberg, J. (1977). Hemi-attention in rehabilitation: The evaluation of a rationale remediation program. In R. Friedland (Ed.), *Advances in neurology* (pp. 179–202). New York: Raden.

Geschwind, N. (1982). Disorders of attention: A frontier in neuropsychology. In D.E. Broadbent & L. Weiscrantz (Eds.), *The neuropsychology of cognitive function* (pp. 173–185). London: Royal Society.

Head, H. (1926). The conception of nervous and mental energy. II vigilance: A physiological state of the nervous system. *British Journal of Psychology, 14*, 126–147.

James, W. (1890). *The principles of psychology.* New York: Holt.

Kahneman, D. (1973). *Attention and effort.* Englewood Cliffs. NJ: Prentice-Hall.

Kahneman, D., & Treisman, A. (1984). Changing views of attention and automaticity. In R. Parasurman (Ed.), *Varieties of attention* (pp. 29–61). London: Academic Press.

Kuhlman, E. (1904). Experimental studies in mental deficiency. *American Journal of Psychology, 15*, 391–446.

Luria, A.R. (1961). *The role of speech in the regulation of normal and abnormal behavior.* New York: Livingston.

Luria, A.R. (1982). *Language and cognition.* New York: Wiley.

Mack, J.L. (1986). Clinical assessment of disorders of attention and memory. *Journal of Head Trauma Rehabilitation, 1*(3), 22–34.

Meichenbaum, D.M. (1974). *Cognitive-behavior modification.* New York: Plenum Press.

Newcombe, F. (1985). The neuropsychology of consciousness. In D.A. Oakley (Ed.), *Brain and mind* (pp. 97–112). London: Methuen.

Nissen, N.J. (1986). Neuropsychology of attention and memory. *Journal of Head Trauma Rehabilitation, 1*(3), 13–22.

Parasurman, R. (1984). Sustained attention in detection and discrimination. In R. Parasurman (Ed.), *Varieties of attention* (pp. 243–271). London: Academic Press.

Ponsford, J.L., & Kinsella, G. (1988). Evaluation of a program for attention deficits following head injury. *Journal of Clinical and Experimental Neuropsychology.*

Posner, N.I., & Boies, S.W. (1971). Components of attention. *Psychological Review, 78*, 391–408.

Posner, N.I., & Rafal, R.D. (1987). Cognitive theories of attention and the rehabilitation of attentional deficits. In M. Meier, A. Benton, & L. Diller (Eds.), *Neuropsychological rehabilitation* (pp. 182–202). New York: Churchill Livingstone.

Reason, J. (1984). Lapses of attention in everyday life. In R. Parasurman (Ed.), *Varieties of attention* (pp. 515–549). London: Academic Press.

Schneider, W., Dumais, S., & Shiffrin,

R. (1984). Automatic and control processing and attention. In R. Parasurman (Ed.), *Varieties of attention* (pp. 95–107). London: Academic Press.

Shiffrin, R.M., & Schneider, W. (1977). Controlled and automatic human information processing. *Psychological Review, 84*, 127–190.

Strauss, A., & Kephart, N. (1947). *Psychopathology and education of the brain injured.* New York: Grune & Stratton.

Stuss, D.T., & Benson, D.F. (1986). *The frontal lobes.* New York: Raven Press.

Trexler, L. (1987). Neuropsychological rehabilitation in the United States. In M. Meier, A. Benton, & L. Diller (Eds.), *Neuropsychological rehabilitation* (pp. 437–460). London: Churchill Livingstone.

Van Zomeren, E., & Deelman, B. (1978). Long-term recovery of physical reaction time after closed head injury. *Journal of Neurology, Neurosurgery, and Psychiatry, 41*, 452–457.

Webster, J., & Scott, R. (1983). The effects of self-instructional training on attentional deficits following head injury. *Clinical Neuropsychology, 4*, 69–74.

Whyte, J. (1986). Outcome evaluation in the remediation of attention and memory deficits. *Journal of Head Trauma Rehabilitation, 1*(3), 64–72.

Wilson, B. (1984). Memory therapy in practice. In B. Wilson & N. Moffatt (Eds.), *Clinical management of memory problems* (pp. 89–112). London: Croom Helm.

Wood, R.L. (1986). Rehabilitation of patients with disorders of attention. *Journal of Head Trauma Rehabilitation, 1*(3), 43–54.

Wood, R.L. (1987). *Brain injury rehabilitation: A neurobehavioral approach.* London: Croom Helm.

Wood, R.L., & Fussey, I. (1987). Computer-based cognitive retraining: A controlled study. *International Disability Studies* (formerly *International Journal of Rehabilitation Medicine*), 9, 149–153.

16

Acquisition of Domain-Specific Knowledge in Patients with Organic Memory Disorders

ELIZABETH L. GLISKY

DANIEL L. SCHACTER

Memory disorders are among the most prevalent consequences of various kinds of cerebral trauma (for reviews, see Cermak, 1982; Hirst, 1982; Parkin, 1987; Schacter & Crovitz, 1977; Squire, 1987; Weiskrantz, 1985). Although memory impairments are typically associated with poor performance on standard laboratory tests of recall and recognition, they can also seriously affect an individual's ability to lead an independent life (Schacter, Glisky, & McGlynn, in press). With increasing numbers of people surviving closed head injury and other brain insults that produce memory problems, the need for effective rehabilitation techniques has increased and research activity has expanded correspondingly. Yet memory deficits have remained largely resistant to remedial efforts.

One reason for this is that most research concerning remediation of organic memory disorders has attempted either to restore memory function through the use of repetitive drills and exercises, or to teach patients how to use mnemonic strategies (i.e., visual imagery) that can be broadly applied in everyday life. Unfortunately, neither of these approaches has yet produced any clinically significant effects: The use of repetitive drills and exercises, which is based on the misguided notion that memory is like a muscle that can be strengthened through practice (e.g., Harris & Sunderland, 1981), has failed to provide any evidence of memory improvement; and attempts to teach mnemonic strategies have foundered because brain damaged patients have proven unable to use such strategies spontaneously in their daily lives (for more detailed discussion, see Glisky & Schacter, 1986a, 1986b; O'Connor & Cermak, 1987; Schacter & Glisky, 1986; Wilson, 1987).

In view of the lack of evidence for general improvements of memory function in various patient groups, we decided to focus on a more limited goal that seemed somewhat more realistic and perhaps useful: to help patients acquire specific knowledge and skills that could enable them to function more productively in a particular area or domain of everyday life. Accordingly, our approach to memory remediation is concerned with the acquisition of *domain-specific knowledge*—knowledge pertaining to a specific task, function, or subject that is or could be relevant to a patient's ability to function independently in the real world (Schacter & Glisky, 1986). This approach is based in part on recent theoretical and empirical developments concerning preserved memory abilities in amnesic patients, which have provided new insights into the nature of both normal and pathological memory processes.

The main purposes of the present paper are to review briefly the foundations of our approach to memory remediation, to describe a number of studies that have yielded positive outcomes both in the laboratory and in the real world, and to consider some promising new directions for future investigations.

EMPIRICAL AND CONCEPTUAL FOUNDATIONS OF THE DOMAIN-SPECIFIC APPROACH

Preserved Learning in Amnesic Patients

In recent years, it has become clear that memory impaired patients are capable of acquiring new facts about their everyday world. For example, patients have learned names of people in their environment (Dolan & Norton, 1977; Glasgow, Zeiss, Barrera, & Lewinsohn, 1977; Jaffe & Katz, 1975), appropriate hospital behaviors (Dolan & Norton, 1977; Seidel & Hodgkinson, 1979), details about their illness (McGlynn & Schacter, in press; Wilson, 1987), and information about daily living activities (Cermak, 1976). For the most part, however, knowledge acquired in these studies has been relatively simple, consisting of just a few discrete facts. More critically, in most instances, although they were able to learn the information, patients were unable to apply it in their daily lives. The newly acquired information seemed to remain isolated from the rest of their world knowledge (cf. O'Connor & Cermak, 1987).

Other studies have demonstrated that severely amnesic patients can acquire various perceptual, motor, and cognitive skills in a normal or nearly normal fashion. For example, patients have learned to perform rotary pursuit tasks (Milner, Corkin, & Teuber, 1968), read mirror-inverted text (Cohen & Squire, 1980; Moscovitch, 1984), and solve jigsaw puzzles (Brooks & Baddeley, 1976) at the same rate as normal subjects, although they may have no explicit recollection of the learning experience.

Preserved learning by amnesic patients has also been demonstrated in repetition priming tasks (e.g., Cermak, Talbot, Chandler, & Wolbarst, 1985; Diamond & Rozin, 1984; Graf & Schacter, 1985; Jacoby & Witherspoon, 1982; Schacter & Graf, 1986; Warrington & Weiskrantz, 1968, 1974), in which performance with respect to a stimulus is facilitated as a result of a single prior exposure to the same stimulus. For example, Warrington and Weiskrantz (1974) reported that after studying a list of words such as *chair, flame*, and so forth, amnesic patients were as likely as normal subjects to complete word stems such as *cha*_____ and *fla*_____ with words from the studied list, even though they could not explicitly remember that the words had been previously presented.

The foregoing findings have important implications for the remediation of memory disorders. The various demonstrations of preserved learning by amnesic patients suggest that it may be possible for patients to acquire knowledge in domains relevant to everyday life even though the knowledge may not be explicitly retrievable. Additionally, the results of the priming studies suggest that a possibly effective teaching method may be one that capitalizes on patients' positive responses to fragment cues. The goal of our research program was to explore these possibilities—to determine whether amnesic patients could acquire complex domain-specific knowledge that was applicable to everyday life and to assess the effectiveness of fragment cuing techniques in facilitating the acquisition of that knowledge. In addition, we hoped to establish whether such knowledge could be retained over long periods of time, and most importantly, whether the knowledge acquired in the laboratory could ultimately be used in real-world contexts.

Method of Vanishing Cues

Initial studies focused on the domain of knowledge relevant to the understanding and operation of a microcomputer. We selected this domain both for its practical relevance and for its theoretical significance. The computer has the potential to serve as a powerful compensatory device if memory impaired patients can learn how to operate it (e.g., Harris, 1984; Jones & Adam, 1979; Skilbeck, 1984; Wilson & Moffat, 1984). Additionally, computer knowledge represents a well-specified domain of interrelated facts and information that is well suited to the experimental study of complex learning (cf. Norman, 1978).

Our first study (Glisky, Schacter, & Tulving, 1986b) investigated whether memory impaired patients could acquire some of the vocabulary associated with the use of a microcomputer. Relatively little is known about vocabulary learning by amnesic patients and the little evidence that exists is negative (Gabrielli, Cohen, & Corkin, 1983). For this rcason, learning of vocabulary seemed like an ideal task in which to test the effectiveness of a new teaching technique. The teaching method that we developed was designed to tap patients' preserved memory abilities, specifically the ability to produce previously studied material in response to fragment cues. The basic idea of this technique, which we have called the *method of vanishing cues*, is to provide sufficient cue information on an initial learning trial to ensure elicitation of the correct response, and then to withdraw that information gradually across learning trials until the target is produced in the absence of cues.

The method of vanishing cues is similar to a procedure that Skinner (1958) found useful in developing programs for his teaching machines and to techniques that have been applied to teach normal and autistic children difficult discriminations (e.g., Schreibman & Charlop, 1981). Cue fading methods have also been used in cognitive rehabilitation programs to facilitate problem-solving behavior (e.g., Ben-Yishay et al., 1985) and to teach new behaviors to mentally handicapped individuals (e.g., Schaefer & Martin, 1975). There is also at least one report of the successful use of a first-letter cuing and fading technique with an amnesic Korsakoff patient who learned the location of his locker and the names of two hospital staff members (Jaffe & Katz, 1975). Many of the reports, however, are anecdotal, and administration of the techniques has lacked systematic control.

Our study compared the method of vanishing cues with a standard repetition procedure in which definitions and words were simply presented repeatedly without cues. Four memory impaired patients (three with closed head injuries and one postencephalitic) attempted to learn the definitions of 30 computer-related vocabulary items. In the vanishing cues condition, a definition was presented on Trial 1, for example, *to store a program*, and was followed by an ever-increasing fragment of the target word (i.e., *s*_____, *sa*____, *sav*___) until the subject was able to respond correctly with the word *save*. On subsequent trials, letters were gradually withdrawn from the fragment (i.e., *sav*___, *sa*____, *s*_____, ______) until eventually the definition was presented alone without any letter cues. If at any time patients were unable to produce the correct response, letters were added one at a time until the target was generated.

Results of this study demonstrated that (a) memory impaired patients were able to acquire 20 to 30 items of new vocabulary and produce them without letter cues, (b) learning was faster by the method of vanishing cues than by the standard repetition procedure, (c) the rate of learning for memory impaired patients was much slower than that for normal subjects, and (d) learning was durable with little forgetting over a 6-week retention interval. This evidence for learning and retention of vocabularly is particularly impressive in view of the fact that one of our patients was so severely amnesic that he could not even remember ever having performed the task—yet he was able to learn and retain almost all of the vocabulary items.

Two positive features of the method of vanishing cues are noteworthy. First, the procedure permits a systematic tracking of performance over time in terms of the number of letter cues required for correct responding. In the present study, as training continued, subjects needed progressively fewer letters to identify targets. This steady reduction of letter cues implied that learning was taking place even though patients were unable in the early trials to produce the correct responses when no cues were present. Second, all patients enjoyed learning by this method. Because a correct response is generated on every trial, training is a positive experience that is much less frustrating for patients than simple repetition.

Having demonstrated that memory impaired patients could acquire the basic vocabulary associated with a microcomputer, we embarked on a series of studies to explore whether patients could use this knowledge to learn how to operate a microcomputer. In all of these experiments, the method of vanishing cues served as the principal training technique.

Computer Learning in Memory Impaired Patients

Three interactive computer lessons were constructed to teach patients some of the basic operating procedures for an Apple IIe microcomputer. In the initial study (Glisky, Schacter, & Tulving, 1986a) four head injured patients with memory disorders of varying severity constituted the experimental group; a matched control group also participated. The three lessons were graded in complexity and required patients to learn and use correctly a total of nine different computer commands. For example, Lesson 1 focused on the PRINT command, which is used to display information on the computer screen, and the HOME command, which is used to clear the screen. Patients were instructed regarding the meanings of these commands, and then performed various tasks that required use of them. In Lesson 2, patients had to learn many new commands such as LIST, SAVE, CATALOG, and others; they were also introduced to the idea of a "program" and were taught to write brief programs that increased in complexity as training progressed. Lesson 3 introduced additional commands and taught patients how to edit their programs by adding, deleting, or changing lines. In each of the three lessons, learning proceeded via the method of vanishing cues. If patients failed to type the appropriate command, they pressed the RETURN key on the computer and were presented with letter-fragment cues. As in the vocabulary study, patients' progress was charted by tracking the number of letter cues required for successful performance.

All four head injured patients in our initial computer learning study successfully completed the three computer training programs. At the end of that time they could display messages on the screen, clear the screen, perform disk storage and retrieval functions, and write and edit simple programs. Even the most severely amnesic patient, who never remembered ever working on a computer despite more than 100 hours of training, nonetheless was able to learn all of the basic operations. Furthermore, the training techniques seemed to be broadly applicable. In a subsequent experiment (Glisky & Schacter, in press) similar findings were obtained with memory impaired patients of other etiologies, including ruptured aneurysm and encephalitis. In addition, it was demonstrated that the computer knowledge acquired by patients in these studies was retained, with little evidence of decay, over long periods of time (7 to 9 months).

Although patients learned to perform all of the procedures within the context of the training programs, their learning was far from normal. They required many more training trials (26 to 154) to achieve criterial levels of performance than did controls (10 to 28) and the knowledge that they acquired seemed to be qualitatively different. Patients' new learning could be characterized as "hyperspecific": It was bound to the stimulus characteristics of the training situation and was relatively inaccessible to cues other than those present during original learning. Patients had considerable difficulty responding to open-ended questions about what they had learned and could not specify appropriate computer commands when the wording of instructions was altered. Control subjects, on the other hand, had no particular problems with these tasks.

The results of these experiments provide some reasons for optimism concerning possibilities for the rehabilitation of memory disorders but they also suggest some caveats. First, on the positive side, patients with memory disorders of varying severity and etiology can acquire some complex knowledge and skills in the laboratory, including procedures necessary to perform basic operations on a microcomputer. It therefore seems reasonable to speculate that patients could be trained to use a microcomputer as an external aid outside of the laboratory to assist them in everyday living. Second, the vanishing cues technique could be used to teach patients complex knowledge in other domains (e.g., educational, vocational, domestic) that might enable them to handle problems of daily life independently. However, the inflexibility or hyperspecificity of learning achieved by patients implies that difficulties of transfer from the laboratory to the real world are likely. It is important therefore to test directly whether knowledge acquired in the laboratory can be used by patients in the real world and under what conditions. The next section describes a case study in which we attempted to teach a memory impaired patient knowledge and skills that had to be applied in an important domain of everyday life: the workplace.

VOCATIONAL TRAINING: EMPIRICAL CASE STUDIES

Computer-Related Work

Numerous studies of brain injured patients have cited memory impairment as a major obstacle to re-entry into the work force (Bond, 1975; Bruckner & Randle, 1972; Levin, Grossman, Rose, & Teasdale, 1979; Prigatano & Fordyce, 1986; Weddell, Oddy, & Jenkins, 1980). Because of their inability to remember the procedures required in even the simplest jobs, patients are often unable to obtain any kind of meaningful employment. We recently had the opportunity to investigate whether the vanishing cues procedure could be used to help a patient with serious memory problems acquire domain-specific knowledge necessary to perform a complex job (Glisky & Schacter, 1987).

The patient, H.D., was a 32-year-old woman who became severely amnesic as a result of herpes simplex encephalitis. Following her illness, H.D. was retained by her employer in a simple clerical position. When this job was subsequently eliminated from the company, however, the patient was considered to be untrainable for any of the remaining available jobs. On our recommendation, the employer agreed to allow us to attempt to train this patient for a part-time job within the corporation.

H.D. has a severe memory disorder; her memory quotient on the Wechsler Memory Scale is 65, which reflects substantial impairment. In addition she has a somewhat depressed IQ (84 on the Wechsler Adult Intelligence Scale–Revised) (Wechsler, 1981) and a slight dysnomia. However, she possesses excellent attentional abilities and is strongly motivated to learn new information and skills. H.D. had participated in our computer learning studies and had demonstrated that she was capable of learning complex material using the method of vanishing cues; she also had very good keyboard skills that she had acquired many years earlier as a typist. For these reasons we recommended a computer data-entry job as being well suited to her capabilities.

The job required a data-entry clerk to extract information from company documents called "meter cards" and enter it into a computer display consisting of nine columns with coded headings. Meter cards were all similar in appearance and relevant information appeared on all cards in the same location. However, varying amounts of irrelevant information also appeared on the cards and had to be ignored, and the mapping between cards and computer display was not straightforward. For example, the last six numbers of the eight-digit SERIAL NO. on the meter card had to be entered into the DOC # column of the computer display, and the date was entered in the reverse order to which it appeared on the card. The task was thus relatively complex, but once learned it remained invariant across trials and cards.

Performance of the job required learning of (a) the general terminology associated with the job, (b) the meaning of each of the nine coded headings in the computer display, (c) the document and operation codes, (d) the location and meaning of the information on the cards, (e) the mapping between cards and display, (f) the use of specific function keys on the computer keyboard, (g) the meaning of the correct response to error messages, and (h) the integration of all of these components into the correct sequence. In addition, the actual data-entry task had to be performed quickly; experienced clerks at the company required approximately 10 to 15 seconds to enter data from a single card into the computer.

The first three phases of job training were conducted in the laboratory, where we constructed a detailed simulation of the real-world job. In the first phase of training, H.D. attempted to learn, using the method of vanishing cues, the basic facts and concepts associated with the task. During this *knowledge acquisition* phase of training, 28 incomplete sentences were presented on the computer screen and H.D. was required to type the correct completions on the keyboard. For example, *Information from one document is entered into a single row and is called a* (blank) was to be completed with the word *record.* Sentences defined terms and concepts, explained column headings, and outlined card/computer mappings. Hints were provided, when needed, in the form of initial letters of the target word and were gradually vanished over trials.

On the first training trial, H.D. needed 60 hints and took 55 minutes to complete all sentences correctly. By the end of the 25th trial, however, she was performing perfectly without hints in approximately 9 minutes. She then entered the *skill acquisition* phase of training during which she actually performed the data-entry task with real meter cards. The purpose of this phase of training was to improve speed and efficiency of data entry. Across 15 training sessions (2 to 3 per week) and 2,440 meter cards, H.D.'s time to enter data from a single card declined from 63 seconds to 13 seconds, well within the range of speeds achieved by experienced operators. The third segment of laboratory training was concerned with the teaching of *special procedures* such as error-handling routines. Once again, H.D. showed steady learning across six training sessions.

The final phase of the experiment took place in the real world, where we assessed whether and to what extent the knowledge and skills acquired in the laboratory could be used on the job. Following an initial adjustment to minor differences between the laboratory simulation and the actual task, H.D. rapidly achieved error-free performance at speeds equivalent to those attained in the laboratory. Furthermore, despite spending only 2 to 3 days per month on the task, her speed continued to improve on the job over 3 months until performance asymptoted at approximately 10 seconds per card. H.D., at the time of this writing, is still performing this job on a regular part-time basis at a high level of efficiency. Interestingly, although her ability to recount some aspects of the job has improved with time and experience, she is still unable to report many details of the task despite her ability to perform it flawlessly.

Extending the Domain of Vocational Training: A Microfilming Job

Because of our success in training H.D. for the part-time data-entry job and because of her skill and efficiency in performing the task, H.D.'s employers were interested in having us teach H.D. another part-time job so that she could eventually be employed on a full-time basis. The new job required that H.D. learn to operate a microfilming machine for the purpose of filming several thousand medical records that were occupying much-needed space in filing cabinets.

This job differed from the data-entry job in that laboratory simulation of the task was impossible because of equipment requirements. For this task, therefore, we used labeled pictures of the apparatus and attempted to teach all aspects of the procedures in propositional form—similar to the knowledge acquisition phase of the previous study. Forty-five incomplete sentences that explained information, concepts, and operations required by the task were presented on the computer screen one at a time. H.D. had to type the correct completions on the computer keyboard with initial letter cues of the target responses being provided as cues if needed. Some sample sentences are illustrated in Figure 16.1.

H.D. once again started slowly; she required 73 minutes to complete the first trial and needed 129 hints to produce the correct responses. However, as shown in Table 16.1, performance improved steadily and after 31 trials across 11 training sessions, H.D. achieved error-free performance in 21 minutes.

At the same time as H.D. was learning the facts and procedures associated with the performance of the microfilming job, she was also involved in another aspect of job preparation that attempted to teach her the names and occupations of her new coworkers. Having observed in our previous study

Picture A shows the machine that you will be operating. The machine is called a ________. (MICROFILMER)
Picture B is a close-up diagram of the ________. (COPYBOARD)
At the right front of the copyboard, there are three switches or ________. (BUTTONS)
The button labeled #1 is called an ________. (INDICATOR LIGHT)
The indicator light is (color) ________. (RED)
When the film has reached the end of the roll, the red indicator light ________. (FLASHES)
Picture C is a close-up diagram of the ________. (CAMERA)
The part of the camera indicated by the number 1 is called the ________. (WINDING HANDLE)
When loading or unloading film from the camera, you turn the winding handle ________. (CLOCKWISE)
The number of turns you make is at least ________. (TEN)

Figure 16.1. Sample sentences from the microfilming training sessions with the correct completions shown in parentheses.

TABLE 16.1
Number of Hints and Time per Trial to Complete Correctly 45 Sentences Concerning the Microfilming Job

Sessions (3 trials/session)	Hints	Time (min)
1	129–109	73.2–41.4
2	97– 64	39.8–29.2
3	52– 28	40.0–34.6
4	23– 13	36.7–30.5
5	12– 8	29.1–27.4
6	7– 4	29.0–26.6
7	4– 2	28.1–24.2
8	2– 1	28.4–24.6
9	2– 1	24.6–22.0
10	2– 1	21.8–20.3
11	0	21.0

that H.D. was somewhat embarrassed by her inability to remember details about her work environment, we included this segment of training in an attempt to facilitate her social adjustment to her new surroundings. For the same reason, we included three sentences in the basic training program concerning the department and building in which the job was located.

To teach H.D. information about each of seven fellow employees, we presented her with a company photograph of the person, and three sentences on the computer screen. Sentences were as follows: *The first name of the person in photograph # 5 is* ____. When this sentence had been completed correctly with the name *Anne*, for example, the following sentence was displayed: *ANNE'S last name is* ____. After correct completion of this sentence, the final sentence read, *ANNE BLACK is the* ____, which was to be completed with the response *nurse*. The method of vanishing cues was again used to provide letter hints for the correct responses. The procedure was modified slightly from its usual format. To prevent random guessing of proper names on the initial trial, complete names were provided on Trial 1 and vanished a letter at a time on subsequent trials. The minimum possible number of hints on the first trial was therefore 78, which included all letters in the names. Occupations were generated as in previous experiments with letters being added on the first trial until a correct response was produced and then withdrawn across trials.

Results of the name/face learning study are presented in Table 16.2. Steady learning over trials is again evident with hints decreasing from 94 on

TABLE 16.2
Number of Hints and Time Taken to Complete 21 Sentences Concerning the Names of Fellow Employees and Their Jobs

Sessions (3 trials/session)	Hints	Time (min)
1	94–65	15.1–8.4
2	57–39	12.2–8.8
3	32–18	10.4–7.2
4	15–12	9.9–9.1
5	13– 5	8.1–7.2
6	8– 4	7.7–7.1
7	6– 4	9.0–7.5
8	4– 3	7.9–6.8
9	4– 3	7.8–6.8
10	2– 0	6.6–5.9
11	0	5.0

Trial 1 to zero by the end of 30 trials. Times decreased correspondingly. H.D. had some difficulty discriminating between three similar female faces, which she could not remember until she was given the first letter of the first name. This pattern of responding can be seen in Table 16.2 by the flat levels of performance in Sessions 8 and 9. Until that point in training, photographs had always been presented in a different random order on each trial. During the 10th session, this procedure was changed in an attempt to overcome her problems. On each of the three trials of Session 10, photographs were displayed on the table in a hierarchical order according to job description. This organizational framework appeared to eliminate the confusion that she had been experiencing. In Session 11, photographs were again presented in a random order, and performance was perfect.

It remained to be demonstrated whether such laboratory training would benefit on-the-job performance given that the actual job had never been performed except in the laboratory. Because the laboratory and real-world tasks were so different, we were not able to obtain direct measures of transfer. However, we provided two days of on-the-job practice on the microfilming task and then monitored H.D.'s performance continuously for 6 days and twice a week for 2 weeks thereafter. Our observations indicated that the patient was initially confused by the actual job situation and did not recognize various aspects of the task as being related to those learned in the laboratory. For example, she appeared not to be familiar with the microfilming equipment although it was identical to the apparatus in the photographs with which she had been trained. In addition, many features of the job were new to H.D.: the location of her work space, the procedures involved in removing and replacing files from the cabinets, some record-keeping chores, and so on.

However, she appeared to learn the task relatively quickly. Across the first 6 days, H.D.'s filming speed increased from approximately 12.3 seconds to 7.3 seconds per document. By this time, performance appeared to be relatively automatic and the patient was filming approximately 2,500 records per day, a number that the company considered to be more than satisfactory. She also learned to monitor for the end-of-film signal and to load and unload film from the camera without help. Although we could not be certain that on-the-job performance was enhanced by prior laboratory training (no control conditions were possible), the fact that she learned the task so readily is strongly suggestive of that conclusion.

Summary of Training Studies

The two foregoing studies demonstrate that it is possible to teach a patient with a severe memory disorder different kinds of complex domain-specific knowledge that can be applied in an important segment of everyday life.

Although we have demonstrated success with two different vocational tasks, we have as yet trained only a single patient. Generalizability of our findings to other patient groups, therefore, is uncertain until further investigations are conducted. On the basis of our research to date, however, we have reached some tentative conclusions concerning the types of jobs that are most likely to be appropriate for memory impaired patients and some of the potential pitfalls that might be encountered in vocational contexts.

First, suitable jobs are likely to be those that require a set of relatively invariant procedures. Patients appear able to learn complex tasks but are unable to cope with novel situations. Any variations on basic procedures thus disrupt performance unless the means of handling such variations are taught specifically. Second, it appears that complex tasks can be most easily learned if they are broken down into component steps with each component being taught explicitly and directly. This approach is well documented as an effective instructional technique with learning disabled individuals (e.g., Smith & Robinson, 1986) and similar task analysis approaches have been used in vocational training of severely retarded persons (e.g., Mithaug, 1979; Wacker & Hoffman, 1984; Wehman & Hill, 1981). Third, laboratory training should mimic the actual job situation as closely as possible in order to minimize transfer problems. Although much has yet to be discovered about the factors affecting transfer of training, we know that memory impaired patients experience serious difficulties when called upon to apply information learned in one setting to similar problems that occur in a different setting.

CONCLUDING COMMENTS

The research reported in this chapter represents an initial attempt to explore some of the conditions under which patients with memory disorders can acquire complex knowledge and skills in domains relevant to everyday life. Only a few domains have been investigated as yet and those with only a few patients. Nevertheless, the results are encouraging. In the domains that we have studied, we have not yet observed any limit on the amount or complexity of knowledge that can be acquired by amnesic patients. It is conceivable that although the learning process is slow, a great deal of knowledge can be acquired and retained by memory impaired patients that could significantly improve their ability to function independently in the real world.

Many directions for further research can be envisioned. Other domains of knowledge need to be explored—vocational, educational, social, and so on—and opportunities for nonsheltered employment might be considered for individuals with other kinds of handicaps (cf. Brown et al., 1986). The method of vanishing cues has proven to be an extremely effective technique for teaching new information to patients with memory deficits. Other intellectually or cognitively disabled populations, including children with cerebral trauma, may benefit similarly.

Problems involved in transfer will continue to occupy investigators concerned with training handicapped individuals to function in the real world. Until more is known about the factors affecting generalization to new contexts, the methods of training that seem most likely to be successful are those that focus on teaching each skill, fact, or procedure directly and explicitly in a context as similar as possible to that in which the information will ultimately be used. A major challenge for research will be to discover methods by which such learning can be made more flexible and thereby more useful in the endless variety of situations presented in everyday life.

REFERENCES

Ben-Yishay, Y., Rattok, J., Lakin, P., Piasetsky, E.G., Ross, B., Silver, S., Zide, E., & Ezrachi, O. (1985). Neuropsychological rehabilitation: Quest for a holistic approach. *Seminars in Neurology, 5*, 252–259.

Bond, M.R. (1975). Assessment of the psychosocial outcome after severe head injury. In *Outcome of severe damage to the C.N.S. Symposium 34* (pp. 141–153). London: Ciba Foundation.

Brooks, D.N., & Baddeley, A.D. (1976). What can amnesic patients learn? *Neuropsychologia, 14*, 111–122.

Brown, L., Shiraga, B., Ford, A., Nisbet, J., VanDeventer, P., Sweet, M., York, J., & Loomis, R. (1986). Teaching severely handicapped students to perform meaningful work in nonsheltered vocational environments. In R.J. Morris & B. Blatt (Eds.), *Special education: Research and trends* (pp. 131–189). New York: Pergamon.

Bruckner, F.E., & Randle, A.P.H. (1972). Return to work after severe head injuries. *Rheumatology and Physical Medicine, 11*, 344–348.

Cermak, L.S. (1976). The encoding capacity of a patient with amnesia due to encephalitis. *Neuropsychologia, 14*, 311–322.

Cermak, L.S. (Ed.). (1982). *Human memory and amnesia.* Hillsdale, NJ: Erlbaum.

Cermak, L.S., Talbot, N., Chandler, K., & Wolbarst, L.R. (1985). The perceptual priming phenomenon in amnesia. *Neuropsychologia, 23*, 615–622.

Cohen, N.J., & Squire, L.R. (1980). Preserved learning and retention of pattern-analyzing skill in amnesia: Dissociation of "knowing how" and "knowing that." *Science, 210*, 207–209.

Diamond, R., & Rozin, P. (1984). Activation of existing memories in the amnesic syndrome. *Journal of Abnormal Psychology, 93*, 98–105.

Dolan, M.P., & Norton, J.C. (1977). A programmed training technique that uses reinforcement to facilitate acquisition and retention in brain-damaged patients. *Journal of Clinical Psychology, 33*, 496–501.

Gabrielli, J.D.E., Cohen, N.J., & Corkin, S. (1983). The acquisition of lexical and semantic knowledge in amnesia. *Society for Neuroscience Abstracts, 9*, 238.

Glasgow, R.E., Zeiss, R.A., Barrera, M., & Lewinsohn, P.M. (1977). Case studies on remediating memory deficits in brain-damaged individuals. *Journal of Clinical Psychology, 33*, 1049–1054.

Glisky, E.L., & Schacter, D.L. (1986). Remediation of organic memory disorders: Current status and future prospects. *Journal of Head Trauma Rehabilitation, 1*(3), 54–63.

Glisky, E.L., & Schacter, D.L. (1987). Acquisition of domain-specific knowledge in organic amnesia: Training for computer-related work. *Neuropsychologia, 25*, 893–906.

Glisky, E.L., & Schacter, D.L. (in press). Long-term retention of computer learning by patients with memory disorders. *Neuropsychologia.*

Glisky, E.L., Schacter, D.L., & Tulving, E. (1986a). Computer learning by memory-impaired patients: Acquisition and retention of complex knowledge. *Neuropsychologia, 24*, 313–328.

Glisky, E.L., Schacter, D.L., & Tulving, E. (1986b). Learning and retention of computer-related vocabulary in memory-impaired patients: Method of vanishing cues. *Journal of Clinical and Experimental Neuropsychology, 8*, 292–312.

Graf, P., & Schacter, D.L., (1985). Implicit and explicit memory for new associations in normal and amnesic subjects. *Journal of Experimental Psychology: Learning, Memory, and Cognition, 11*, 501–518.

Harris, J. (1984). Methods of improving memory. In B.A. Wilson & N. Moffat (Eds.), *Clinical management of memory problems* (pp. 46–62). Rockville, MD: Aspen Systems.

Harris, J.E., & Sunderland, A. (1981). A brief survey of the management of memory disorders in rehabilitation units in Britain. *International Rehabilitation Medicine, 3*, 206–209.

Hirst, W. (1982). The amnesic syndrome: Descriptions and explanations. *Psychological Bulletin, 91*, 435–460.

Jacoby, L.L., & Witherspoon, D. (1982). Remembering without awareness. *Canadian Journal of Psychology, 36*, 300–324.

Jaffe, P.G., & Katz, A.N. (1975). Attenuating anterograde amnesia in Korsakoff's psychosis. *Journal of Abnormal Psychology, 34*, 559–562.

Jones, G.H., & Adam, J.H. (1979). Towards a prosthetic memory. *Bulletin of the British Psychological Society, 32*, 165–167.

Levin, H.S., Grossman, R.G., Rose, J.E., & Teasdale, G. (1979). Long-term Neuropsychological outcome of closed head injury. *Journal of Neurosurgery, 50*, 412–422.

McGlynn, S.M., & Schacter, D.L. (in press). Unawareness of deficits in neuropsychological syndromes. *Journal of Clinical and Experimental Neuropsychology.*

Milner, B., Corkin, S., & Teuber, H.L. (1968). Further analysis of the hippocampal amnesic syndrome: 14 year follow-up study of H.M. *Neuropsychologia, 6*, 215–234.

Mithaug, D. (1979). The relation between programmed instruction and task analysis in the prevocational training of severely and profoundly handicapped persons. *American Association for the Education of the Severely/Profoundly Handicapped Review, 4*, 162–178.

Moscovitch, M. (1984). The sufficient conditions for demonstrating preserved memory in amnesia: A task analysis. In L.R. Squire & N. Butters (Eds.), *Neuropsychology of memory* (pp. 104–114). New York: Guilford.

Norman, D.A. (1978). Notes toward a theory of complex learning. In A.M. Lesgold, J. Pellegrino, S. Fokkema, & R. Glaser (Eds.), *Cognitive psychology and instruction* (pp. 39–48). New York: Plenum.

O'Connor, M., & Cermak, L.S. (1987). Rehabilitation of organic memory disorders. In M.J. Meier, A. Benton, & L. Diller (Eds.), *Neuropsychological rehabilitation* (pp. 260–279). New York: Guilford.

Parkin, A.J. (1987). *Memory and amnesia*. London: Basil Blackwell.

Prigatano, G.P., & Fordyce, D.J. (1986). Cognitive dysfunction and psychosocial adjustment after brain injury. In G.P. Prigatano and Others, *Neuropsychological rehabilitation after brain injury* (pp. 1–17). Baltimore: Johns Hopkins University Press.

Schacter, D.L., & Crovitz, H.F. (1977). Memory function after closed head injury: A review of the quantitative research. *Cortex, 13*, 150–176.

Schacter, D.L., & Glisky, E.L. (1986). Memory remediation: Restoration, alleviation, and the acquisition of domain-specific knowledge. In B. Uzzell & Y. Gross (Eds.), *Clinical neuropsychology of intervention* (pp. 257–282). Boston: Martinus Nijhoff.

Schacter, D.L., Glisky, E.L., & McGlynn, S.M. (in press). Impact of memory disorder on everyday life: Awareness of deficits and return to work. In D. Tupper & K. Cicerone (Eds.), *The neuropsychology of everyday life. Vol. I. Theories and basic competencies*. Boston: Martinus Nijhoff.

Schacter, D.L., & Graf, P. (1986). Preserved learning in amnesic patients: Perspectives from research on direct priming. *Journal of Clinical and Experimental Neuropsychology, 8*, 727–743.

Schaefer, H.H., & Martin, P.L. (1975). Teaching new behaviors to the mentally retarded. In H.H. Schaefer & P.L. Martin (Eds.), *Behavioral therapy* (pp. 242–253). New York: McGraw-Hill.

Schreibman, L., & Charlop, M.J. (1981). S+ versus S− fading in prompting procedures with autistic children. *Journal of Experimental Child Psychology, 31*, 508–520.

Seidel, H., & Hodgkinson, P.E. (1979). Behavior modification and long-term learning in Korsakoff's psychosis. *Nursing Times, 75*, 1855–1857.

Skilbeck, C. (1984). Computer assistance in the management of memory and cognitive impairment. In B.A. Wilson & N. Moffat (Eds.), *Clinical management of memory problems* (pp. 112–133). Rockville, MD: Aspen Systems.

Skinner, B.F. (1958). Teaching machines. *Science, 128*, 969–977.

Smith, D.D., & Robinson, S. (1986). Educating the learning disabled. In R.J. Morris & B. Blatt (Eds.), *Special education: Research and trends* (pp. 222–248). New York: Pergamon.

Squire, L.R. (1987). *Memory and brain*. New York: Oxford University Press.

Wacker, D.P., & Hoffman, R.C. (1984). Vocational rehabilitation of severely handicapped persons. In C.J. Golden (Ed.), *Current topics in rehabilitation psychology* (pp. 139–171). Orlando, FL: Grune & Stratton.

Warrington, E.K., & Weiskrantz, L. (1968). New method of testing long-term retention with special reference to amnesic patients. *Nature, 217*, 972–974.

Warrington, E.K., & Weiskrantz, L. (1974). The effect of prior learning on subsequent retention in amnesic patients. *Neuropsychologia, 12*, 419–428.

Wechsler, D. (1981). *Wechsler adult intelligence scale–Revised* (manual).

New York: Psychological Corp.

Weddell, R., Oddy, M., & Jenkins, D. (1980). Social adjustment after rehabilitation: A two year follow-up of patients with severe head injury. *Psychological Medicine, 10*, 257–263.

Wehman, P., & Hill, J.W. (1981). Competitive employment for moderately and severely handicapped individuals. *Exceptional Children, 47*, 338–345.

Weiskrantz, L. (1985). On issues and theories of the human amnesic syndrome. In N. Weinberger, J. McGaugh, & G. Lynch (Eds.), *Memory systems of the brain: Animal and human cognitive processes* (pp. 380–415). New York: Guilford.

Wilson, B. (1987). *Rehabilitation of memory.* New York: Guilford.

Wilson, B., & Moffat, N. (1984). Rehabilitation of memory for everyday life. In J.E. Harris & P. Morris (Eds.), *Everyday memory: Actions and absent-mindedness* (pp. 207–233). London: Academic Press.

PART IV

OUTCOME ISSUES

17

Chronic Emotional, Social, and Physical Changes After Traumatic Brain Injury

MURIEL D. LEZAK

KEVIN P. O'BRIEN

The presence of emotional, behavioral, and personality change after head injury has been long recognized (Goldstein, 1942; Harlow, 1868; Luria, 1966). More recently, the effects of these characterological changes on family, occupational, and social relationships have increasingly been receiving attention (Bond, 1975; Brooks, 1984; Brooks & McKinlay, 1983; Levin, Benton, & Grossman, 1982; Lezak, 1978; Oddy, Humphrey, & Uttley, 1978; Rosenbaum & Najenson, 1976). The findings from these studies suggest that traumatically brain injured (TBI) patients are much more seriously handicapped by emotional and personality disturbance than by their residual cognitive and physical disabilities.

Many of the more frequently observed characterological changes following brain injury have been identified (see Table 17.1). Recently, Prigatano and his colleagues (Prigatano and Others, 1986) presented a schema for classifying personality disorders after brain injury. They described three overlapping and

This research was supported in part by VA Medical Research Service Grant No. 648-5243.

TABLE 17.1
Summary of Personality Changes Reported After Brain Injury

Symptom	Studies[a]
Agitation	8
Aggressiveness	3,5
Anger (increased)	3,7,8
Anxiety	3,5,6,8
Apathy	1,3,4,5,6,7,8
Blunted or restricted affect	1,5
Childishness	2,4,8
Denial of illness	1,8
Depression	2,3,4,5,6,8
Diminished self-awareness	1,8
Disinhibition	2,3,5
Euphoria	2,3,5
Facetiousness/fatuousness	1,2
Helplessness/increased social dependency	4,8
Hopelessness	8
Impatient/more easily frustrated	3,4,7,8
Impulsivity	1,3,4,8
Indifference	2
Irritability	1,2,3,4,5,6,7,8
Lability	1,4,5,8
Misperception of the intentions or actions of others	4,8
Paranoid/delusional thinking	3,4,8,9
Phobias	3,5,6,8
Restlessness	2,4,7
Sexual interest (more/less)	4
Socially inappropriate comments	8
Suspiciousness/distrustfulness	8,9
Withdrawal	1,8

[a]1. Alexander (1982); 2. Heilman & Satz (1983); 3. Leigh (1979); 4. Lezak (1978); 5. Lishman (1978); 6. Merskey & Woodforde (1972); 7. Oddy, Humphrey, & Uttley (1978); 8. Prigatano and Others (1986); 9. Prigatano, O'Brien, & Klonoff (in press).

broad categories that encompass most of the behavioral problems frequently encountered in the clinical setting: *reactionary* (involves disturbances reactive to alterations in perceptions, capacities, and situations due to the brain injury); *neuropsychologically based* (refers to those mental and behavioral disturbances directly associated with tissue damage and physiological abnormalities); and *characterological* (involves dysfunctional behaviors arising from premorbid personality predispositions). Such distinction may be useful in formulating appropriate clinical interventions (Crosson, 1987; Prigatano and Others, 1986).

Until recently most studies have provided information about the psychosocial and emotional problems of TBI patients based on one or two follow-up assessments (Dikmen, McLean, & Temkin, 1986; Elsass & Kinsella, 1987; Van Zomeren & Van den Burg, 1985), although there are some exceptions (Crawford, 1983; Oddy, Coughlan, Tyerman, & Jenkins, 1985). Serial longitudinal studies of the emotional and personality status of TBI patients have been lacking. Yet increased understanding regarding the course of neuropsychologically based personality changes or the development of reactionary emotional and psychosocial problems may lead to more effective clinical management, as well as improvement of long-term planning for many TBI patients. The study reported here is offered as one effort toward enhancing this understanding.

The findings reported here come from a long-term study of the psychological consequences of brain injury that originally was planned to measure cognitive changes (Lezak, 1987). However, as the study proceeded, the importance of social competency to the TBI patient's quality of life and capacity for rehabilitation or employment became increasingly obvious. For example, of 39 TBI patients who were examined during their third post-accident year, only 18 were working or attending school; and of that 18, just 6 were functioning at levels consonant with their premorbid educational or vocational status.

The overall losses in vocational status reflect only one aspect of these patients' psychosocial dislocations. Five years posttrauma, 5 of these patients had had psychiatric hospitalizations, 6 were in aftercare facilities (e.g., nursing homes, domiciliaries), 1 had served a jail sentence, and 11 were known to have been involved in subsequent accidents, nearly all motor vehicle accidents. Significant speech problems were rare; most patients exhibited grossly intact levels of cognitive functioning in most areas (Lezak, 1979; O'Brien & Lezak, 1982) and displayed a practically adequate motor competency. However, emotional and social disturbances persisted for many.

Therefore this study soon took on the additional objective of documenting sequentially the emotional and psychosocial consequences of head trauma. A questionnaire, the Portland Adaptability Inventory (PAI) (Lezak, 1987), was developed following the broad outlines of a similar behavioral inventory offered by Bond (1975), but it was modified to deal with both the short- and long-term behavioral and social adjustment problems of our patients and with the psychometric requirements of such an instrument (see Appendix). An instrument specifically designed to examine problems relevant to head injured persons avoids the potential biases of objective tests, which typically have been standardized on normal (Alexander, 1982) or psychiatric samples (Levin & Grossman, 1978). Moreover, PAI scores may be based on reports by patients and family members—subject to the judgment of the interviewer—as well as trained observers. Situational data determine some PAI scores (e.g., Is the patient working? Driving a car?). Thus a wider range of information is available than can be obtained by self-report alone (e.g., Merskey & Woodforde, 1972) or by relative or caregiver ratings (e.g., Oddy et al., 1978; Prigatano and Others, 1986). The PAI made it possible to trace systematically the course of, and to some extent, the interrelationships among, personality dimensions, social consequences, and some perceptual, motor, and language competencies of a group of TBI patients.

METHOD

Clinical Sample

Subjects were 42 unselected white male patient volunteers with a history of TBI (see Table 17.2). Two-thirds of them had received their injuries in motor vehicle accidents. At the time of injury their mean age was 27.1 years ($SD = 7.4$), and on average they had completed 12.4 years ($SD = 2.2$) of formal education. Seventeen were unconscious less than 2 weeks and 25 were unconscious longer than 2 weeks. None had a prior psychiatric history.

Each patient had been injured less than a year when first examined. Most patients received a neuropsychological examination within the first 6 months ($n = 33$), at 6 to 12 months postinjury ($n = 39$), and in the second and third years. Some patients missed one or two follow-up examinations, which accounts for the differences in the number of patients evaluated in each time period. Nearly two-thirds of the total sample ($n = 26$) received fourth-year examinations and over half were also seen 5 years postinjury. Thus this study covers the six examination periods beginning with two in the first year posttrauma and once in each of the 4 subsequent years.

Procedure

Material: The Portland Adaptability Inventory (PAI). A detailed description of the administration, scoring, and item content of the PAI is available elsewhere (Lezak, 1987). Each item in the PAI is based on a 4-point scale in which 0 reflects no impairment or disturbance. Scores of 1, 2, and 3 represent mild, moderate, and severe degrees of difficulty, respectively. Judgments of severity on the Temperament and Emotionality (T/E) section are keyed to

TABLE 17.2
Descriptive Data
(N = 42)

Variable		
Age	Mean:	27.1
	SD:	7.4
Education	Mean:	12.4
	SD:	2.2
Sex	males:	100%
		N
Unconsciousness (duration)	< 1 day:	8
	< 2 weeks:	9
	> 2 weeks:	23
	> 1 month:	2
Etiology	MVA[a]:	28 (67%)
	blow to head:	7 (17%)
	fall:	5 (12%)
	other:	2 (5%)

[a]Motor vehicle accident.

observations. Patients' complaints for which there are no supporting observations merit a score of only 1; scores of 2 or 3 are based on the examiner's observations or reports from third persons (e.g., family members, medical personnel). The criteria for most of the Activities of Social Behavior (ASB) and Physical Capabilities (PC) scale items refer to objectively verifiable events, situations, or behaviors.

Data Collection. At the time that each patient volunteer was given his regularly scheduled cognitive examinations, the neuropsychological technician obtained the information covered by the PAI items, using all available resources to get as complete and accurate reports as possible. Since the PAI portion of the study was initiated after the earliest entered patients had been examined—a few as many as three times—the technician's extensive notes and reports, hospital records, correspondence, and reports from other sources provided the information for scoring the PAI in these instances.

Data Analysis. All PAI items were included in this analysis except ASB 8, 9, and 10 (Law Violation, Drugs, and Alcohol, respectively), for which too few positive scores were obtained for meaningful evaluation. For the remaining 21 items, the proportion of patients obtaining scores of 2 or 3 (i.e., those exhibiting moderate to severe impairment) were computed for each of the six time periods. These data were then visually inspected for patterns and trends. Changes over time were evaluated by means of nonparametric statistical tests (i.e., Fisher Exact Probability or X^2 test for k independent samples). Third-year relationships between measures of independence (Self-care, Residence, and Driving) and measures of psychosocial functioning (Work/School, Leisure, and Significant Relationships) also were evaluated nonparametrically.

Analyses of items that compared patients with no problems (i.e., scores of 0) to those with mild or greater difficulty (i.e., scores of 1, 2, or 3) also were conducted and have been reported elsewhere (Lezak, 1987). This report examines the course of aspects of temperament and emotion, social behavior, and physical status in which a significant degree of difficulty (i.e., moderate or greater) emerged.

RESULTS

Patterns of Change

Table 17.3 shows considerable variability among items with respect to change over time. (Some of the very small differences between time periods reflect changes in sample sizes rather than number of patients with problems.) For patients showing moderate to severe impairment (i.e., scoring 2 or 3), three patterns emerged over the six time periods.

First, a pattern of continuing difficulty was very common. Seven Temperament and Emotionality and Activities and Social Behavior areas (Anger, Anxiety, Significant Relationships, Social Contacts, Work/School, Driving, and Appropriate Social Interaction) continued as significant problems for more than one-third of the patients through the fifth year. Two of them (Social Contacts, Work/School) remained problem areas for the majority of patients. Anger was an enduring problem for 31% to 64% of the sample at any given time period. Problems with Significant Relationships were evident in 22% to 36% of the patients throughout the study.

The only exception to this picture of continuing impairment was provided by a subgroup of eight men with relatively minor injuries (i.e., length of unconsciousness less than 24 hours, if at all). Five of them had returned to work by the end of the fifth year and three were working at or near premorbid levels.

A second pattern was characterized by rapid or marked improvement over time. For example, initially, more than 60 of the patients had significant difficulty with Initiative, living independently (Residence and Self-care), Leisure activities, and Ambulation. Forty-five percent had significant difficulties with aphasia. However, by the fifth year, the proportion of patients showing problems in each of these areas had decreased threefold. For all items, change over time was statistically significant (i.e., X^2 for independent samples, $p < .05$).

A third pattern emerged in which improvement was slower, more variable over time, or of less magnitude. For example, the proportion of patients with driving problems or inappropriate social interaction decreased by 5% or more for nearly all time periods during the first 5 years postinjury. In contrast, the proportion of patients showing significant problems with Anxiety and Depression actually *increased* initially (i.e., from the 6-month to 12-month follow-up evaluations) before decreasing. However, these areas were significant problems for less than one-third of the sample by the third year. For Anxiety, Depression, Driving, and Appropriate Social Interaction items, change was statistically significant ($p < .05$). A trend for improvement for Anger did not reach statistical significance ($p < .10$).

Patients' Status at 3-Year Follow-up

In the third year, only those relatively few patients who enjoyed a full return to independence as indicated by zero scores on Residence, Self-care, and Driving were likely to have resumed normal family relationships and a premorbid level of work or school activities. For the rest, although many had improved over time, their increased capacities for independence were generally not associated with concomitant success in maintaining close relationships, holding a job or going to school, or for effective use of leisure time (see Table 17.4). However, there were two exceptions: ability for Driving was associated with a better Work/School outcome, and Self-care skills were associated with the ability to engage in Leisure activities satisfactorily.

Psychiatric Disorders

In any given time period, 12% to 28% of these patients exhibited behavior for which they received psychiatric diagnoses. At one time or another, 19 (45%) displayed symptoms of Delusions and Hallucinations, Paranoia, or both kinds of ideational disturbance. Eight patients (29%) experienced these problems for three or more time periods. Since none of the group had prior psychiatric histories, these data suggest that posttraumatic psychiatric prob-

TABLE 17.3
Percentage of Patients Obtaining Scores of 2 to 3 on Items of the Portland Adaptability Inventory (PAI) over Six Time Periods[a]

PAI Subtests	Time Since Injury (mo) 0–6 (N = 33)	7–12 (N = 38)	13–24 (N = 36)	25–36 (N = 40)	37–48 (N = 26)	49–60 (N = 23)	X^2
Temperament and Emotionality							
Anger	64	63	61	54	31	39	+[b]
Anxiety	51	58	44	31	45	39	*
Indifference	5	0	0	0	0	0	+
Depression	48	66	50	33	19	22	***
Delusions and Hallucinations	21	21	14	5	4	13	
Paranoia	15	13	14	13	8	13	
Initiative	64	53	36	21	19	22	***
Activities of Social Behavior							
Significant Relationships	22	32	36	31	27	35	
Residence	88	26	22	15	15	22	***
Social Contacts	84	74	70	56	65	74	
Self-care	68	42	22	10	12	13	***
Work/School	94	90	75	74	73	83	
Leisure	76	55	33	15	19	22	***
Driving	88	76	61	54	38	44	***
Law Violation	0	0	0	3	4	0	
Appropriate Social Interaction	73	58	44	41	31	39	*

TABLE 17.3 (cont.)

PAI Subtests	0–6 ($N = 33$)	7–12 ($N = 38$)	13–24 ($N = 36$)	25–36 ($N = 40$)	37–48 ($N = 26$)	49–60 ($N = 23$)	X^2
	Time Since Injury (mo)						
Physical Capabilities							
Ambulation	61	40	28	18	23	17	**
Hands	18	10	11	10	8	25	
Auditory	0	3	0	0	0	0	
Vision	33	37	33	38	31	35	
Dysarthria	27	18	16	13	15	17	
Aphasia	45	34	19	18	12	4	**

Note. Adapted from "Relationships Between Personality Disorders, Social Disturbances, and Physical Disability Following Traumatic Brain Injury" by M.D. Lezak, 1987, *Journal of Head Trauma Rehabilitation, 2,* 57–69.

[a]Scores of 2 and 3 represent moderate and severe impairment (see text).

[b]Based on X^2 test for k independent samples (proportion of patients scoring 0,1 versus 2,3 across six time periods).

$+p < .10$; $^*p < .05$; $^{**}p < .01$; $^{***}p < .001$.

TABLE 17.4
Relationship Between Indicators of Independence and Components of Psychosocial Functioning

Indicators of Independence	Components of Psychosocial Functioning: Significant Relationships X^2	Work/School X^2	Leisure X^2
Residence	0.222[a]	0.002	0.271
Self-care	0.050	0.543	7.601*
Driving	1.044	8.166*	1.277

Note. Adapted from "Relationships Between Personality Disorders, Social Disturbances, and Physical Disability Following Traumatic Brain Injury" by M.D. Lezak, 1987, *Journal of Head Trauma Rehabilitation, 2,* 57–69.

*p <.01. [a]Comparisons were between scores of no or mild impairment and those of moderate or severe impairment (i.e., 0,1 vs. 2,3).

lems, including full-blown posttraumatic psychoses requiring hospitalization, may be relatively common sequelae of traumatic brain injuries.

Physical Impairment

In general, two patterns of change appeared to characterize the Physical Capabilities items over time. First, as noted for the Temperament and Emotionality, and for Activities and Social Behavior items, there was a pattern of continuing difficulty. In the fifth year, more than one-third of the sample had persistent disturbances of vision (e.g., diplopia), and one-fourth had diminished or altered use of hands. Although changes in Ambulation and Dysarthria were less significant problems, these were still areas of difficulty for 17% of the sample. In contrast, significant Auditory impairment was reported in just one time period by only one patient.

On a positive note, two items documented a second pattern of rapid or marked improvement. During the initial evaluation, approximately one-half to two-thirds of the sample had moderate to severe difficulties with Ambulation or Aphasia. However, these problems improved significantly over time for the majority of patients. For example, by the fifth year postinjury just 17% had moderate and/or severe difficulty walking and only one patient had moderate to severe deficits in communicating or understanding language. Physical disability did not figure prominently among the patients showing serious emotional/social disturbances.

DISCUSSION AND CONCLUSIONS

A relatively high incidence of emotional, social, and physical problems was observed in this unselected group of patients. Recall that many had suffered what would be considered mild brain injuries (i.e., loss of consciousness less than 24 hours). Consequently, it would be expected that the incidence of emotional, social, and physical difficulties would be higher in samples composed of more severely injured patients.

For our sample, in all time periods the areas in which impairments were most frequently noted were related to social adjustment (i.e., Work/School, Social Contacts, Driving, and Appropriate Social Interaction). These difficulties reflect widespread and persistent social dislocation and social withdrawal among traumatically brain injured patients. Furthermore, diminished social contact and frank social isolation remained persistent problems for many patients despite improvement trends for such emotional and behavioral disturbances as depression, anxiety, capacity to take the initiative, and general social competency. It is noteworthy that feelings of loneliness, dissatisfaction with interpersonal relationships, and loss of interest in premorbid leisure and recreational pursuits are common complaints of brain injured victims, even among those who may not be significantly depressed or obviously impaired.

Some areas of difficulty persisted for many patients, while improvement was noted in others, though the rate of progress varied. Since none of these patients had participated in a formal brain injury rehabilitation program (although a number had received speech, physical, or occupational therapy, mostly while still hospitalized), in general these data reflect spontaneous (i.e., untreated) improvement. It is interesting to speculate whether rehabilitative intervention could reduce the likelihood or severity of postinjury emotional/behavioral changes.

Contrary to what was observed for most areas of emotional, social, and physical functioning, the proportion of patients exhibiting difficulty with anxiety, depression, and significant relationships actually increased during the first 12 to 24 months postinjury. Then, continued improvement was generally seen through the third or fourth year. This pattern suggests that although patients typically improve most rapidly during the first 6 to 12 months postinjury, increased awareness of their altered status may be accompanied by emotional distress, at least initially. Similar observations have been reported by Prigatano and his colleagues (Prigatano and Others, 1986).

Working in a rehabilitation setting, Prigatano observed that many patients tend to misjudge the severity of their deficits. Consequently, many patients attempt to return to work and resume previous social activities relatively soon after release from the hospital. If occupational and social demands exceed postinjury cognitive and physical capacities, patients typically become frustrated and unable to cope. Faced with this failure in the environment, patients tend to withdraw to a safer or more constricted milieu. This hypothesis may account for the pattern observed in our patient sample: Although there was improvement over time with regard to anxiety and depression, problems with social isolation and diminished social contact persisted.

The observation of increased disturbance and disruption of social relationships 6 to 12 months postinjury also has been documented in reports by family members (Oddy, 1984; Vigouroux et al., 1971). Patients and family members alike do not expect the patient's personality to change. Initially, family members tend to overlook or downplay the patient's altered, inappropriate, or irritable behavior. It may take 6 months to a year or more for family members to begin to realize the extent and possible permanence of the patient's cognitive, emotional, and/or behavioral difficulties. Moreover, aspects of the patient's postinjury functional status have been linked to the emotional adjustment of family members 1 to 4 years postinjury. O'Brien (1986), for example, reported a statistically significant association between offspring psychosocial impairment (which includes emotional and social behavior) and the degree of parental anxiety, depression, and emotional distress.

Given that nearly 40% of the sample evaluated in the fifth year postinjury experienced moderate to severe problems with anger, it is not surprising that many reported significant difficulty in forming or maintaining social relationships. The socially destructive role of anger also was suggested by Oddy et al. (1978), who found similar social problems in a sample of generally younger patients seen 6 months postinjury. However, poor anger control alone does not account for the extensive social maladaptations suffered by so many of these patients. Rather, it appears to be one of many personality and temperament characteristics that contribute to their social failures (Lezak, 1978; Prigatano and Others, 1986).

All in all, these findings suggest that the most significant behavioral sequelae of traumatic brain injury involve capacities for getting and keeping a job, making constructive use of one's time, and forming and maintaining satisfying interpersonal relationships. Moreover, these sequelae are not transient phenomena for many head injured patients. Persistent emotional, social, and physical difficulties were seen in many patients as long as 5 years postinjury with no indication that they would improve spontaneously.

REFERENCES

Alexander, M.P. (1982). Traumatic brain injury. In D.F. Benson & D. Blumer (Eds.), *Psychiatric aspects of neurologic disease: Vol. II* (pp. 239–341). New York: Grune & Stratton.

Bond, M.R. (1975). Assessment of psychosocial outcome after severe head injury. *Ciba Foundation Symposium, 34*, 141–157.

Brooks, D.N. (1984). Head injury and the family. In D.N. Brooks (Ed.), *Closed head injury* (pp. 123–147). Oxford: Oxford University Press.

Brooks, D.N., & McKinlay, W. (1983). Personality and behavioral change after severe blunt head injury—A relative's view. *Journal of Neurology, Neurosurgery, and Psychiatry, 46*, 336–344.

Crawford, C. (1983). Social problems after severe head injury. *New Zealand Medical Journal, 96*, 972–974.

Crosson, B. (1987). Treatment of interpersonal deficits for head-trauma patients in inpatient rehabilitation settings. *The Clinical Neuropsychologist, 1*, 335–352.

Dikman, S., McLean, A., & Temkin, N. (1986). Neuropsychological and psychosocial consequences of minor head injury. *Journal of Neurology, Neurosurgery, and Psychiatry, 49*, 1227–1232.

Elsass, L., & Kinsella, G. (1987). Social interaction following severe closed head injury. *Psychological Medicine, 17*, 67–78.

Goldstein, K. (1942). *Aftereffects of brain injuries in war*. New York: Grune & Stratton.

Harlow, J.M. (1868). Recovery after severe injury to the head. *Publication of the Massachusetts Medical Society (Boston), 2*, 327–346.

Heilman, K.M., & Satz, P. (1983). *Neuropsychology of human emotion*. New York: Guilford.

Leigh, D. (1979). Psychiatric aspects of head injury. *Psychiatry Digest, 40*, 21–33.

Levin, H.S., Benton, A.L., & Grossman, R.G. (1982). *Neurobehavioral consequences of closed head injury* (pp. 172–188). New York: Oxford University Press.

Levin, H.S., & Grossman, R.G. (1978). Behavioral sequelae of closed head injury. *Archives of Neurology, 35*, 720–727.

Lezak, M.D. (1978). Living with the characterologically altered brain injured patient. *Journal of Clinical Psychiatry, 39*, 592–598.

Lezak, M.D. (1979). Recovery of memory and learning functions following traumatic brain injury. *Cortex, 15*, 63–70.

Lezak, M.D. (1987). Relationships between personality disorders, social disturbances, and physical disability following traumatic brain injury. *Journal of Head Trauma and Rehabilitation, 2*, 57–69.

Lishman, W.A. (1978). *Organic psychiatry*. Oxford: Blackwell Scientific Publications.

Luria, A.R. (1966). *Higher cortical functions in man* (2nd ed.). New York: Basic Books.

Merskey, H., & Woodforde, J.M. (1972). Psychiatric sequelae of minor head injury. *Brain, 95*, 521–528.

O'Brien, K.P. (1986). *Parental mood, emotional distress, and coping in families with a head-injured offspring*. Unpublished doctoral dissertation, University of Victoria, Victoria, BC.

O'Brien, K.P., & Lezak, M.D. (1982,

June). *Long-term improvements in intellectual function following brain damage.* Paper presented at the Fourth European Meeting of the International Neuropsychological Society, Bergen, Norway.

Oddy, M. (1984). Head injury and social adjustment. In N. Brooks (Ed.), *Closed head injury* (pp. 108–121). Oxford: Oxford University Press.

Oddy, M., Coughlan, T., Tyerman, A., & Jenkins, D. (1985). Social adjustment after closed head injury: A further follow-up seven years after injury. *Journal of Neurology, Neurosurgery, and Psychiatry, 48,* 564–568.

Oddy, M., Humphrey, M., & Uttley, D. (1978). Subjective impairment and social recovery after closed head injury. *Journal of Neurology, Neurosurgery, and Psychiatry, 41,* 611–616.

Prigatano, G.P., and Others (1986). *Neuropsychological rehabilitation after brain injury.* Baltimore: Johns Hopkins University Press.

Prigatano, G.P., O'Brien, K.P., & Klonoff, P.S. (in press). *The clinical management of delusions in patients with traumatic brain injuries.*

Rosenbaum, M., & Najenson, T. (1976). Changes in life patterns and symptoms of low mood as reported by wives of severely brain-injured soldiers. *Journal of Consulting and Clinical Psychology, 44,* 881–888.

Van Zomeren, A.H., & Van den Burg, W. (1985). Residual complaints of patients two years after severe head injury. *Journal of Neurology, Neurosurgery, and Psychiatry, 48,* 21–28.

Vigouroux, R.P., Baurand, D., Naquet, R., Chament, J.H., Choux, M., Benayoun, R., Bureau, M., Charpy, J.P. Clamens-Guey, M.J., & Guey, J. (1971). *A series of patients with craniocerebral injuries studied neurologically, psychometrically, electroencephalographically, and socially.* Proceedings of the International Symposium on Head Injuries (pp. 335–341). Edinburgh: Churchill Livingstone.

APPENDIX
Portland Adaptability Inventory

Temperament and Emotionality (T/E)

T/E-1 Irritability to aggression: 0 Socially appropriate; 1 Self-report only; 2 Mild to moderate irritability and verbal aggression; 3 Physical or severe verbal aggression.

T/E-2 Anxiety to agitation: 0 Socially appropriate; 1 Self-report only; 2 Mild to moderate anxiety; 3 Severe anxiety to agitation.

Note: Adapted from "Relationships Between Personality Disorders, Social Disturbances, and Physical Disability Following Traumatic Brain Injury" by M.D. Lezak, 1987, *Journal of Head Trauma Rehabilitation,* 2, 57–69.

T/E-3 Indifference: 0 Socially appropriate; 1 Indifferent to problems; 2 Denies existence or seriousness of problems; unable to comprehend them; 3 Euphoric.

T/E-4 Depression: 0 Appropriate; 1 Self-report; 2 Apparent to observer but not disruptive for practical purposes; 3 Disruptive for practical purposes.

T/E-5 Delusions and hallucinations: 0 None; 1 Self-report only; no hallucinations; 2 Apparent to observer but not disruptive for practical purposes; 3 Disruptive for practical purposes.

T/E-6 Paranoia: 0 None; 1 Self-report only; 2 Apparent to observer but not disruptive for practical purposes; 3 Disruptive for practical purposes.

T/E-7 Initiative: 0 Within normal limits; 1 Slow to get started; initiates less (conversation, activity) than premorbidly but sufficient for practical purposes; 2 Initiates some (conversation, activity) but insufficient for practical purposes; 3 Initiates no conversation or planned activity; totally dependent in this respect.

Activities and Social Behavior (ASB)

ASB-1 Significant relationships; 0 Unchanged, established, or re-established; 1 Dissatisfactions; significant relationships mildly to moderately disturbed; 2 Disrupted or very deteriorated significant relationships; 3 Total separation; no significant relationships.

ASB-2 Residence: 0 Single or family residence, self-supporting or at least full self-care (e.g., handles own finances); 1 Single or family residence, neither self-support nor full self-care; 2 Structured living in community (e.g., boarding house, half-way house) or no regular place of residence; 3 Institution.

ASB-3 Social contact: 0 No loss; 1 Mild to moderate decrease in social contacts; 2 Severe decrease in social contacts; 3 Total isolation.

ASB-4 Self-care: 0 Full self-care—adequate; 1 Self-care—not fully adequate; 2 Partial self-care—more than token efforts; 3 Needs full care and supervision.

ASB-5 Work/school: 0 Same work, different work—same level or same work—higher level; 1 Lower level but same general work classification; 2 Much lower level but same general work classification or sheltered workshop (including domiciliary program) or assumes and maintains regular chore schedule at home; 3 Does not work or go to school; idle.

ASB-6 Leisure activities: 0 No loss of self-initiated activities; 1 Mild to moderate loss of active pursuits; increase in passive pursuits (e.g., watching TV, people, drinking coffee); 2 Severe loss since injury; only passive pursuits; 3 No self-initiated activity ("sits and stares," sleeps a lot).

ASB-7 Driving: 0 No change; 1 Driving infractions, minor accidents (including self-reports); 2 Suspended automobile license but continues to drive; accidents involving damage or injury (without lawsuit or hospitalization); 3 Incapable of driving; does not drive; jailed, sued, or injured because of driving.

ASB-8 Law violations: 0 None; 1 Misdemeanors (including self-report); 2 Felony conviction with probation or misdemeanor conviction, serves time; 3 Felony conviction, serves time.

ABS-9 Alcohol: OA Nonuse; OB Occasional to moderate use (social); 2 Problem drinking.

ASB-10 Drugs: OA Nonuse; OB Occasional to moderate use (social); 3 Problem drug use.

ASB-11 Appropriate social interaction: 0 Socially appropriate; 1 Infrequent inappropriate behavior (but more than an occasional faux pas); 2 Frequent inappropriate behavior (childish, silly, out-of-place); 3 Practically complete lack of social awareness.

Physical Capabilities (PC)

PC-1 Ambulation: 0 No detectable impairment; 1 Walks unaided but with a limp; 2 Walks with cane, crutches, or walker; 3 Cannot walk even with aids.

PC-2 Use of hands: 0 Neither hand impaired; 1 Only nonpreferred hand impaired; 2 Only preferred hand impaired; 3 Both hands impaired.

PC-3 Sensory status: audition: 0 No impairment or additional impairment; 1 Slight impairment relative to premorbid impairment but within socially useful range; 2 Lacks reliable or useful social hearing; 3 Practically deaf.

PC-4 Sensory status: vision: 0 No impairment or increase in premorbid impairment; 1 Slight impairment relative to premorbid impairment but does not require glasses or a change in premorbid prescription; 2 Impairment sufficient to require glasses or change in premorbid prescription or to interfere with ordinary activities; 3 Practically blind.

PC-5 Dysarthria: 0 None; 1 Mild—easy to understand; 2 Moderate—difficult for strangers to understand; 3 Severe—incomprehensible or no speech.

PC-6 Aphasia: 0 None; 1 Mild—has adequate communication skills for most conversation and practical purposes; 2 Moderate—some communication ability, insufficient for many practical purposes; 3 Severe—insufficient for practical purposes or absent.

18

Family Issues in Traumatic Brain Injury

DARLENE AULDS MARTIN

Traumatic brain injury (TBI) has been identified as one of the largest contributors to death and disability among children and adolescents in the United States (Frankowski, 1985; Goldstein & Levin, 1987). An estimated 1 million children sustain closed head injuries annually (Eiben et al., 1984), and a large majority of that group will develop physical, intellectual, or behavioral deficits (Fisher, 1985; National Head Injury Foundation, 1985). While these statistics are staggering, they do not convey the full magnitude of the tragedy. In reality, the actual number of victims is much larger because an injury to a child also represents an injury to a family.

Although it may not be possible to fully comprehend the effect of the injury on the family system, it is vitally important for educators and health professionals who work with head injured children to understand the nature of the family's experience and their special perspective. It is also important to acknowledge the pivotal role that families can play in the rehabilitation process, including the development of effective educational programming.

Unfortunately, there has been limited research examining the specific effects of traumatic brain injury in children upon the family. The lack of research in this area can be partially attributed to the poor survival rate of children prior to the recent development of sophisticated trauma care and advanced life-saving technologies for those with brain injuries. Of necessity, much of the basic research related to head injury has focused on the physiological, intellectual, and behavioral effects of the injury on the child as well as comparative results of various medical, surgical, and neuropsychological interventions. There has been increasing recognition, however, that an equal emphasis must be given to the study of the impact of TBI upon the family and to analysis of family coping and adaptation patterns (Bond, 1983; Rosenthal & Geckler, 1986). The family's ability to survive intact and to adapt to the trauma is crucial since they often are the key to the child's successful rehabilitation and re-entry into society.

Although family-oriented research with brain injured children has been limited, there are related studies of coping patterns among families of adults with TBI as well as children with other serious disabilities and chronic illness that can provide a framework for analysis. Many of these studies suggest that families progress through general stages as they attempt to adapt to the initial crisis and long-term care of a child with a serious chronic health problem such as traumatic head injury (Blacher, 1984; Drotar, Baskiewicz, Irvin, Kennell, & Klaus, 1975).

STAGES IN FAMILY ADAPTATION

Shock

The most common initial stage that families experience is one of overwhelming shock as they are confronted with the news that their child has sustained a severe, and potentially lethal, head injury. The shock is often intensified by the specter of a child who is comatose and appears to be lifeless and totally unresponsive. The intensive care unit setting with all of its high-tech equipment and noisy monitors may further add to the parents' feelings of shock. They often experience a sense of numbness and disorientation and may not be able to think or respond rationally. The family may feel a tremendous sense of helplessness and fear as they see their child struggle for life. Very few of life's experiences prepare us to grapple with "life in the balance."

Denial or Disbelief

As the shock about the trauma gradually fades, parents often move into a phase of denial or disbelief about their child's injury. They may deny the actual existence of an injury or the extent or permanence of the disability.

Denial has generally been considered to be dysfunctional; Pueschel (1986), however, argues that initial denial may actually serve as a protective mechanism that allows families time to gradually absorb the reality of their child's injury. The temporary disavowal of reality can help them master the devastating early period of loss and threat.

Persistent denial about the injury, however, can prevent the family from adapting to the child's actual losses and from participating in needed rehabilitation and educational programming. In addition, the inability to accept the permanence of disability may cause family members to develop unrealistic expectations about the child and, unfortunately, to set up a cycle of failure for both the child and family. It may also drive them to constantly search for treatment that they believe could totally reverse the brain injury and restore their child to his or her former, intact self.

Sorrow

As parents begin to develop an awareness of the magnitude of the injury, they may experience a profound sense of sorrow and despondency. While much of the sadness comes from witnessing the acute pain and suffering of their child, it also derives from a realization that their child is forever changed. A lifetime of hopes and dreams about the future may seem to have vanished in an instant. The sense of loss and despair that parents may feel was eloquently expressed by Pearl Buck, whose child was severely disabled:

> To learn how to bear the inevitable sorrow, is not easily done. I can look back at it now, the lesson I learned, and see the steps; but when I was taking them, they were hard indeed, each apparently insurmountable. For in addition to the practical problem of how to protect the child's life which may last beyond the parents', there is the problem of one's own self-in-misery. All the brightness of life is gone, all the pride in parenthood. (Pueschel, 1986, p. 177)

The sorrow may endure for weeks and months as the family tries to come to terms with the trauma and resultant physical and psychological changes in their child. The process of understanding and accepting a child with severe disabilities while at the same time clinging to the memories of experiences with that child before the injury can be excruciating. It may be analogous to a process described by Solnit and Stark (1961) in their pioneering research with family adaptation to the birth of a handicapped newborn. Families reported that they had to mourn the loss of the expected, idealized infant before they could become attached to the actual new baby with congenital handicaps. There certainly may be similar elements of mourning for the losses that the brain injured child has sustained, especially if there are substantial intellectual and personality changes. Bond (1983) notes that it may take families a period of 1 to 2 years following the injury to become emotionally stabilized and realistically oriented to the needs of the brain injured child.

Even when the family has been able to adapt to the child with traumatic head injury, they may always have some residual feelings of sadness, which Olshansky (1970) has characterized as "chronic sorrow." That sorrow was poignantly expressed by one mother who stated that "Even now, years after the accident, I still feel the heartache that someone has stolen my child's future. I don't think that feeling ever completely goes away" (personal communication, 1988). The sadness may lie dormant for long periods of time only to resurface when the child and family encounter new difficulties in achieving educational or vocational goals or when new social-behavioral problems develop.

Anger

In addition to feelings of sadness, families may experience a diffuse sense of anger about the seeming injustice of their child's traumatic injury. The anger may be directed toward the persons or circumstances that led to the injury, but more often than not, there is no clear "enemy" on whom they can vent their outrage. The unexpressed anger may then be turned inward, in which case they may blame themselves for not being able to protect their child from harm, or their anger may be directed toward the medical team, other family members, and, later, toward the rehabilitation and educational team. While anger may initially energize the parents and allow them to release some of their frustrations, it can become destructive if it persists over an extended period of time. The family may need counseling to help them overcome angry feelings and move toward more positive, effective adaptation.

Adaptation

This stage represents a time in which the family is reaching some form of emotional equilibrium and is developing constructive adaptation to the child's disabilities. Over time they have gathered more data about the child's injury and may have developed more realistic expectations about recovery and the nature of residual disabilities. Frequently, the family has gone through a process of reorganization and redefinition of roles in order to accommodate the needs of the brain injured child.

This last stage is unquestionably the most difficult one for families to achieve. Adaptation is a very complex and time-related process that appears to be related not only to the type and severity of the child's residual disabilities but also to a variety of other factors, including the family's intrinsic coping abilities and the degree of external social support (Featherstone, 1980; Holaday, 1984; McCubbin, Cauble, & Patterson, 1982).

Other factors that have been identified as potentially influencing family adaptation include age of the child who has the disability, number of other siblings in the family, length and stability of the marital relationship, parents' educational and religious background, and ethnicity (Darling & Darling, 1982). It is not clear, however, what degree of influence each of these variables has, singly or in combination, upon the family's ability to adapt to the needs of a handicapped child.

Research and clinical data do strongly suggest that adaptation is not a static, one-time event, but is rather a very fluid process that may fluctuate over long periods of time (Blacher, 1984; Elkins & Brown, 1986; Klaus & Kennell, 1982; Pueschel, 1986). In fact, there are probably levels of acceptance or adaptation within each stage; families may experience varying degrees of adaptation as their child progresses through different developmental stages.

Darling and Darling (1982) conclude from their research that the most prevalent attitude of parents toward their congenitally handicapped children is one of realistic acceptance in which "parents acknowledge and are unhappy about their child's limitations; yet they are able to appreciate whatever abilities their children do possess and to love their children in spite of their handicaps" (p. 68).

In summary, clinical observations and available research data do suggest that many families of children with various types of developmental disabilities and chronic illness progress through similar stages as they try to come to terms with and adapt to the disabled child. However, it is important to note that there may be substantial differences between and within families in terms of the rate and sequence of progression through these stages. Some families, or individual family members, for example, may not necessarily go through every stage. Some stages may also be repeated as families encounter new developmental or situational crises with their disabled child. Although the concept of stages can be very useful in helping to assess families' level of adaptation and readiness for various types of intervention, it should be used as a guide rather than as a mechanism to rigidly categorize family behaviors.

It is also important to note that while clinical observations suggest that parents of children with traumatic brain injury proceed through similar stages in adaptation, there is a need for research to validate those observations. There may be qualitative differences in parents' responses due to factors such as the sudden onset of the head injury, the relative uncertainty about the degree of recovery, and the frequently dramatic changes that can occur in cognitive abilities and personality.

SOURCES OF FAMILY STRESS

The ability of the family to maintain its integrity and adapt to the child with a severe disability or chronic illness is often contingent on its ability to cope effectively with stress. Clearly, the occurrence of a traumatic head injury to a child creates upheaval and stress within the family. The crisis begins almost immediately after the injury and may continue for months and years as the family tries to adapt to substantial changes in the child and in the family system (Blayzk, 1983; Rosenthal & Geckler, 1986). While the sources of stress may vary from family to family, certain patterns of stress seem to be related to distinct features of brain injury. These specific features include prognostic uncertainty as well as the possibility that the child will sustain substantial residual changes in physical abilities, intellectual functioning, and personality characteristics. Each of these potential sources of stress is briefly discussed below.

Uncertainty About Recovery

The large degree of ambiguity and uncertainty about a traumatically brain injured child's prognosis and degree of recovery creates one of the most prevalent sources of stress for families. While it is evident that physical, cognitive, and behavioral deficits are directly related to the severity and specific site of the injury, it is equally clear that eventual recovery and outcome are quite variable and dependent upon a complex set of interrelated factors that are not fully understood (Ewing-Cobbs & Fletcher, 1987; Prigatano, 1987). Some children appear to make fairly rapid and remarkable "spontaneous" recoveries while others may languish in coma or survive the initial trauma but be left with substantial permanent impairments.

Although uncertainty about the child's survival in the early stages of the injury may produce the most acute distress, it is the general uncertainty about long-term recovery that perhaps creates a more pervasive, lingering type of stress. While the most substantial recovery of physical and cognitive abilities tends to occur within the first 6 months after the injury, the continuing process of recovery may proceed at a much slower rate with extended plateaus for several years (Bond, 1983). The unevenness and unpredictability of recovery can thrust parents onto an emotional roller coaster ride that seems to have no end.

Panting and Merry (1972) found that the substantial lack of information about prognosis and general uncertainty about what families should prepare for in the future were major factors that created stress in families with brain injured members. McCubbin et al. (1982) note that such ambiguity can increase the risk of family crisis by causing disagreement among family members and professionals about the most effective and appropriate course of action to take on behalf of the child.

Cognitive and Personality Changes

As the child moves out of the acute phase of the injury into the rehabilitative phase, the family usually begins to develop a painful awareness of cognitive and behavioral changes that have occurred. The marked changes in these two areas have been identified as the most stressful for children with traumatic brain injuries and their families (Chadwick, 1985; Rosenthal & Geckler, 1986).

Although cognitive deficits vary with each child, some of those that may be present include memory impairment, with difficulty in storing and retrieving information; reduced ability to process information and problem solve; distractibility; and a reduced ability to concentrate. Other related problems may include an inability to adapt to change and new situations, including new environments and people.

Personality and behavioral changes may include inappropriate behavior in social situations, mood swings, poor impulse control, poor anger control, and aggressiveness. The older child or adolescent may actually regress to the developmental level of a much younger child and exhibit behaviors such as bedwetting, temper tantrums, and fear of being left alone. While some of these children may return to age-appropriate developmental levels during recovery and rehabilitation, some may stay at the regressed level and require extensive assistance and monitoring in areas such as daily living tasks and safety.

Stress frequently occurs as the family, who may already be emotionally drained from the child's early struggle for survival, tries to adjust to and care for a child who may seem radically different from the way he or she was before the injury. This process of adaptation is extremely difficult and complex and may require, as noted earlier in the discussion, a form of rebonding or reconnecting with the postinjury child. Ironically, the process may be made more difficult if the child has no discernible physical disabilities, because the family may be reluctant to accept the reality of the cognitive-behavioral changes. There may be a strong belief that the youngster can be returned to his or her former self through intensive rehabilitation and the passage of time.

The salience of cognitive and behavioral changes as family stressors has been supported by a number of researchers. Bond (1983) found that residual mental deficits among severely head injured adults were more closely correlated with family cohesion and functioning than was the presence of permanent physical deficits.

The work of McKinlay, Brooks, Bond, Martinage, and Marshall (1981), who investigated the occurrence of stress in wives and mothers of men who had sustained severe head injury, suggested that levels of stress varied according to the specific types of residual problems and that the nature of these problems changed over time. During the first 3 months after injury, families reported that the most significant problems were related to memory impairment and emotional-behavioral changes. At 6 months postinjury, emotional and behavioral changes in the injured member remained significant sources of family stress, but another variable, patient dependency, also emerged as a substantial stressor.

In a related study of the impact of head injury upon family members in Great Britain, Oddy, Humphrey, and Uttley (1978) found a high incidence of depression among wives of men who had sustained a closed head injury. The depression appeared to be closely associated with substantial personality changes in the TBI spouse. It was most acute during the first month following the injury, but continued to persist in various forms during the first year.

Long-term Rehabilitation

In addition to the stress that may be generated by changes in the child's cognitive abilities and behavior, the family may be overwhelmed by the demands of an intensive, long-term rehabilitation program. Although the programs vary according to the nature and severity of the child's injuries, rehabilitation generally continues for several years, and some components may be necessary for the remainder of the child's life as he or she grows to adulthood.

Children with TBI frequently require a wide range of services including physical, occupational, and speech therapy, psychological counseling, and neurological monitoring. Parents often spend an enormous amount of time in transporting their child to and from health clinics as well as in repeating and reinforcing the therapies while the child is at home.

The sheer volume of time and energy expended by the family during rehabilitation can be physically and emotionally exhausting. It can become a major source of stress if the family cannot receive some type of respite and time-out from daily responsibilities. Mothers may be especially susceptible to burnout if they have provided the bulk of care for the child. DeMyer and Goldberg (1983) have noted the fatigue of "perpetual parenthood" that can occur among parents who are the predominant caregivers.

Economics of Care

The economic costs of acute care and long-term rehabilitation can also be a substantial source of stress for the family. Although some of these costs may be covered by private insurance or federally funded programs such as Medicaid, families often have to expend large sums of money for medical and medically related services. In addition, parents may be faced with travel and lodging costs if they are required to transport their child to a rehabilitation center outside of their own community.

Other related expenses may include costs for educational services if the child is not in a public school program covered by P.L. 94-142. These private programs can be very expensive, particularly if the child is in residence during the school year. Parents may have to pay additional fees for educational or child care services during the summer.

Additional economic pressures can develop if one of the spouses is required to discontinue employment in order to provide full-time care of the child with traumatic brain injury. If the family has been dependent on two incomes, the reduction in funds may substantially alter their life-style. Frequently, the employed spouse or siblings have to assume other jobs in order to help pay for household costs as well as for medical costs for the injured child. Economic burdens can be especially problematic for single-parent families, who may have limited incomes and resources.

COPING WITH STRESS

Although there are numerous factors that can potentially create stress and crisis in families with a traumatically brain injured child, there appear to be wide variations in the responses of families to such stress. While some families become largely dysfunctional and may even disintegrate as a unit, others remain remarkably intact and are able to adapt effectively to the needs of their disabled child. Clearly, some patterns of coping are more successful than others in mediating the possible negative effects of stress on the family system. This section will briefly examine some of the key factors that are related to successful coping and adaptation.

Family Stress Theory

Family stress theory provides a meaningful framework for analysis of family coping with a child who has a serious disability such as a traumatic brain injury. The classic work conceptualizing family stress and the variability of families in adjusting to life stressors was conducted by Hill (1949) among families who had been separated by war and then later reunited. This led to the development of the ABCX family crisis model:

> A (the stressor event)—interacting with B (the family's crisis meeting resources)—interacting with C (the definition the family makes of the event)—produces X (the crisis). The second and third determinants—the family resources and definition of the event—lie within the family itself and must be seen in terms of the family's structures and values. The event, which goes to make up the first determinant, lies outside the family and is an attribute of the event itself. (Hill, 1958, p. 141)

Hill (1958) defined crisis in terms of a dramatic change that could not be effectively dealt with by the use of old coping patterns or strategies. Crisis can exist on a continuum and cause varying amounts of disruption and disorganization within a family system. Hill's original model has been expanded by McCubbin and Patterson (1983) to include the pile-up of other problems or life events that influence the family's ability to adapt as well as the type of active coping strategies that families use over time. Thus, it is the interaction between the family's resources and the stressful event that determines the degree of family stress (Turk & Kerns, 1985).

Although Hill's model of family crisis has not been extensively tested with families of brain injured children, it has been utilized in studies of children with other serious chronic illnesses and disabilities, including cystic fibrosis (McCubbin & Patterson, 1983), spina bifida (Nevin & McCubbin, 1979), and autism (Bristol & Schopler, 1984). Results drawn from these and related studies (Gallagher, Cross, & Scharfman, 1981) suggest that there are characteristic family resources and family definitions of illness that positively influence coping and adaptation.

Crisis-Meeting Resources

Several aspects of family resources, including family environment, informal social support, and specific coping responses, appear to be closely related to successful coping and adaptation. Certain important characteristics within the psychosocial environment seem to help families develop more resistance to crisis or more restorative powers following crisis. These include family cohesion and support for individual members, ability of family members to express their feelings and emotions, maintenance of an optimistic attitude about the child's condition, and ability of families to be flexible and adaptable when faced with change (Holaday, 1984; McCubbin et al., 1982; Patterson, 1985). Two additional factors that have been associated with effective family coping are religious affiliation (Simeonsson & McHale, 1981) and family participation in recreational and social activities outside of the home (Bristol & Schopler, 1984; Nevin & McCubbin, 1979).

In addition to positive psychosocial environments and internal supports, families who are more adaptive tend to have access to an informal network of social support. This network may include members of the extended family, neighbors, friends from work or church, and parents who have children with similar disabilities. Parent support groups provide families with an avenue for sharing their feelings and problems with other families who have had similar experiences. The groups serve as a major source of information about practical aspects and approaches to caring for a child with severe disabilities. The support and networking provided by these groups appear to reduce the parents' feelings of isolation and despair (Lieberman & Borman, 1979) and increase their feelings of parental competence (Holaday, 1984). One of the most helpful support groups for families with children who have traumatic brain injury is the National Head Injury Foundation, which has local branches in most communities across the country.

Another important characteristic that has been linked to successful coping is the family's active engagement in problem solving and stress reduction. McCubbin (1979) has noted that families who take an active role in trying to modify, minimize, or tolerate stressful situations may increase their ability to endure stress. Over time, the family develops skills and success as a problem-solving unit, which in turn can increase their sense of control and mastery over their own environment (Holaday, 1984).

Family Definition of the Stressful Event

Based on Hill's theory of family stress, one of the most important factors that influences the family's response to a stressful event is the subjective definition and meaning that they give to that event (e.g., a traumatic head injury). There is a need to make sense out of a traumatic situation that has left family members feeling powerless and out of control.

A family's perceptions of events and the meaning of the experience evolve over time and are shaped by a complex array of factors. These factors may include the quality and quantity of information that families receive about their child's condition, their personal religious and philosophical beliefs about handicapping conditions, and perceived attitudes of other family members, friends, and professionals toward the child and his or her disability.

Darling and Darling (1982) argue that from an interactionist point of view, the meaning that parents ascribe to their experience with a handicapped child and their ability to adapt are more a function of interaction with the social system than of individual coping abilities. Darling and Darling (1984, p. 68) believe that an "ideology of acceptance" evolves as families care for and become attached to their child and interact with others.

SUMMARY AND CONCLUSIONS

The occurrence of a traumatic brain injury to a child has the potential for creating substantial disruption and stress within a family system. The primary sources of family stress appear to be related to the sudden and often dramatic changes in the child's cognitive abilities and personality, the large degree of ambiguity about recovery, and the increased dependency and long-term care needs of the brain injured child. Other stress-producing factors may include lack of financial resources to cover extensive costs of medical care, lack of respite care, and lack of appropriate rehabilitation and educational programs within the family's community.

As families attempt to adapt to the brain injured child and cope with his or her special needs, they may progress through stages that are similar to those of the grieving process—shock, denial, anger, sorrow, and acceptance—but their rate of progression may vary according to the severity of the child's injury and the extent of recovery. Parents may have to go through a process of mourning for the "loss" of the preinjury child and reattach or rebond to the postinjury child.

Adaptation is clearly not a static, one-time event, but rather is a very complex, fluid process that may fluctuate over time as the child progresses through different rehabilitative and developmental stages. For example, entry of a young brain injured child into the school system for the first time may precipitate a crisis both for the child and family as they try to adjust to a new environment and new demands. Similarly, adolescence may create new types of family stress due to the teenager's needs for independence and sexual expression.

The ability of the family to cope with stress and adapt to the brain injured child appears to be related to a complex set of internal and environmental variables. Internal factors include family cohesiveness and support, active involvement in problem solving, and participation in recreation activities outside of the home. Environmental variables include access to and utilization of informal support networks as well as availability of rehabilitation and educational services within the community.

REFERENCES

Blacher, J. (Ed.). (1984). *Severely handicapped young children and their families—Research in review.* San Francisco: Academic Press.

Blazyk, S. (1983). Developmental crisis in adolescents following severe head injury. *Social Work in Health Care, 80,* 55–59.

Bond, M.R. (1983). Effects on the family system. In M. Rosenthal, E.R. Griffith, M. Bond, & J.D. Miller (Eds.), *Rehabilitation of the head injured adult* (pp. 209–217). Philadelphia: F.A. Davis.

Bristol, M.M., & Schopler, E. (1984). A developmental perspective on stress and coping in families of autistic children. In J. Blacher (Ed.), *Severely handicapped young children and their families* (pp. 91–141). San Francisco: Academic Press.

Chadwick, O. (1985). Psychological sequelae of head injury in children. *Developmental Medicine and Child Neurology, 27,* 69–79.

Darling, R.B., & Darling, J. (1982). *Children who are different.* St. Louis: C.V. Mosby.

Deaton, A.V. (1987). Behavioral change strategies for children and adolescents with severe brain injury. *Journal of Learning Disabilities, 20*(10), 581–589.

DeMyer, M., & Goldberg, P. (1983). Family needs of the autistic adolescent. In E. Schopler & G.B. Mesibov (Eds.), *Autism in adolescents and adults* (pp. 75–90). New York: Plenum.

Drotar, D., Baskiewicz, A., Irvin, N., Kennell, J.H., & Klaus, M.H. (1975). The adaptation of parents to the birth of an infant with a congenital malformation: A hypothetical model. *Pediatrics, 56,* 710–717.

Eiben, C.F., Anderson, T.P., Lockman, L., Matthews, D.J., Dryja, R., Martin, J., Burrill, C., Gottesman, N., O'Brien, P., & Witte, L. (1984). Functional outcome of closed head injury in children and young adults. *Archives of Physical Medicine Rehabilitation, 65,* 168–170.

Elkins, T.E., & Brown, D. (1986). An approach to Down's syndrome in light of infant Doe. *Issues in Law and Medicine, 1,* 419–440.

Ewing-Cobbs, L., & Fletcher, J.M. (1987). Neuropsychological assessment of head injury in children. *Journal of Learning Disabilities, 20*(9), 526–535.

Featherstone, M.A. (1980). *A difference in the family.* New York: Basic Books.

Fisher, J.M. (1985). Cognitive and behavioral consequences of closed head injury. *Seminars in Neurology, 5,* 197–204.

Frankowski, R.F. (1985). Head injury mortality in urban populations and its relation to the injured child. In B.F. Brooks (Ed.), *The injured child* (pp. 20–29). Austin: University of Texas Press.

Gallagher, J.J., Cross, A.H., & Scharfman, W. (1981). Parental adaptation to a young handicapped child. *Journal of the Division for Early Childhood, 3,* 3–14.

Goldstein, F.C., & Levin, H.S. (1987). Epidemiology of pediatric head injury: Incidence, clinical characteristics, and risk factors. *Journal of Learning Disabilities, 20,* 518–525.

Hill, R. (1949). *Families under stress: Adjustment to the crisis of war separation and reunion.* New York: Harper.

Hill, R. (1958). Generic features of families under stress. *Social Casework, 49,*

139–150.

Holaday, B. (1984). Challenges of rearing a chronically ill child. *Nursing Clinics of North America, 19,* 361–368.

Klaus, M.H., & Kennell, J.H. (1982). *Parent-infant bonding.* St. Louis: C.V. Mosby.

Lieberman, M., & Borman, L. (1979). *Self-help groups for coping with crisis.* San Francisco: Jossey-Bass.

McCubbin, H. (1979). Integrating coping behavior in family stress theory. *Journal of Marriage and the Family, 42,* 237–244.

McCubbin, H.I., Cauble, A.E., & Patterson, J.M. (1982). *Family stress, coping, and social support.* Springfield, IL: Thomas.

McCubbin, H., & Patterson, J. (1983). Family transitions: Adaptation to stress. In H. McCubbin & C. Figley (Eds.), *Stress and the family* (Vol. 1, pp. 5–25). New York: Brunner/Mazel.

McCubbin, M. (1984). Nursing assessment of parental coping with cystic fibrosis. *Western Journal of Nursing Research, 6,* 407–422.

McKinlay, W.W., Brooks, D.N., Bond, M.R., Martinage, D.P., & Marshall, M.M. (1981). The short-term outcome of severe blunt head injury as reported by relatives of the injured person. *Journal of Neurology, Neurosurgery, and Psychiatry, 44,* 527–533.

National Head Injury Foundation. (1985). *An educator's manual: What educators need to know about students with traumatic brain injury.* Framingham, MA: Author.

Nevin, R.S., & McCubbin, H.J. (1979). *Parental coping with physical handicaps: Social policy implications.* Paper presented at the National Council of Family Relations Annual Meeting, Boston.

Oddy, M., Humphrey, M., & Uttley, D. (1978). Stresses upon relatives of head injured patients. *British Journal of Psychiatry, 133,* 507–513.

Olshanky, S. (1970). Chronic sorrow: A response to having a mentally defective child. In R.L. Noland (Ed.), *Counseling parents of the mentally retarded—A sourcebook.* Springfield, IL: Thomas.

Panting, A., & Merry, P. (1972). The long term rehabilitation of severe head injuries with particular reference to the need for social and medical support for the patient's family. *Rehabilitation, 38,* 33–37.

Patterson, J. (1985). Critical factors affecting family compliance with home treatment for children with cystic fibrosis. *Family Relations, 34*(1), 79–89.

Prigatano, G.P. (1987). Recovery and cognitive retraining after craniocerebral trauma. *Journal of Learning Disabilities, 20*(10), 603–613.

Pueschel, S.M. (1986). The impact on the family: Living with the handicapped child. *Issues in Law and Medicine, 2*(3), 171–187.

Rosenthal, M., & Geckler, C. (1986). Family therapy issues in neuropsychology. In D. Wedding, A.M. Horton, Jr., & J. Webster (Eds.), *The neuropsychology handbook* (pp. 325–344). New York: Springer.

Simeonsson, R.J., & McHale, S. (1981). Review: Research on handicapped children in sibling relationships. *Child Care, Health, and Development, 7,* 153–171.

Solnit, A.J., & Stark, M.H. (1961). Mourning and the birth of a defective child. *Journal for the Psychoanalytic Study of the Child, 16,* 523–537.

Turk, D., & Kerns, R. (1985). The family in health and illness. In D. Turk & R. Kerns (Eds.), *Health, illness and families* (pp. 1–22). New York: Wiley.

19

Legal Challenges in Traumatic Brain Injury

REED MARTIN

Students with a disability that adversely affects educational performance have a right to certain special education services through their public schools. The vast majority of traumatic brain injured (TBI) students would presumably have not been in special education prior to the trauma causing their injury. Their entitlement to special services, their parents' role in securing those services, and the school district's perception of them as disabled will all be new and very sudden. In this writer's experience, the parents of a TBI student are much less likely to be able to advocate effectively for their youngster's special educational needs than the parents of a child born with disabilities, who have learned over time how to work with the educational system. In fact, both parents and regular school personnel may be resistant to special education services.

OVERVIEW OF LEGAL ENTITLEMENT

The basic entitlement comes through two federal statutes. In 1973, the United States Congress amended the Rehabilitation Act by adding a final section (commonly referred to as Section 504) to prohibit recipients of federal financial assistance from discriminating against program beneficiaries on the basis of handicap.[1] Federal financial assistance and the regulatory authority that runs with it reach virtually every school setting in the United States today. Section 504 has had a shaky application to special education: Regulations of this 1973 act were not issued until June 1977, and from July 1984 to August 1986, the United States Supreme Court said Section 504 did not apply to special education.[2] But it is quite clear now, through the Handicapped Children's Protection Act,[3] effective August 5, 1986, and the enforcement by the federal Office of Civil Rights, that Section 504 definitely applies. The importance of the Section 504 protection is that its breadth clearly encompasses the TBI student. Another federal act (detailed below) has specific eligibility criteria that are sometimes hard to apply to those with TBI, but Section 504 clearly reaches anyone with a mental or physical injury that adversely affects education.[4]

The second major statute, and the one that school districts are most familiar with and most responsive to, is the 1975 amendment to the Education of the Handicapped Act, known as Public Law 94-142 or the Education for All Handicapped Children Act.[5] That act places a duty upon public schools to (a) identify eligible students, (b) provide sufficient evaluation (including medical diagnostic work) upon which to base a program, (c) meet with parents to plan a special educational offering, (d) reduce that plan to writing with annual goals and short-term measurements to determine if the program is moving toward the attainment of those goals, and (e) propose changes in the program as necessary to meet the individual child's needs.[6] The act, and the language of the United States Supreme Court in interpreting it, make it clear that the program has to be responsive to the individual student's needs; it has to be "personalized," "specially designed," "meet the unique needs of the individual handicapped child," and "tailored."[7]

---

[1]29 U.S.C. 794, 34 CFR 104. (Note: U.S.C. contains federal statutes in the U.S. Code and CFR contains federal regulations in the Code of Federal Regulations.)

[2]Smith v. Robinson, 468 U.S. 992 (1984)

[3]Public Law 99–372, 20 U.S.C. 1415(f)

[4]See 34 CFR 104.3(j)

[5]20 U.S.C. 1401 et seq., 34 CFR 300.1 et seq.

[6]20 U.S.C. 412(2)(C), 34 CFR 300.128 and .200, 34 CFR 300.530–.543, 20 U.S.C. 1414(a)(5), 34 CFR 300.343, 34 CFR 300.340–.349, 20 U.S.C. 1401(19), and 34 CFR 300.346

[7]Board of Education v. Rowley, 458 U.S. 176 (1982)

These two acts have redefined education, as we know it, in public schools. The parent of a TBI youngster who, prior to the injury, was in regular education is ill-equipped to argue for special services. The lay approach to education assumes that the student will fit into ongoing public school programs (for example, a regular eighth-grade math classroom) and that if a youngster is not ready to be in school his or her place is out of school. Prior to these federal acts, children who were not toilet trained, who could not sit still, could not walk, could not speak, and so forth, were simply told to stay at home until they were ready for what the school offered. Now, however, schools must offer special educational services to children as early as age 3, who cannot self-toilet, speak, respond to instructions, sit in neat rows, and so forth. Education includes the full scope of skills that we used to assume would be developed by the time the child reaches school age: The program must be made to fit the needs of the individual; the individual does not have to wait to reach the entry criteria of the school program.

The vital importance of this to the TBI student is that during the perhaps lengthy period of recovery from a head injury, the youngster may not appear to be ready for school. Further, the parents may assume that their injured child should simply stay at home until he or she recovers to near preinjury level and can then return to school. This delay can be quite damaging to the stimulation and educational development the student probably needs.

These acts also contain one additional entitlement that parents would find unusual: an entitlement to services in most states through the age of 22.[8] When Congress deliberated on Public Law 94-142, they determined that many children with handicaps learned more slowly. Therefore, graduating them at age 17 or 18, after approximately 12 years of school, left many adolescents with disabilities ill-equipped for any transition to adult life. Congress determined that those students should be served through the school year in which they turn 22 in order to give them that extra amount of time and education. Many head injuries occur in the teen years, and it is not unusual to see a youngster about to graduate from high school receiving a head injury. Ordinarily, his or her parents would presume that their child's educational days had run out; it is doubly important to realize that the youngster may be eligible to receive special education services for a number of additional years.

The entitlement to services through age 22 does not mean that a student would sit through 4 more years of high school. The educational offering would be tailored to the unique needs of that one adolescent. So the student can seek, through the local school district, medical and other diagnostic services sufficient to tailor an educational offering, counseling, retraining in academics

[8]20 U.S.C. 1412(2)(B), 34 CFR 300.122. The only exception is if state law forbids the use of state funds for services to youth beyond the age of 18.

lost through memory loss, physical therapy needed to enable the student to benefit from the educational offering, sensory motor integration therapies, training in independent living skills (if those have been lost), and so forth. Some of the above services might not be offered by the local high school the youth was attending, so the local school district must locate, arrange for, and provide transportation to such services.

Further, through Public Law 94-142 the entitlement is to services offered by any state agency to youth with disabilities. Perhaps for a 20-year-old the appropriate service would be intensive work with the state rehabilitation agency, placement in a job site, and one-to-one services of a job coach. Through the federal statute, all that is to be arranged through the local school district. Otherwise parents and youth would be running from agency to agency trying to piece together services, and that is exactly what Congress sought to end.

ELIGIBILITY FOR SERVICE

There is an understandable reluctance on the part of regular education personnel, parents, and even TBI students themselves to recognize that they are different enough to need special education. This effort to treat TBI children as more normal than different is laudable and can be beneficial in some ways. But it can also destroy children if they, in fact, have a disability that will prevent successful educational performance. Youngsters with even mild head injuries will undoubtedly go through a fairly long period of recovery, and the tendency to say "Let's just wait until he fully recovers" is understandable—similar to the way a physical education teacher might approach a youngster recovering from a complicated leg fracture. But the problem with head injured students is that as we wait for that total recovery that we all hope for, we may be irreparably passing up personalized stimulation necessary for as full a recovery as possible, and the regular educational environment may be torture for a youngster with even as mild a residual problem as short-term memory loss.

An additional complication of determining eligibility, and marshaling appropriate services, is the transience of the disability. This writer has seen, for example, a young adolescent progress over a 5-year period from functioning at a lowered level of mental ability with severe mobility problems; to recovery of cognitive function and mobility during a phase of serious emotional instability, with potential for seizures and such weakened stamina and shortness of attention span that he could tolerate only short periods of educational intervention; to eventual recovery of cognitive abilities but with residual problems of a slight hearing distortion that causes distractibility in classrooms with normal noise levels, a visual processing problem, and short-term memory loss; and finally to success in all regular classes with resource room assistance and participation in an extracurricular sport with increased social interaction. That youngster was clearly entitled to special education services each step of the way, but the school district has to be highly flexible and responsive in determining eligibility and continuing programming for that type of child. It would have been easy for a school to have locked him into an MR, ED, or LD label.

A final problem in determining eligibility is the expected parental resistance to special education labeling. It is very important emotionally for parents to remain optimistic during the years of recovery that may occur after an injury, and with that hope will predictably come refusal to see their youngster labeled, or programmed for, as retarded or emotionally disturbed or even health impaired or learning disabled. Therefore, part of the school's educational (and legal) duty to the child will include parent counseling, focusing specifically on the implications of the child's disability for functioning at school—both in the classroom and in other settings.

DIAGNOSTIC AND ASSESSMENT SERVICES

Public Law 94-142 requires the school to evaluate the student sufficiently to be able to program educationally. This includes medical diagnostic services, if necessary, at school expense[9] to form the basis for educational programming. Schools do not mind educational diagnoses that are relatively easy to confirm, such as having a staff person administer individual intelligence and adaptive behavior tests to determine mental retardation, or classroom observation to report on possible learning disabilities. But a full assessment of a TBI student is almost always going to be beyond the combined competence of the staff of the public school. The specialties needed may include neurology, psychiatry, neuropsychology, physiatry, physical therapy, occupational therapy, audiology, ophthalmology, and sophisticated cognitive rehabilitation therapies. Since those evaluators are frequently not on the staff of the public school, and their services are typically expensive, the expense is likely to exceed the school's budget.

This writer's experience is that schools often question the necessity to obtain or pay for neurological studies. Worse, because the spontaneously recovering TBI student will predictably go through several phases, a single assessment will probably not be enough, and repeated neurological and other examinations may well be required—far beyond the typical evaluation sched-

[9]20 U.S.C. 1401(17), 34 CFR 300.13(a)

ule of schools, which is to re-evaluate every 3 years. In fact, the necessity for re-evaluations every 3 to 6 months is not uncommon.

The parents of a recently injured student would not expect the school to have to pay for medical diagnostic work. If school personnel tell them, "Go to Dr. X and get the diagnostic work done and bring it to us," the parent would not necessarily expect the school to reimburse the cost, although this is the school's duty. This writer often hears of situations in which the parent does not feel the student has been fully diagnosed but cannot afford further work, and the school has illegally withheld from them the information that the school would be responsible for paying the costs of sufficient diagnostic work to form the basis of an appropriate educational program. The reader should not misinterpret these comments: No one is suggesting that the school is responsible for all the medical bills, all the medical diagnostic work, and all the therapies that may ensue from a brain injury. But the school clearly is responsible for sufficient medical diagnostic work to form the basis for a program and also for the therapies and other related services needed in order for that program to confer reasonable educational benefit.

A final problem with diagnostic services is that the assessment should yield more than a simple diagnosis. It should also yield a prescription for services needed to address the remediation of the disability. The evaluator who has noted, for example, a short-term memory loss should recommend what should be done educationally to deal with such a loss. Schools, however, are very resistant to prescriptions that seem to tell them where to place the youngster and what to do after the student is in the placement. This writer is often told by assessment professionals that the school has contracted with them to do an evaluation but has indicated to them that they are not to make a prescription, especially one that recommends a particular placement or array of services. Worse, those "outside" professionals are often not invited to the Individualized Education Program (IEP) conference at which their diagnoses are discussed, which leaves the resulting IEP very vulnerable to attack. A school may not legally limit the assessment professional from offering prescriptions and placement recommendations, nor may the school legally refuse to consider, at the IEP conference, all the available information.

EDUCATIONAL SERVICES BEFORE RETURN TO SCHOOL

Because of their injuries, students may be physically unable to return to school for a period of time, and the school faces the challenge of providing appropriate services delivered other than in the traditional school environment. Public Law 94-142 recognizes services to hospital-bound and homebound students.[10] Traditionally, those services are limited by the school to only a few days and a few hours per week. The model that schools fall back on is the visiting teacher who takes classroom assignments to the youngster and picks up completed homework to take back to the teacher. That is an absolutely unacceptable model for the recovering TBI student.

The student may need a full school day of programming that may be even more than the usual 6 hours of instruction per day. The person interacting educationally with the child may need to have much more specialization and training than the typical visiting teacher. Materials may need to be substantially modified and tailored for that child's unique needs. A variety of related therapies and services may need to accompany the instructional offering in order for the individual to be able to benefit from the total educational program. All of those needs—length of daily services, competency of personnel, modification of materials, and related services—are required by Public Law 94-142 but are often missing from what the school district is prepared to offer a student who is not yet able to return to the full-time educational environment at school.

RESISTANCE TO SPECIAL EDUCATIONAL PROGRAMMING

An expected attitude of both school persons and parents is that the youngster should stay at home until he or she is well. If a student previously served in regular education is now functioning at a level of severe mental retardation or exhibiting somewhat bizarre behaviors, it is not unusual to find well-meaning school persons counseling the parents to keep the student at home rather than place him or her in classes with emotionally disturbed or mentally retarded students. Parents may be told by well-meaning staff, "You wouldn't want your child in with those kids." It is recognized by specialists in the rehabilitation of TBI children that the recovering student should be around appropriate rather than inappropriate peer models, and that placing a youngster who temporarily functions as if retarded in a group of exclusively retarded children would hardly spur recovery. On the other hand, placing that student back into the regular class, at this particular stage of recovery, can destroy social interaction with peers and teachers and destroy the student's self-esteem.

[10] 20 U.S.C. 1412(5)(B), 34 CFR 300.551(b)(1)

The key is that a segregated special education class or a return to the regular classroom is not the only alternative the school must offer. The school must be prepared to have a continuum of services, including substantial modifications to a regular class. School personnel and parents are often resistant to making the modifications needed to enable an individual currently functioning well below the level of the other students in a regular classroom to function in that environment. The term this writer often hears is that it would be "coddling" the youngster and would be unfair to the other students.

In developing needed modifications, one must be mindful of the difference between accommodation and remediation. Certain obvious modifications can be made to accommodate a student: A wheelchair ramp can be built to the room to enable the currently orthopedically impaired youngster to enter; material can be read to the student with current visual processing problems; mimeographed material can be given to the student who can no longer take notes rapidly; homework assignments can be given in writing by the teacher to the student who has difficulty getting them orally; extended time on tests can be given to the student who can master the material but not repeat it as rapidly as others.

A problem occurs if accommodations are so substantial that they stigmatize the student and remove the educational reason for being in the class. One example, offered by an expert witness in a recent trial, was to have one student in a high school French class receive and return the information in English. That could certainly be a successful accommodation for that student, but it makes one wonder why the student would be in the French class to begin with. One must make sure that accommodations do not become a crutch that slows or prevents remediation. To continue the example, a youngster who could eventually function successfully in a French class might re-enter it with a lowered volume of material, with much of that material in English, as he or she phased back into the full French curriculum. It is easy to see, however, that if the student were offered material only in English and never expected to perform in French, the accommodation would actually become a barrier to the intellectual stimulation needed to aid with both the student's overall recovery and his or her ability to function in the class at a reasonable level.

Similarly, untimed tests might be an absolutely vital accommodation to a re-entering TBI student, but schools must be aware of when rehabilitation would encourage reimposing limitations on the total amount of time allowed to perform a particular task. For example, one common enemy of the recovering TBI student is the "pop" test. An understandable accommodation offered by schools would be simply not to have that student take pop tests. However, at some time during the youngster's recovery, one might want to use pop tests as a diagnostic tool to determine whether other aspects of the program are remediating his or her deficits sufficiently that he or she can begin to attempt taking pop tests again.

DIFFICULTIES IN GOAL SETTING

Public Law 94-142 requires goals to be set annually, in each area needing special attention, at the IEP meeting. These areas are not simply academic or cognitive but include developmental, physical, social, emotional, and vocational areas as well. How does one set a goal for a recovering TBI student and say that by this time next year Johnny will be able to perform a certain task at a certain level or no longer exhibit a certain inappropriate behavior? Obviously, competent diagnostic and prescriptive advice is necessary. The IEP meeting must also establish a schedule for short-term measures of progress so that it can be determined during the year whether the desired result has been obtained. In setting interim objectives and determining how they will be assessed, competent diagnostic and prescriptive advice must be sought as well.

Finally, when goals are set, resources must be allocated sufficiently so that the program can be reasonably expected to confer the desired educational benefit. A school cannot agree that Johnny will have an educational goal of performing a certain task at a particular level of skill and then ignore the prescriptive advice that this will require a certain kind of therapy or a certain frequency and duration of therapy sessions. It is not unusual to see a school set a goal to remediate a physical disability and then place Johnny in the same twice-a-week, 20-minute group physical therapy slot in which it places all children who need physical therapy. Once a reasonable goal has been set, sufficient instructional and related services must be made available to lead Johnny to that goal, or it is not an appropriate educational program. Similarly, when short-term measures indicate that Johnny is not making progress toward achieving the expected goal, the school district must be prepared to reallocate resources. If Johnny is not meeting his goal in the twice weekly, 20-minute group sessions offered, then the school must be able to offer Johnny individual sessions, or longer duration or greater frequency of sessions.

RIGHT TO MORE THAN THE REGULAR SCHOOL DAY OR YEAR

Cases interpreting Public Law 94-142 make it clear that the student's entitlement is to appropriate educational services, not just whatever the school can offer during a regular 6-hour day, 5 days per week, 175 days per year. One recent Texas Federal Court case[11] underscored the right of the youngster to receive services beyond 6 hours per day, on weekends if needed, and throughout the summer. The school vigorously resisted any notion of services beyond

[11]Garland I.S.D. v. Wilks, 657 F.Supp. 1163 (N.D. Tex 1987)

6 hours, but the mother protested that her child was not only not receiving educational benefit but was doing so badly after school hours and on weekends that the overall effect was one of deterioration. The nature of his disability was such that he required continuous structured programming in order to be able to achieve anything educationally. The mother hired a tutor to work at home with the child in the evening, on weekends, and during the 2½-month summer recess. The federal court found that the school should have been offering that kind of service to the child and ordered the school to pay the mother back all the money she had spent privately to procure those services.

The logical extension of this right is that some students may need 24-hour-per-day continuity of structure in order to move forward educationally. Further, the educational personnel that interact with them during that 24-hour structured day may be needed at a skill level beyond that of parents or school personnel. To talk about 24 hours per day is no exaggeration for some TBI youngsters; disruptions in sleep patterns, including both frequency and duration, may be dramatic for extended periods of time, and a highly skilled individual for intervention may be as needed at 1:00 a.m. as at 1:00 p.m. The result may be the need to place some students for some portion of time in residential facilities where they can receive both continuous care and competent instructional programming.

When it is necessary to place the student in a residential facility in order to receive educational benefit, then all the costs, including room and board, would be a public expense under Public Law 94-142.[12] With any such placement in an alternative setting, the key is to make sure that a goal is developed to assist the youngster in reintegrating into more normal environments. One does not want goals that are aimed at institutionally appropriate behaviors that would be a barrier to the student ever returning to school. Such residential programs can be enormously expensive, and even though the right is clear under the law, one can always expect resistance from under-budgeted school districts.

DISCIPLINE PROBLEMS

Not all TBI students will exhibit behaviors that run afoul of disciplinary codes, but many will. Since the student was previously seen by the school district as normal, there will be an understandable tendency on the part of school personnel to expect that youngster to once again conform to regular rules of student conduct. Modifications have to be made in the management of

---

[12] 20 U.S.C. 1413(a)(4)(B), 34 CFR 300.302

behavior just as they do in the academic area if desired behavioral results are to be achieved.

Federal courts have made clear that before disciplining a student who has broken a school rule, the group of individuals who have planned the student's special educational program must first ask and answer whether the misbehavior was the result of the handicapping condition and/or the result of an inappropriate educational program or placement.[13]

Signs that a TBI student is beginning to misbehave can provide very significant diagnostic information, showing either a change in condition or a need for a change in the program. It may be that the youngster, once an exemplary citizen, no longer comprehends that a certain behavior is prohibited. Similarly, even if he or she comprehends the prohibited nature of the conduct, his or her disability may prevent the student from exercising the impulse control needed to prevent exhibiting the behavior. This writer has had reported to him typical incidents of shouting out in class, using obscene or abusive language, and totally refusing to comply with simple instructions such as "get back into your seat" or "go to the principal's office." Even sexual acting out or drug-related misconduct might be reported to shocked parents by shocked school personnel. It is hard, in that environment, to imagine appropriate disciplinary modifications without seeming to condone the misconduct, yet that is exactly what Public Law 94-142 requires.

This does not mean that the misbehavior is to be excused or forgotten. Misbehavior significant enough to warrant discipline is important diagnostic information that must be fed back into the IEP planning process to determine that at all times appropriate educational services are being offered. Where the conduct in question is so disruptive that it raises a concern for the safety of the student or others, the federal law certainly allows that the individual may be immediately removed from the educational environment. But even then the planning committee must reconvene as soon as possible to determine what, given this new misbehavior, constitutes appropriate educational programming, including modifications to address the behavior.[14]

When a TBI student is returning to school and to an environment of both peers and professionals who have viewed him or her differently prior to the accident, this writer likes to see the IEP planning conference produce a plan that includes information that would help others in the environment understand that behavior may be different for a while, but that with proper, informed responses by school staff and nonpunitive interventions, the student may recover the ability to conform to norms of conduct, just as it is hoped he or she will recover abilities to perform academically. This kind of counseling is certainly appropriate for the IEP.[15]

---

[13] S–1 v. Turlington, 635 F.2d 342 (5th Cir. 1981)

[14] Ibid.

[15] 20 U.S.C. 1401(17), 34 CFR 300.13

In summary, although any student receiving special educational services poses a challenge to a school district, the TBI youngster, both during initial recovery and long afterwards, poses a unique challenge. While TBI youngsters may seem normal and look normal in most aspects, they may be the most troubled and disabled students in the entire school district.

PART V

CONCLUSIONS AND FUTURE DIRECTIONS

20

Conclusions/Synthesis

ERIN D. BIGLER

This special series and edited text have addressed the current research and clinical status of traumatic brain injury. This epilogue is intended to review and synthesize what has been discussed and to focus on future directions in our understanding and treatment of acquired cerebral trauma.

TECHNOLOGICAL ADVANCES

Oftentimes with a period of rapid progress, future progress may outstrip its predecessor. Let us hope that this is the case with acquired cerebral trauma. Less than two decades ago it was almost unimaginable that we would be able to noninvasively image the central nervous system (Bigler, Yeo, & Turkheimer, 1989). But within the last 10 years we have witnessed not only the refinement of computerized tomographic (CT) scanning but also the introduction of magnetic resonance imaging (MRI) techniques that provide even greater detail than that obtained with CT scanning (Ruff, Cullum, & Luerssen, 1989), so that each image approximates a gross anatomic specimen (see Figure 20.1). Simultaneous with these advances are improvements in electrodiagnostics (Duffy & McAnulty, 1985; see Figure 20.2) and metabolic imaging (Positron Emission Tomography; PET; Pawlik & Heiss, 1989; see Figure 20.3) methods that offer windows into the underlying physiology of the brain. These past 10 years have literally been unprecedented in the technological progress that has been achieved in brain imaging (see Andreasen, 1988).

As a by-product of these imaging and electrophysiological methods, we now have a much better understanding of the mechanics of brain injury (Bigler, 1987a, 1987b). We can now visualize the acute structural effects of brain injury via CT and MRI, and these same procedures allow follow-up studies to evaluate the chronic structural residual deficits. These improved anatomic methods have led to greater understanding of brain and behavior relationships.

The technological improvements of the past two decades also have been matched by steady improvements in medical management of the brain injured victim. This has been particularly true with respect to regional trauma centers' improved neurosurgical techniques, including microsurgery and pharmacological methods to better treat acute cerebral edema, the major morbidity factor associated with traumatic brain injury (Lewis, 1976). Prior to these advances, the majority of patients with moderate to severe head injury died. Because of this fact, there was little emphasis on treatment. If the patient survived, then one hoped for spontaneous improvements in the cognitive and behavioral areas, but if improvements did not occur, treatment was often not sought because of the old philosophy that there was nothing you could do if you were brain damaged. Part of this can be attributed to the outdated thinking in psychology, neurology, and psychiatry that there was a clear delineation between normal and organic and that organic brain damage was untreatable (Goldstein, 1986).

TREATMENT

Fortunately, we now know that there are numerous treatment and intervention procedures that can be undertaken with the traumatically brain injured individual. Prigatano's chapters in this book demonstrated the positive effects that cognitive retraining (CR) may have on improving certain aspects of cognition in the brain injured individual. However, as Prigatano points out, there are many limitations to this new area of cognitive retraining, and this field is just emerging. Glisky and Schacter, in Chapter 16, demonstrated the effectiveness of a computer-based CR memory training program. It is anticipated that this type of methodology will continue to provide an exceptional opportunity for treating certain cognitive disorders. But it needs to be noted that Glisky and Schacter's work is the *first* to demonstrate the effectiveness of

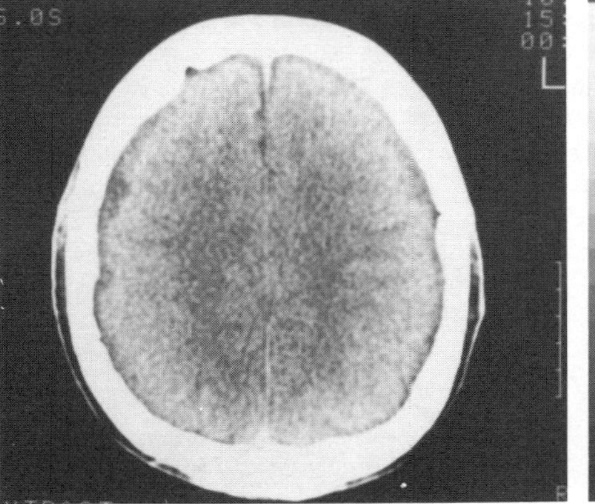

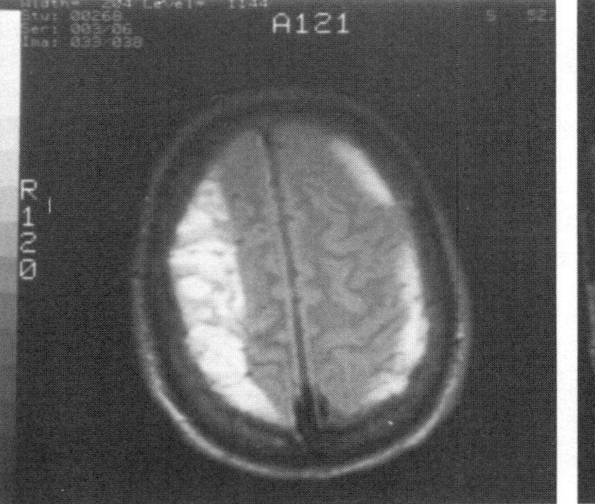

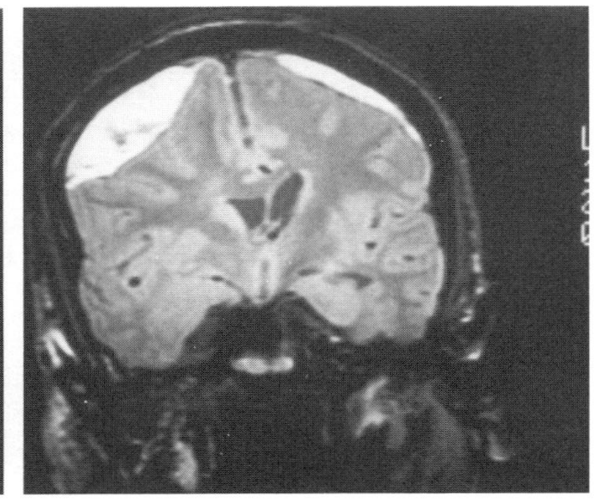

Figure 20.1. The CT scan on the left was interpreted as normal. However, the patient, a 67-year-old rancher, continued to complain of headache and impaired balance/coordination following a head injury incurred when he fell off of his moving tractor. Although the CT scan adequately depicts the major anatomic structures of the brain, it failed to detect the bilateral presence of a chronic subdural hematoma. (In retrospect, the thin, dark outer rim bilaterally is actually subdural fluid collecting.) However, MRI scans exquisitely depict the presence of the bilateral hematomas and the massive displacement of cerebral structures. The MRI scans were obtained 10 days after the CT and approximately 2 weeks postinjury. The MRI technology is permitting a much greater precision in the study of the structural effects of traumatic brain injury. Because of this, the next decade should see the evolution of improved understanding of neuroanatomic factors associated with brain injury, their detection, and outcome significance.

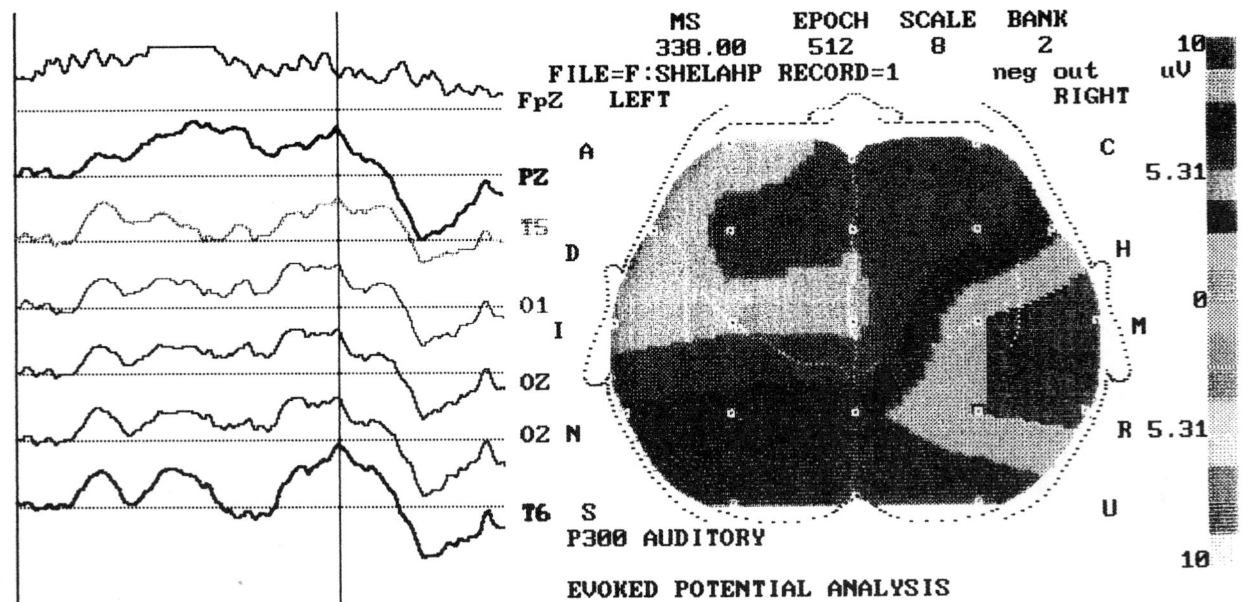

Figure 20.2. Computerized electroencephalography (EEG) map (Brain Map) from a 17-year-old male who had sustained severe brain injury 18 months prior. The dark area in the right hemisphere is indicative of abnormal activity in that region consistent with the area damaged when the patient sustained significant right temporal lobe contusion and secondary damage associated with a large epidural hematoma that was subsequently surgically removed. This is the same patient who was discussed in Figure 2.14 of Chapter 2 (this volume). The "Brain Map" method of evaluating the EEG provides a much-improved method of objective analysis of the electrophysiological abnormalities that may accompany traumatic brain injury, particularly in terms of chronic effects. Many times, the routine EEG will either be normal or display some minor irregularities, as it did for this patient, whereas the Brain Map results may portray a much more graphic and clinically descriptive picture of underlying electrophysiological abnormalities. It is anticipated that over the next decade we will have a much-improved understanding of the electrophysiological abnormalities associated with brain injury because of these computerized data analysis improvements.

such a program and its generalization to an actual work situation. This research is based on only one patient. It goes without saying that group studies and studies involving and comparing different etiologies (e.g., trauma, tumor, stroke, infection) are sorely needed. Treatment protocols need to be designed and tested and treatment standards need to be developed in the area of cognitive rehabilitation (Kreutzer & Boake, 1987; Rimmele & Hester, 1987).

As initial cognitive treatment programs for brain injured individuals were being reported in the late 1970s and early 1980s, some astounding improvements were noted (Rimmele & Hester, 1987). However, much of this early clinical research was fraught with many methodological problems, the most formidable of which has been the process of spontaneous improvement and recovery of function following a brain injury. To date, this problem has been best studied in aphasic patients who have suffered an acute cerebral vascular accident (i.e., stroke) that has damaged language centers of the brain but left other areas intact. Several studies have demonstrated significant improvement due solely to spontaneous recovery (Hartman & Landau, 1987; Wertz et al., 1986). These studies also have suggested that a variety of language treatment methods may bring about identical improvement. Thus, the key variable may be some level of language stimulation and training, irrespective of the treatment method used (i.e., speech therapists, trained volunteers, family members as therapists, or group counseling). From these studies it is apparent that any task that brings about cognitive stimulation may assist in recovery of function; this process obviously interacts with the spontaneous recovery processes as well. Thus, the jury is still out on the efficacy of *specific* cognitive retraining programs in the rehabilitation of the patient with acquired cerebral trauma, and more research is needed in this area.

Thus, the initial optimism of cognitive rehabilitation programs (cf. Rao & Bieliauskas, 1983) has now been met with the reality of how multifaceted and complex this problem is (Rimmele & Hester, 1987). Likewise, many cognitive deficits may be resistant to change with any of the currently available technologies. Another shortcoming is that these cognitive rehabilitation strategies have not found their way into many of the classroom settings where children with traumatic brain injury are being taught. It is likely that the child with significant brain injury, to receive optimal educational treatment, will require a comprehensive program very different from what is currently being offered (see Cohen, 1986).

Deaton's chapter (Chapter 10) reviewed various effective behavioral treatment strategies for improving the child's behavior in the classroom, outpatient treatment program, or home. Similarly, Telzrow's chapter (Chapter 11) provided specific guidelines for the school to aid in dealing with the academic deficiencies encountered by brain injured children. What is needed in the future is an integration of this information and an incorporation of cognitive rehabilitation strategies with the behavioral and academic deficits

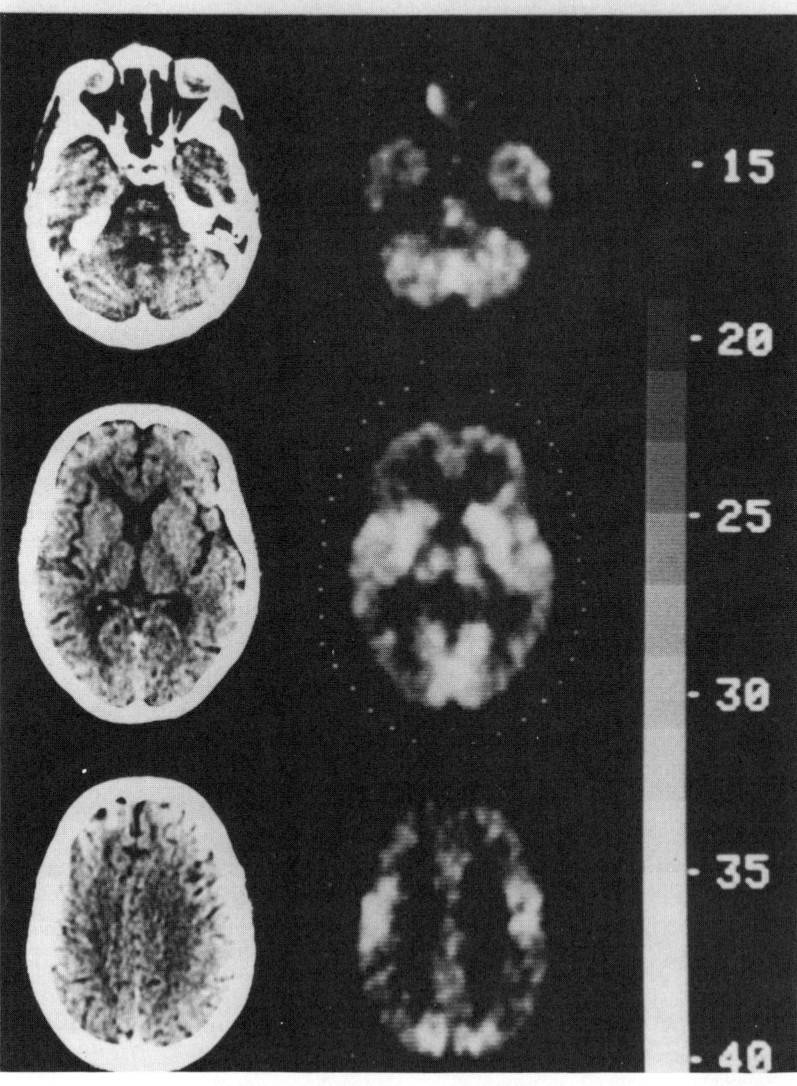
CT
PET
CMRglu
(μmol/100g/min)
15
20
25
30
35
40

seen in traumatic brain injured children. It is hoped that the guidelines offered by the authors in this series will be a catalyst for the implementation of such guidelines.

It is likely that some of the future advances in the treatment of the patient with acquired brain injury will come from a totally innovative approach that breaks with tradition. Much of our current understanding of human brain function has been molded by research that has been dominated by lesion-localization and hemispheric specialization theories (Orbach, 1982). However, we are still in the infancy of understanding human brain function, and some of our past neuropsychological traditions may actually hamper new insights into treatment. A case in point is the work by Helm-Estabrooks, Emery, and Albert (1987), who demonstrated improved language function in poststroke aphasic patients by focusing on perseverative behavioral deficits rather than specific language deficits. By utilizing behavioral strategies to reduce or eliminate perseverative behaviors, there was a concomitant improvement in overall language function, even though treatment of the language disorder was not the specific focus of the therapy, per se. Thus, eliminating one aberrant behavior (perseveration) had a very positive effect in improving a somewhat unrelated behavior (i.e., language). By stepping out of the bounds of traditional therapy (i.e., in this case not limiting the treatment to traditional speech therapy), an effective behavioral treatment method may assist in language recovery. It is hoped that similar improvements can be attained when innovative treatment strategies are applied to other neurobehavioral problems of those with acquired cerebral trauma.

Similarly, the research by Wood reviewed in Chapter 15 has significant implications for such nonspecific improvements. Since attention is so fundamental to all aspects of cognition, it seems reasonable to assume that

---

Figure 20.3. (facing page) The CTs presented on the left are from an 18-year-old male who had severe closed head injury. The CTs depict diffuse cortical atrophy, particularly in frontal and temporal lobe regions. The Positron Emission Tomography (PET) scans taken at a similar level demonstrate the marked changes in brain metabolism (i.e., the dark areas are regions of hypometabolism or less than normal activation) that accompany such severe brain injury (from Pawlik & Heiss, 1989). Although CT and MRI scanning techniques have reached such a level of technological advancement that the image generated approximates an actual anatomic specimen, such anatomic precision does not yield direct information about function. With the advent of PET scanning, we now have in vivo imaging techniques that provide some index of function. PET scanning is sensitive to regional changes that may accompany certain cognitive operations, and it is hoped that future research with PET will provide further understanding of the physiological changes that accompany brain injury. CMRglu stands for cerebral metabolic rate for glucose. As can be seen by comparing PET findings with CTs, the resolution with PET does not permit precise structural localization of metabolic activity. However, as resolution techniques improve, there should be corresponding improvement in our understanding of brain-behavior relationships.

techniques that improve attention in the brain injured individual may have generalized effects on numerous other behaviors. This further underscores the need to treat the whole individual and not just a single deficit area (Ben-Yishay et al., 1985).

Historically, there are a number of parallels between the development of school-based services for the congenitally brain injured individual (e.g., cerebral palsy) and program development for the learning disabled (LD) student (Rattan & Dean, 1987). Actual empirically derived and clinically proven programs that are integrated into public education are a rather recent phenomenon (Cohen, 1986). For most of this century, children with LD were taught with traditional methods and received no specialized educational treatment. Fortunately, over the past three decades we have witnessed an explosion of programs for the child with LD. It is hoped that this will be mirrored in terms of specific services and programs for the child/adolescent with acquired cerebral injury (Bengali, 1987).

ASSESSMENT

Although advancements have been made in the assessment of cognitive and behavioral effects of brain injury, it should be noted that the basic neuropsychological methods currently used in clinical practice were developed from the 1940s to the 1960s. Clinical assessment, in many ways, has not kept pace with developments in the cognitive sciences. For example, the Halstead-Reitan Battery (Reitan & Wolfson, 1985) was developed in the 1950s, based on Halstead's (1947) work on the functioning of the frontal lobes. The battery was standardized long before the use of brain imaging methods and does not have a theoretical basis (see Bigler et al., 1989). As reviewed in this text by Ewing-Cobbs and Fletcher (Chapter 5), the Halstead-Reitan tests are sensitive to cognitive deficits in brain injury, but it appears that there is need for much improvement. A number of researchers have been examining innovative assessment strategies that appear to have promise (Incagnoli, Goldstein, & Golden, 1986). It is also likely that computer-based assessment strategies hold great promise as assessment tools in this area.

The same criticisms raised over the somewhat outdated neuropsychological assessment methods can be raised with psychoeducational methods as they are used in assessing children with acquired cerebral trauma. As Obrzut and Hynd (Chapter 7) demonstrated in this text, educational tests can be either adapted or interpreted in ways that can lead to rich clinical information. But psychoeducational methods are steeped in rich tradition, and many may have little relationship to the cognitive or behavioral deficits associated with brain injury. Further, they may not provide a foundation from which to design fully effective treatment programs. It is not uncommon for the psychoeducational assessment to be quite unrepresentative of the deficit of a particular child who has sustained a brain injury. The brain injured child will often be examined in a sound-attenuated room in a one-to-one assessment situation. The examiner controls the pace of administration and assists with keeping the child's attention focused. However, none of this approximates what is seen in the classroom or home, where there are a multitude of competing stimuli and tasks that the child may be required to do or is exposed to. Thus, current clinical assessment has many limitations. This problem needs to be addressed through further research on the interrelationship between psychoeducational methods and neuropsychological techniques, along with innovative assessment methods that will meet the needs of the brain injured child. Similar statements can be made about language deficits and their assessment as has been outlined by Marquardt, Stoll, and Sussman in Chapter 8.

As pointed out by Wood in Chapter 15, one of the most common deficits encountered in acquired brain injury is in the area of attentional deficits. Yet few of the current assessment methods address attention. Along these lines Wilson and Moffat (1984a, 1984b) have demonstrated the greater effectiveness of a memory assessment battery that incorporates a naturalistic setting (see also Baddeley, 1986). Considerable innovativeness needs to be directed to this entire area of assessment.

POTENTIAL INNOVATIVE THERAPIES

Recent advances have been made in the pharmacologic treatment of the cognitive and behavioral deficits associated with traumatic brain injury. McGuire and Sylvester reviewed the current status in this area in Chapter 9 of this text. Unfortunately, clinical research in the area of pharmacologic treatment in brain injury has lagged behind the general use of medications in the treatment of emotional disorders (Cope, 1987). Various case studies and small group studies now have demonstrated beneficial results in brain injured individuals with a wide spectrum of psychoactive agents (Cardenas, 1987; Childs, 1987; Evans & Gualtieri, 1987; Glenn & Joseph, 1987; Hayes, Stonnington, & Lyeth, 1987; Horn, 1987; McLean, Stanton, Cardenas, & Bergerud, 1987; Mysiw & Jackson, 1987; O'Shanick, 1987; Parmalee & O'Shanick, 1987; Weinberg, Auerbach, & Moore, 1987). The net effect of brain injury may be depletion of certain critical neurotransmitter levels for normal cognitive and behavior functioning. This is particularly true for the catecholamines because their projection from the midbrain region ascends via the frontal lobes (Robinson, Lipsey, & Price, 1985). Since the frontal lobes are so often involved with traumatic brain injury (Bigler, 1987b), it would be expected that there could be neurotransmitter dysregulation in many cases of acquired cerebral trauma.

Pharmacologic intervention in the future may also play a major role in the acute recovery process. Feeney and his colleagues (Feeney & Hovda, 1985; Hovda & Feeney, 1984, 1985; Sutton, Weaver, & Feeney, 1987) have demonstrated that amphetamine treatment early in the course of recovery from experimentally induced brain damage in rats and cats enhances recovery. It appears that there is an important interactive effect with postinjury treatment experience with drug administration, since pharmacologic treatment in isolation does not result in the desired outcome. It is also important to note that this improvement can be blocked by pharmacological treatment with haloperidol (Haldol®), a major antipsychotic drug (Feeney, Gonzalez, & Law, 1982). Since haloperidol is one of the more commonly used tranquilizers for behavioral management (Cardenas, 1987), it may actually hinder cognitive recovery if used early in rehabilitation. No definitive human clinical research is available yet, but the issue is the topic of intense research at a number of centers. For example, Crisostomo, Duncan, Propst, Dawson, and Davis (1988) recently demonstrated modest clinical improvement in motor function in eight poststroke (cerebral infarction) patients who were treated with amphetamine and traditional physical therapy methods. It needs to be underscored that this is very preliminary work, and extensive clinical trials with double-blind cross-over research methods need to be carried out.

Nonetheless, this preliminary research with pharmacologic treatment appears to hold tremendous promise for the brain injured individual. The amphetamine medication, per se, will probably not be the answer, because it has a variety of potentially negative side effects, particularly in terms of hypertensive vascular properties and effects on seizure threshold, both of which represent important problems for the brain injured patient. Thus, various amphetamine analogs are being evaluated (Sutton et al., 1987). If this research continues to show promise, it is likely that human clinical trials will be forthcoming with catecholamine agonists being administered throughout the acute and initial recovery phases.

Animal models studying the neurologic recovery from an embolic stroke (i.e., cerebral vascular accident that occurs because of a foreign particle creating a clot in a vessel) have made significant progress in developing pharmacologic agents that may reduce the clot and restore appropriate blood flow (Zivin et al., 1988). These studies have indicated that significant neurologic improvement can occur up to 45 minutes poststroke, with the improvement occurring as a by-product of restored blood flow. Since one of the main damaging effects of edema associated with traumatic brain injury is reduced blood flow, further pharmacologic treatment advances in the management and early treatment of cerebral edema and improved blood flow should lead to improved outcome in acquired cerebral injury. Thus, advances in stroke research should be closely monitored, because they may have significant implications for improving recovery in traumatic brain injury.

Other preliminary research has suggested that there may be a role of pharmacologic treatment in patients with unilateral neglect syndromes. Neglect is the phenomenon usually associated with right hemisphere damage, particularly in posterior regions, where the patient may display one or a combination of the following behaviors (Bigler, 1988a, 1988b): (a) failure to cross midline opposite to the side of the cerebral lesion, (b) failure to perceive auditory, tactile, or visual stimulation contralateral to the area of brain damage, or (c) lack of awareness of the opposite body side (usually the left) altogether, so that the patient may not even be aware of the opposite-side body deficits (i.e., not appreciating the presence or significance of left-side paralysis). Fleet, Valenstein, Watson, and Heilman (1987) demonstrated that by using a medication that functions as a dopamine agonist (i.e., a medication that facilitates release of dopamine, an important brain neurotransmitter), the degree of left-side neglect could be minimized. Although this is preliminary case study research, it does suggest that there may be potential medication breakthroughs in the treatment of various chronic residual deficits associated with acquired cerebral trauma.

Considerable research is directed toward a better understanding of regenerative properties of neurons once they have been injured, but not irrevocably damaged (Benowitz & Routtenberg, 1987). It may be that pharmacologic intervention will play a role in regeneration of partially damaged neurons. Research in this area is just beginning.

Recently, there have been amazing advances in the treatment of Parkinson's disease, with the first grafting/transplanting of tissue into the brain of patients severely afflicted with this degenerative disease (Björklund et al., 1987). In Parkinson's disease there is a loss of dopamine, a brain neurotransmitter critical for background motor control, which occurs as a result of degeneration of the basal ganglia. At least in the early stages of this disease, the degeneration is specific to the nigro-striatal system involving the basal ganglia, and the remainder of the brain is unaffected (Bigler, 1988b). Because of the depletion of dopamine, a resting tremor develops that results in the movement disorder characteristic of Parkinson's disease. Replacement of dopamine partially restores normal motor control; hence the tremendous success of this procedure. It needs to be emphasized that in these cases there is not generalized damage to the central nervous system, and that the grafting/transplantation is directed to treating a specific deficit—the tremor associated with the loss of appropriate levels of dopamine in the brain.

At least in the short term it does not appear that this method holds any promise for acquired brain injury, unless it is in a traumatically induced Parkinsonism-type condition, without generalized brain injury. The reason for this limitation is that with acquired brain injury, the damage is usually diffuse, affecting multiple areas of the brain along with numerous neurotransmitter systems (Bigler, 1987a, 1987b). The complexity of disrupted neuronal and pharmacologic interconnections with brain injury is literally unfathomable. It has been estimated that a single neuron may have as many as 10,000 separate inputs from other neurons (Nauta & Feirtag, 1986). Since there are 10^{12} neurons within the central nervous system, the number of potential interconnections is almost limitless. Thus, even minor damage probably disrupts millions of cells and tens of millions of interconnections. Since neural interconnections develop over time and in response to experience (Cowan, 1979), it is unlikely that brain grafting, in its present form, will play a role in treating acquired cerebral injury. This remains a major basic research area, and potential applications are certainly a possibility.

LONG-TERM OUTCOME

As pointed out by Lezak and O'Brien in Chapter 17, the potential cognitive-behavioral and characterological problems of the individual with acquired brain damage are many and may be permanent. Table 20.1 reviews the major residual deficits in this domain that may accompany cerebral trauma. Because of the degree and severity of these deficits, a number of individuals with chronic brain injury will require some form of long-term placement. Until recently this was a neglected patient population, but numerous residential programs have been developed over the past decade. These are typically structured community programs that utilize behavioral principles in managing the organic behavior problems. Many of the methods outlined by Deaton (1987) in this series are useful in the care and treatment of the brain injured patient in this setting. These programs have demonstrated considerable effectiveness in managing many of the behavior problems, particularly the impulsivity and amotivational syndromes that so often accompany brain injury (Burke, 1987).

A main factor related to the success of these residential programs is that they provide the external structure that many individuals with chronic brain injury require (Kozloff, 1987; Harrington & Levandowski, 1987). Most of the problems outlined in Table 20.1 relate in some fashion to poor monitoring and control of internal states and the inability to effectively interact and adapt to the environment. These programs provide stability by reducing the complexity of the surrounding environment and the coping demands placed upon the brain injured individual. In such residential settings the environment is made more predictable and less ambiguous by following routines and schedules along with simple behavior reinforcement schedules. In a residential treatment environment, task complexity can be gradually increased to determine

TABLE 20.1
The Most Common Cognitive-Behavioral Sequelae Associated with Traumatic Brain Injury

Impaired Orientation	Slow Rate of Performance
Impaired Attention	Decreased Flexibility
Impaired Concentration	Increased Perseveration
Dysfunctional Memory	Difficulty Staying on Task
Poor Impulse Control	Impaired Initiation
Overly Concrete	Diminished Capacity to Generalize
Impaired Language Processing	Impaired Judgment
Slowness in Thinking	Impaired Problem-Solving Skills
Slow Rate of Processing	Poor Frustration Tolerance
Inconsistent Performance	Fatigability

Note. Adapted in part from Thomsen (1987).

the patient's highest level of adaptive functioning and degree of independence that can be attained. The majority of individuals with brain injury who will require residential care will be in such placements for 18 to 36 months, and in some cases much longer. There is also a subgroup of brain injured patients who will require permanent residential placement because the degree of their behavioral-personality disturbance does not permit independent functioning and the family cannot meet the level of care required to keep their behavior under control.

As R. Martin points out in Chapter 19 of this text, these brain injured individuals are entitled to certain legal rights and treatment opportunities. Over the past half century we have witnessed the growth of programs for many debilitating conditions, such as cerebral palsy, muscular dystrophy, diabetes, and so forth. With the creation of the National Head Injury Foundation (NHIF),[1] along with its local programs, there is now a focus on greater community awareness for the needs of the brain injured individual. This has resulted in the development of community-based therapeutic programs for the chronically brain injured individual. These are important developments because the comprehensive hospital-based or extended treatment programs are labor intensive and accordingly very expensive (i.e., $50,000 to $100,000 per year or more). Only a minority of acquired brain injury patients have the financial resources or insurance to cover such expenses. This is why it will be so critical to develop community programs to fill this need in the future, as the

[1]NHIF Address: P.O. Box 567, Framingham, MA 01701.

funding problem will likely continue. It should also be noted, as pointed out by Goldstein and Levin (Chapter 3, this volume), that the preponderance of acquired brain injury occurs in individuals 25 years of age and younger. Thus, such individuals are looking ahead at a lifetime and need the opportunity for the most complete recovery possible.

The emotional and stress effects of TBI on the family begin immediately after the family is informed that one of their family members has been injured. Dealing with life and death issues associated with an emergency admission to a hospital following TBI sets the stage for many profound emotions with which most people have not had previous experience. Similarly, most families have never had experience in dealing with the effects of acute or chronic brain injury. Following a traumatic injury to the brain, immediate family members are usually under the mistaken assumption that once the immediate crisis is over their loved one will simply "recover" and be just "like they were." Most families are prepared for neither the acute nor the chronic emotional impact that TBI has.

To illustrate the acute impact effects on emotional coping in the family, excerpts from a mother's diary written during her son's hospital stay following a severe traumatic injury to the brain are presented in Figure 20.4. Clinical comments are also provided for each entry.

FAMILY IMPACT OF CHRONIC BRAIN INJURY

D. Martin reviewed the impact of traumatic brain injury in children and adolescents on the family in Chapter 18 of this text. Obviously, in children and adolescents who are brain injured, the parents are still in a caregiving role. As D. Martin points out, there are similarities between the impact on the family of a chronic illness such as cystic fibrosis and the impact of traumatic brain injury. However, brain injury in the adult individual throws the spouse, parent, or relative into a caregiving role. Brooks, Campsie, Symington, Beattie, and McKinlay (1987) have studied the effects of severe brain injury on the relatives of the victim up to 7 years postinjury. One of the most important findings of their research is that the level or degree of physical disability did not predict psychosocial burden levels in relatives. Rather, the degree of burden was related to the type of behavioral, cognitive (language and/or memory), affective-emotional, and dependency deficits, with the two most prominent being behavioral and emotional deficits. A full 89% of the relatives indicated moderate to high degrees of subjective burden imposed by changes in the areas of violence, aggression, childishness, and dependency. Livingston (1987) demonstrated that these burden effects are recognized relatively early in the course of recovery and change little over the first year. The

Brooks, McKinley, Symington, Beattie, and Campsie (1987) work covered a time span up to 7 years, suggesting that many of these psychosocial changes may affect the family permanently.

The impact that TBI has upon a spouse is particularly great. What follows is the personal account of the behavioral and cognitive changes from the perspective of a spouse who was 30 years of age when she wrote the following statement. Her 35-year-old husband of 11 years had been a patient of mine for the past 18 months since sustaining a severe closed head injury which had resulted in significant cognitive deficits and changes in behavior. She came in one day and confided to me that she did not know if she could withstand the pressures of dealing with a brain injured spouse and all the accompanying changes. She was coming to grips with the conclusion that her husband was truly a "different" person and that life would not return to the way it had been before he was injured. To help her focus on her loss, so as to understand it better, I asked her to take some time and write out her perception of how things had changed. She was given no other instruction than this, and the report that follows was spontaneously generated by this spouse in approximately 45 minutes. This account is an elegant and poignant personal statement of the emotional challenges that this spouse faced in witnessing and dealing with the behavioral and cognitive changes that occurred (from Bigler, 1989).

Before his injury, Sam (the name has been changed) was an accomplished musician and leader of his own band. He had recently been on a national tour and had just released his first album. He had completed 2 years of college and had no prior history of neurological or psychiatric problems. The spouse's account given in an unabridged form is presented below.

CHANGES IN SAM

Confidence

Before: Was a total professional and perfectionist in his work. He had total confidence in his self, his singing, his writing, his performing and his dealing with his peers, management people and record label people.
After: He has no confidence at all. He doubts everything about himself, *i.e.*, if someone visits with him and mentions collaborating on some material, he avoids the situation because he doesn't think he has the ability or feels the creativeness he once had.

Drive and Energy

Before: Sam was a workaholic. He was always performing or working on his original material. He enjoyed it and worked many odd and long hours.
After: He has lost his drive to do anything. His energy level is very low and takes naps during the day, *i.e.*, he will go to work with me and just sit and then fall asleep. If he's at home he doesn't pick up after his self like he use to, and he'll just sit and do nothing. (*i.e.*, watch TV, but says he doesn't enjoy it as much).

Diary Excerpts	Clinical Comment
April 14 (day of injury) We are talking to him all the time. We don't know what he hears or if his subconscious hears. It's so hard to look at him and not cry. Larry made the newspaper today — such a small article for such a big thing in our lives.	On the day of injury the family is usually in a state of shock and in a short period of time have experienced a bewildering array of emotions. It is very common for family members to misinterpret the significance of the coma and think of it more in terms of a deep sleep and that their loved one will "awaken" at some point and be the person that he or she was before the injury. In addition, most families know very little about brain injury and this further limits their ability to initially comprehend and deal with the acute injury. The mother makes a very poignant statement about how the accident had had such a tragic impact upon their family and instantaneously changed their lives, but only receives passing attention in the newspaper.
Motorcyclist injured in collision with car A 23-year-old motorcyclist received severe head injuries early Wednesday when the motorcycle he was driving collided with an automobile in the 4400 block of South Congress Avenue. In serious condition in Brackenridge Hospital late Wednesday was Larry ■■■■, of 1807½ Fortview Road. The accident occurred at 12:14 a.m., police said. ■■■■ was driving a motorcycle that collided with a car driven by ■■■■, Austin. ■■■■ was not injured.	
April 22 . . . and we know God will eventually put Larry together the way he was before the accident . . . if I can stay thinking clinical, I can keep the emotions of a mother down.	One's religious background often comes into play in helping sustain some degree of hope and optimism during this very trying period.

Figure 20.4. The left-hand column is composed of daily diary excerpts from the mother of a 23-year-old son who had just sustained a severe TBI following a motorcycle-automobile collision. He was rendered deeply comatose. The right-hand column contains the author's comments concerning the mother's emotional reaction and expression at that time. The insert beneath the April 14 entry is the brief newspaper statement that was published the day of the accident. The various excerpts were selected because they demonstrate the typical emotions that a family goes through in the initial stages of a brain injury.

Figure 20.4 (cont.)

The mother also makes a very important observation on how to keep her "emotions" in check. At this point in the recovery process it is usually important for the family member to make this type of adjustment.

May 12

... The coma is so hard for us to live with day in and day out but it's for his protection right now. No pain or memory or full awareness.

The comatose patient does present a difficult situation for the family to deal with and it is common to develop such defensive thoughts as expressed by this mother.

May 14

IT'S NOT FAIR!
IT'S NOT FAIR!

No matter how well a family or family member is coping there is almost always a period of considerable frustration that develops. This may turn into anger that may be directed toward those health care professionals working with the patient or the others involved in the accident.

May 16

... everyone ate supper here tonight — it was so strange for Larry not to be here. I think everyone felt the void in their own way .... This is the first day I've missed since the accident.

The mother had been at the hospital for the entire month from the time of Larry's initial injury and would only leave the hospital to sleep. This was the first day the family had met at home, outside the hospital. As indicated by this entry, each step requires dealing with new and different emotions.

May 25

... Larry said "Hi Mom" — I was so thrilled I cried!

Larry came out of the coma 6½ weeks after being injured and responded with a "Hi Mom." However, this is only the very beginning of the recovery process and the family soon realizes that a very long rehabilitation is in store. Thus, the initial "thrill" of having your loved one respond gives way to the reality of how long the recovery process actually is.

Self-Esteem/Self-Image

Before: Sam used to have a very high self-image and self-esteem. He was his own commodity, his body was his instrument and therefore he had to sell hisself as his business project. He was even known to be somewhat arrogant and cocky. He carried himself in a very business and professional way. He knew his business in and out and spoke with experience and intelligence and was respected by many in the music business.

After: He doesn't think much of his self at all now. He doesn't even like hisself, *i.e.*, He has spoke of wanting to die. He has often said if he lost me and Jimmy he would not want to live. He has feared many times of losing me to someone else or that I would get tired of him and leave him. He very, very seldom (maybe 3 or 4 times since the accident) goes out without me. Even if some one asks him to go to a concert or to the rehearsal hall, he won't go unless I go. He follows me absolutely everywhere I go, *i.e.*, to the grocery store, shopping mall or to run any kind of errand, and he seldom talks. (He NEVER use to go to these places with me.)

Personality/Laughter/Happy/Social

Before: Sam had a great and warm personality and great laugh. He was always bouncing around the house and singing his songs on his guitar. If he wasn't working on his material and the radio was on—he'd be singing very loud and dancing to the song and performing as if he were on a big stage. He was fun to be around and our phone never stopped ringing.

After: He's not aggressive or strong in the personality department. He's not happy often and laughs seldom, *i.e.*, he doesn't socialize hardly at all. When we're around people he seldom talks and sometimes sits in one place off to his self. When he laughs he doesn't push out but sucks it in and has the sound of someone slightly mentally retarded. He never sings around the house or in the car or to me or Jimmy. He never dances.

Fear and Future Aspects

Before: Sam always felt it was meant to be for him to perform and sing and he knew he'd always would make it one day and all our futures would be secured. He was assured of his self.

After: He doesn't know what life has in store for him at all now. He's afraid and can't make many decisions and then he'll start making many (foolish) decisions, *i.e.*, He fears gravely for our future, especially Jimmy's. He talks about buying a boat and going in the Gulf for days at a time to catch fish to make a living (this way he says he would not have to talk or deal with people).

Speech/Voice

Before: Sam communicated and expressed himself eloquently (better than the average person). He had incredible range in his singing voice.

After: Lost his singing voice totally, and talks only when he feels like he has to, *i.e.*, as the day progresses his voice gets weak and it drains his energy. Has poor articulation and has a lot of nasal air loss. He feels uncomfortable talking and *very very very* self conscious of his speech. He seldom answers the phone and has me order for him at restaurants.

Coping/Temper

Before: Sam could handle any given situation and always under total control. Over the years he has taught me how to deal with peole and be independent and self reliant (things I never knew—I was very over-protected and totally taken care of by my parents when I met Sam and married him at 19 years old). I always looked at him as a husband, father and best friend (I still call him Daddy—a term of endearment).

After: Sam lacks the ability to cope in a working or serious world, *i.e.*, He has trouble making simple bank deposits for me. He gets confused when he's trying to explain something and gets mad *very very very very* easy and will cuss me *very very very* ugly (and "*never*" did this before!)

Hearing

Before: Produced and engineered recording sessions with great results.

After: Has high pitch loss of hearing, *i.e.*, Sometimes doesn't hear Jimmy as well. Doesn't hear when a music track is mixed bad. Can't hear the fuzz or cymble problems, etc. Doesn't hear the alarm on his watch. This is an aggrivation to Sam.

Isolated

Before: Sam was in the middle of everything happening musically.

After: Sam feels alienated and left out of everything, *i.e.*, Music people, management, record label, distributors, agents don't call anymore. No one needs his expertise or help anymore.

Smile/Sneezing

Before: Total control of face muscles.

After: Lacks total control of face muscles, *i.e.*, He smiles at inappropriate times. He can't help it and upsets him very much because it usually happens when he's not happy or very serious or mad. He has incredible sneezing attacks. He gets very messy and just hates it. We bought him a bunch of handkerchiefs, but of course he doesn't carry them around with him 24 hrs a day and never knows when he's going to start sneezing uncontrollably.

Weight/Dress

Sam has *never* had a weight problem and always looked great in his clothes and always dressed well. He never had a big appetite and eating was seldom the highlight of his day like it is to many.

After: He has not been able to return to his weight he had before the accident. He's always hungry and looks forward to every meal and then some. Doesn't dress at all the way he use to, *i.e.*, He'll try to leave the house in a wrinkled shirt. He doesn't match his clothes. He'll try and wear pants or shorts that are way too tight and look awful. He dresses very simple and humble.

Eyesite

Before: Perfect 20/20 vision.

After: Has to wear contacts or glasses always. His eyes seem to stay red and bother him. Sometimes he feels he sees much more poorly out of one eye and fears it'll just get worse one day.

Strength

Before: Sam used to be very physical and kept in shape always. Was always active. Around the house he was always doing pull ups, push ups and many chin ups. He was *real good* at all. He would ski on one ski, turn circles and dance on roller skates, was a real good dirt bike rider, loved to play racket ball and beat most of his contenders in tennis. He carried Jimmy around on his shoulders practically everywhere we went. When he was young he had a belt of high rank in either Karate or judo (I don't remember). He was a high school star basketball player and excelled in every sport he did, *i.e.*, pole vaulting.

After: None of the above exist. He'll only do a few sit ups now and then, *i.e.*, Reason being he lacks energy and drive and has a damaged shoulder that cannot stay in the socket, is painful, a constant annoyance and aggrivation. He has trouble doing simple tasks like washing his hair, brushing his teeth or rolling over in bed, because every time the arm moves around, the joint comes out of the socket.

This spouse's account of the significant cognitive and behavioral changes that have occurred since her husband's brain injury personalizes the impact that head injury has on one's life as well as on one's spouse. Based on CT and neuropsychological test results which both indicated frontal-temporal lobe damage/dysfunction, one would expect the development of an organic personality syndrome with corresponding changes in intellect, social skills, judgment, memory, drive, and motivation. All of these changes are eloquently noted by this spouse in her review of how her husband has changed.

Another area that remains a major obstacle in treating patients with acquired brain injury is their impaired awareness of their loss of function; this also impacts the family's ability to deal with the brain injured family member. Brooks et al. (Brooks, Campsie, Symington, Beattie, & McKinlay, 1987; Brooks, McKinlay, Symington, Beattie, & Campsie, 1987) have demonstrated that self-perception in the brain injured individual is typically impaired when compared to relatives' perception of the patient. In their study, Brooks, Campsie, et al. (1987) found that patients with acquired cerebral injury underestimated their level of deficit in all areas when compared to relatives' evaluation (see Table 20.2). The chapter by Prigatano and Klonoff (Chapter 14) argues that this deficit in self-awareness is the major limiting factor in the psychotherapeutic treatment of the traumatically brain injured individual and, accordingly, results in a negative impact on long-term outcome.

PREVENTION

Since we are literally in the genesis of effective treatment modalities for the amelioration of the effects of chronic brain injury, probably the single most

TABLE 20.2
Behavior Problems in the Patient Reported by More Than One-half of the Relatives of Brain Injured Victims and the Corresponding Number of Symptoms Reported by the Patient

Problem	% Relatives Reporting	% Patients Reporting
Slowness	77	
Personality Change	76	
Poor Memory	76	66
Anger/Irritability/Impatience	74	62
Tiredness	70	43
Tension/Anxiety/Worry	65	35
Poor Concentration	64	41
Depression	63	49
Mood Changes	63	
Poor Balance/Coordination	59	23
Restlessness	54	
More Easily Affected by Alcohol	54	

Note. From Brooks et al. (1987).

important method in dealing with acquired brain injury is not to have one or to minimize the degree of injury. The vast majority of brain injuries are accidental and could have been avoided had certain precautions been utilized. Since motor vehicle accidents constitute the number one source of injury (Rivara & Mueller, 1986), improvements in car safety will have a tremendous preventative influence. The public and professional sectors should unequivocally support efforts for improved vehicular safety, road improvements, and laws and ordinances governing safety issues (e.g., seat belts, speed limits, reckless driving, and driving while intoxicated). Rivara and Mueller (1986) have reviewed research in this area suggesting that

> the most successful injury prevention strategies are passive ones in which agents, vehicles, or environments are changed to automatically protect the population at risk. Much less successful are approaches that require the active cooperation of an individual. For example, air bags are more likely to be effective than seat belts, simply because they work automatically and do not require an action every time someone steps into a car. Passive strategies are not easy to implement and for some types of injuries these strategies are not presently available. (pp. 11–12)

The majority of the 15- to 25-year-olds, who have the highest incidence of brain injury (see review in Chapter 3 by Goldstein & Levin), are injured because of reckless driving, driving while intoxicated, or being struck by a driver who was driving while intoxicated (Rivara & Mueller, 1986; Spivack, 1986). This age group should be targeted with an information campaign to increase awareness of the problem.

We should also review and update safety guidelines dealing with athletics. A number of the contact sports, such as football and boxing, place the participant at risk for brain injury (Rivara & Mueller, 1986). Even in these sports areas improvements can be made with safety measures. Also, activities involving skate boards, scooters, and bicycles place the rider at risk if fundamental safety rules are not followed. Educational programs directed toward safety instruction will remain crucial as a preventative measure.

CONCLUSIONS

Courville in 1969 reviewed the current status of craniocerebral trauma at that time. The primary focus of treatment then was on the acute effects of brain injury, and, essentially, Courville's entire text was devoted to that aspect. As for potential residual deficits, based on the knowledge and clinical experience up to that point, Courville concludes that "serious injuries to the head may require one or more years before complete recovery occurs" and that patients should be instructed to "rest until all symptoms have disappeared with the gradual resumption of activities, always staying within the bounds of being symptom free" (p. 201). The implicit message of this statement was that there was little that could be done for the brain injured individual other than to allow the beneficial effects of the passage of time. As can be gathered from the information and current clinical status of patient care for the brain injured individual, we have indeed come a long way in the past two decades. This text has demonstrated that we currently have a much greater understanding of the pathophysiology of brain injury, the acute and chronic structural changes in the brain that may accompany brain injury, and the psychosocial impact that such damage has on the individual and family. Continued clinical research efforts need to be directed toward improved assessment techniques, innovative cognitive and behavioral treatment strategies, and family intervention and coping aids. Focus on long-term outcome and quality-of-life issues needs to be maintained. Basic neuroscience research also may provide potential future treatment options, particularly in the area of psychopharmacologic intervention.

REFERENCES

Andreasen, N.C. (1988). Brain imaging: Applications in psychiatry. *Science, 239*, 1381–1388.

Baddeley, A. (1986). *Working memory.* Cambridge: Oxford University Press.

Bengali, V. (1987). *Head injury in children and adolescents: A resource and review for school and allied professionals.* Brandon, VT: Clinical Psychology Publishing.

Benowitz, L.I., & Routtenberg, A. (1987). A membrane phosphoprotein associated with neural development, axonal regeneration, phospholipid metabolism, and synaptic plasticity. *Trends in Neuroscience, 12*, 527–531.

Ben-Yishay, Y., Rattok, J., Lakin, P., Piasetsky, E.B., Ross, B., Silver, S., Zide, E., & Ezrachi, O. (1985). Neuropsychologic rehabilitation: Quest for a holistic approach. *Seminars in Neurology, 5*, 252–259.

Bigler, E.D. (1987a). The clinical significance of cerebral atrophy in traumatic brain injury. *Archives of Clinical Neuropsychology, 2*, 293–304.

Bigler, E.D. (1987b). Neuropathology of acquired cerebral trauma. *Journal of Learning Disabilities, 20*, 458–473.

Bigler, E.D. (1988a). Acquired cerebral trauma: Attention, memory, and language disorders. *Journal of Learning Disabilities, 21*, 325–326.

Bigler, E.D. (1988b). *Diagnostic clinical neuropsychology* (rev. ed.). Austin: University of Texas Press.

Bigler, E.D. (1989). Behavioral and cognitive changes in traumatic brain injury: A spouse's perspective. *Brain Injury, 3*, 73–78.

Bigler, E.D., Yeo, R.A., & Turkheimer, E. (1989). *Neuropsychological function and brain imaging.* New York: Plenum.

Björklund, A., Lindvall, O., Isacson, O., Brundin, P., Wictorin, K., Strecker, R.E., Clarke, D.J., & Dunnett, S.B. (1987). Mechanisms of action of intracerebral neural implants: Studies on nigral striatal grafts to the lesioned striatum. *Trends in Neurosciences, 10*, 509–516.

Brooks, N., Campsie, L., Symington, C., Beattie, A., & McKinlay, W. (1987). The effects of severe head injury on patient and relative within seven years of injury. *Journal of Head Trauma Rehabilitation*, 2(3), 1–13.

Brooks, N., McKinlay, W., Symington, C., Beattie, A., & Campsie, L. (1987). Return to work within the first seven years of severe head injury. *Brain Injury, 1*(1), 5–19.

Burke, D.C. (1987). Planning a system of care for head injuries. *Brain Injury, 1*, 189–198.

Cardenas, D.D. 31987). Antipsychotics and their use after traumatic brain injury. *Journal of Head Trauma Rehabilitation*, 2(4), 43–49.

Childs, A. (1987). Naltrexone in organic bulemia: A preliminary report. *Brain Injury, 1*, 49–55.

Cohen, S.B. (1986). Educational reintegration and programming for children with head injuries. *Journal of Head Trauma Rehabilitation, 1*, 22–29.

Cope, D.N. 31987). Psychopharmacologic considerations in the treatment of traumatic brain injury. *Journal of Head Trauma Rehabilitation*, 2(4), 1–5.

Courville, C.B. (1969). Trauma to the central nervous system and its envelopes. *Tice's practice of medicine.* New York: Harper & Row.

Cowan, W.M. (1979). The development

of the brain. *Scientific American, 241*, 112–133.

Crisostomo, E.A., Duncan, D.W., Propst, M., Dawson, D.V., & Davis, J.N. (1988). Evidence that amphetamine with physical therapy promotes recovery of motor function in stroke patients. *Annals of Neurology, 23*, 94–97.

Deaton, A.V. 31987). Behavioral change strategies for children and adolescents with severe brain injury. *Journal of Learning Disabilities, 20*, 581–589.

Duffy, F.H., & McAnulty, G.B. (1985). Brain electrical activity mapping (BEAM): The search for a physiological signature of dyslexia. In F.H. Duffy & N. Geschwind (Eds.), *Dyslexia: A neuroscientific approach to clinical evaluation*. Boston: Little Brown.

Evans, R.W., & Gualtieri, C.T. (1987). Psychostimulant pharmacology in traumatic brain injury: *Journal of Head Trauma Rehabilitation*, 2(4), 29–33.

Ewing-Cobbs, L., & Fletcher, J.M. (1987). Neuropsychological assessment of head injury in children. *Journal of Learning Disabilities, 20*, 526–535.

Feeney, D.M., Gonzalez, A., & Law, W.A. (1982). Amphetamine, haloperidol, and experience interact to affect rate of recovery after motor cortex injury. *Science, 217*, 855–857.

Feeney, D.M., & Hovda, D.A. (1985). Reinstatement of binocular depth perception by amphetamine and visual experience after visual cortex ablation. *Brain Research, 342*, 352–356.

Fleet, W.S., Valenstein, E., Watson, R.T., & Heilman, K.M. (1987). Dopamine agonist therapy for neglect in humans. *Neurology, 37*, 1765–1770.

Glenn, M.B., & Joseph, A.B. (1987). The use of lithium for behavioral and affective disorders after traumatic brain injury. *Journal of Head Trauma Rehabilitation*, 2(4), 68–76.

Glisky, E.L., & Schacter, D.L. (1988). Acquisition of domain-specific knowledge in patients with organic memory disorders. *Journal of Learning Disabilities, 21*, 333–339.

Goldstein, G. (1986). The neuropsychology of schizophrenia. In I. Grant & K.M. Adams (Eds.), *Neuropsychological assessment of neuropsychiatric disorders*. New York: Oxford University Press.

Goldstein, F.C., & Levin, H.S. (1987). Epidemiology of pediatric closed head injury: Incidence, clinical characteristics, and risk factors. *Journal of Learning Disabilities, 20*, 518–525.

Halstead, W.C. (1947). *Brain and intelligence*. Chicago: University of Chicago Press.

Harrington, D.E., & Levandowski, D.H. (1987). Efficacy of an educationally-based cognitive retraining programme for traumatically head-injured as measured by LNNB pre- and post-test scores. *Brain Injury, 1*(1), 65–72.

Hartman, J., & Landau, W.M. (1987). Comparison of formal language therapy with supportive counseling for aphasia due to acute vascular accident. *Archives of Neurology, 44*, 646–649.

Hayes, R.L., Stonnington, H.H., & Lyeth, B.G. (1987). Editorial: Pharmacological treatment of head injury —A new challenge. *Brain Injury, 1*(1), 1–2.

Helm-Estabrooks, N., Emery, P., & Albert, M.L. (1987). Treatment of aphasic perseveration (TAP) program: A new approach to aphasia therapy. *Archives of Neurology, 44*, 1253–1255.

Horn, L.J. (1987). "Atypical" medications for the treatment of disruptive, aggressive behavior in the brain-injured patient. *Journal of Head*

Trauma Rehabilitation, 2(4), 18–28.

Hovda, D.A., & Feeney, D.M. (1984). Amphetamine with experience promotes recovery of locomotor function after unilateral frontal cortex injury in the cat. *Brain Research*, *298*, 358–361.

Hovda, D.A., & Feeney, D.M. (1985). Haloperidol blocks amphetamine induced recovery of binocular depth perception after bilateral visual cortex ablation in cat. *Proceedings of the Western Pharmacological Society*, *280*, 209–211.

Hovda, D.A., Sutton, R.L., & Feeney, D.M. (1987). Recovery of tactile placing after visual cortex ablation in cat: A behavioral and metabolic study of diaschisis. *Experimental Neurology*, *97*, 391–402.

Incagnoli, T., Goldstein, G., & Golden, C.J. (1986). *Clinical applications of neuropsychological test batteries*. New York: Plenum.

Kozloff, R. (1987). Networks of social support and the outcome from severe head injury. *Journal of Head Trauma Rehabilitation*, 2(3), 14–23.

Kreutzer, J.S., & Boake, C. (1987). Addressing disciplinary issues in cognitive rehabilitation: Definition, training, and organization. *Brain Injury*, *1*, 199–202.

Lewis, A.J. (1976). *Mechanisms of neurological disease*. Boston: Little, Brown.

Livingston, M. G. (1987). Head injury: The relatives' response. *Brain Injury*, *1*(1), 33–39.

McGuire, T.L., & Sylvester, C.E. (1987). Neuropsychiatric evaluation and treatment of children with head injury. *Journal of Learning Disabilities*, *20*, 590–595.

McLean, A., Stanton, K.M., Cardenas, D.D., & Bergerud, D.B. (1987). Memory training combined with the use of oral physostigmine. *Brain Injury*, *1*, 145–159.

Mysiw, W.J., & Jackson, R.D. (1987). Tricyclic antidepressant therapy after traumatic brain injury. *Journal of Head Trauma Rehabilitation*, 2(4), 34–42.

Nauta, W.J.H., & Feirtag, M. (1986). *Fundamental neuroanatomy*. New York: W.H. Freeman.

Obrzut, J.E., & Hynd, G.W. (1987). Cognitive dysfunction and psychoeducational assessment in individuals with acquired brain injury. *Journal of Learning Disabilities*, *20*, 596–602.

Orbach, J. (1982). *Neuropsychology after Lashley*. Hillsdale, NJ: Erlbaum.

O'Shanick, G.J. (1987). Clinical aspects of psychopharmacologic treatment in head-injured patients. *Journal of Head Trauma Rehabilitation*, 2(4), 59–67.

Parmalee, D.X., & O'Shanick, G.J. (1987). Neuropsychiatric interventions with head injured children and adolescents. *Brain Injury*, *1*(1), 41–47.

Pawlik, G., & Heiss, W.D. (1989). Positron omission tomography (PET) and neuropsychological function. In E.D. Bigler, R.A. Yeo, & E. Turkheimer (Eds.), *Neuropsychological function and brain imaging*. New York: Plenum.

Prigatano, G.P. (1987). Recovery and cognitive retraining after craniocerebral trauma. *Journal of Learning Disabilities*, *20*, 603–613.

Prigatano, G.P., & Klonoff, D.S. (1988). Psychotherapy and neuropsychological assessment after brain injury. *Journal of Head Trauma Rehabilitation*, *3*, 45–56.

Rao, S.M., & Bieliauskas, L.A. (1983). Cognitive rehabilitation two and one-half years post right temporal lobectomy. *Journal of Clinical Neuropsychology*, *5*, 313–320.

Rattan, G., & Dean, R.S. (1987). The neuropsychology of children's learning disorders. In J.M. Williams & C.J. Long (Eds.), *The rehabilitation of cognitive disabilities* (pp. 173–190). New York: Plenum.

Reitan, R.M., & Wolfson, D. (1985). *The Halstead-Reitan neuropsychological test battery.* Tucson, AZ: The Neuropsychology Press.

Rimmele, C.T., & Hester, R.K. (1987). Cognitive rehabilitation after traumatic head injury. *Archieves of Clinical Neuropshchology, 2,* 353–384.

Rivara, F.P., & Mueller, B.A. (1986). The epidemiology and prevention of pediatric head injury. *The Journal of Head Trauma Rehabilitation, 1*(4), 7–15.

Robinson, R.G., Lipsey, J.R., & Price, T.R. (1985). Diagnosis and clinical management of post-stroke depression. *Psychosomatics, 26,* 769–775.

Ruff, R.M., Cullum, C.M., & Luerssen, T.G. (1989). Brain imaging and neuropsychological outcome in traumatic brain injury. In E.D. Bigler, R.A. Yeo, & E. Turkheimer (Eds.), *Neuropsychological function and brain imaging.* New York: Plenum.

Spivack, M.P. (1986). Advocacy and legislative action for head-injured children and their families. *Journal of Head Trauma Rehabilitation, 1,* 41–47.

Sutton, R.L., Weaver, M.S., & Feeney, D.M. (1987). Drug-induced modifications of behavioral recovery following cortical trauma. *Journal of Head Trauma Rehabilitation,* 2(4), 50–58.

Telzrow, C.F. (1987). Management of academic and educational problems in head injury. *Journal of Learning Disabilities, 20,* 536–545.

Thomsen. I.V. (1987). Late psychosocial outcome in severe blunt head trauma. *Brain Injury, 1,* 131–143.

Weinberg, R.M., Auerbach, S.H., & Moore, S. (1987). Pharmacological treatment of cognitive deficits: A case study. *Brain Injury, 1*(1), 57–59.

Wertz, R.T., Weiss, D.G., Aten, J.L., Brookshire, R.H., Garcia-Bunuel, L., Holland, A.L., Kurtzke, J.F., LaPointe, L.L., Milianti, F.J., Brannegan, R., Greenbaum, H., Marshall, R.C., Vogel, D., Carter, J., Barnes, N.S., & Goodman, R. (1986). Comparison of clinic, home, and deferred language treatment for aphasia. *Archives of Neurology, 43,* 653–658.

Wilson, B., & Moffat, N. (1984a). *Clinical management of memory problems.* Rockville, MD: Aspen Systems.

Wilson, B., & Moffat, N. (1984b). Rehabilitation of memory for everyday life. In J.E. Harris & D. Morris (Eds.), *Everyday memory: Actions and absentmindedness.* London: Academic Press.

Wood, R.L. (1988). Attention disorders in brain injury rehabilitation. *Journal of Learning Disabilities, 21,* 327–332.

Zivin, J.A., Lyden, P.D., DeGirolami, U., Kochhar, A., Mazzarella, V., Hemenway, C.C., & Johnston, P. (1988). Tissue plasminogen activator: Reduction of neurologic damage after experimental embolic stroke. *Archives of Neurology, 45,* 387–391.

Glossary

acceleration effects Because the bone and brain tissues are of different densities, rapid acceleration, such as being rapidly vaulted forward in an automobile accident, will cause brain tissue to accelerate at a different rate than bone. There are also differences between white (pathways) and gray (cell bodies) matter regions of the brain. These differences create a gradient that results in shearing forces that may damage brain tissue.

anterograde amnesia Inability to establish new memories or retain new information subsequent to the onset of amnesia, typically traumatically induced.

atrophy Shrinkage of brain tissue due to degeneration.

axon A filament-like structure that projects outward from the cell body of a neuron. The neural impulse is transmitted along the axon.

BEAM Brain electrical activity mapping, a computer assisted EEG evaluation.

cerebrum Brain, cerebral hemispheres.

contralateral On the opposite body side from the reference point.

contusion Bruise.

corpus callosum A large bundle of fibers that interconnects the two cerebral hemispheres. Along this pathway the two hemispheres communicate and integrate information.

CT Computerized tomography. This procedure utilizes computer assisted technology to take X-ray images of the brain and recreate a detailed 2-dimensional view of the brain.

deceleration effects The principle is similar to that described in acceleration effects, only in reverse. Similar brain damage may result from deceleration effects.

diffuse injury Damage that is generalized and nonspecific, affecting areas in both hemispheres and frequently the entire cerebrum.

edema Swelling as a result of an excessive accumulation of fluid.

EEG Electroencephalogram or "brain wave test."

falx cerebri The part of the meninges that folds back upon itself and is located in the interhemispheric fissure.

focal injury Specific injury to one area or region of the brain. Surrounding areas may not be affected and the remainder of the brain may also be unaffected. Focal brain injury may produce a specific syndrome (e.g., expressive aphasia) or specific deficit (e.g., contralateral paralysis).

fossa Cavity, space.

frontal lobe syndrome A variety of aberrant behaviors that typically accompany frontal, frontal and temporal, or generalized cerebral damage. These behaviors include impaired judgment and social reasoning, impulsiveness, emotional lability, and unwanted personality changes.

glial cells Supportive cells of the central nervous system.

gyrus Convolution or ridge of the brain.

hematoma Blood clot.

higher cortical functions These are typically thought to represent the highest order of complex brain function in terms of motor, sensory, language, and perceptual abilities.

hippocampus A structure in the shape of a seahorse that lies in the anterior medial aspect of the temporal lobe. This structure plays a critical role in memory function.

hypoxia Reduced oxygen that may lead to infarction.

infarction A region or area of dead or dysfunctional tissue as a result of a loss or reduction of oxygenated blood to that region.

in situ In the normal anatomic position.

interhemispheric fissure The large cleft that separates the two hemispheres.

ischemia A cutting off or reduction in blood flow.

limbic system The neural systems that line the inside wall of the neocortex. These structures form a "ring" of interconnecting pathways, including the hippocampus, amygdala, septum, cingulate gyrus, and anterior thalamus. Many of these structures are involved in control of affective and memory functions.

MRI Magnetic resonance imaging. This procedure utilizes magnetic fields and their polarization to create the various images of tissue structures. The computer generation of the image is similar to those procedures utilized in CT scanning.

neuron Nerve cell or basic unit of the nervous system.

neuropathology The study of the pathology of the nervous system.

retrograde amnesia Inability to remember events that occurred prior to the onset of amnesia, typically traumatically induced.

sequelae Pathological consequences or residual deficits following brain injury.

sulcus Cleft between gyri.

Sylvian fissure The large cleft on each lateral side of the brain that separates the frontal from the temporal lobes.

ventricles The cavities of the brain that are filled with cerebrospinal fluid, which is under some degree of pressure.

About the Authors

Erin D. Bigler received his PhD from Brigham Young University in 1974. He was the recipient of a National Institute of Health Post-Doctoral Fellowship, which was undertaken at the Barrow Neurological Institute of St. Joseph's Hospital and Medical Center in Phoenix, Arizona. He is currently in practice at the Austin Neurological Clinic and an adjunct professor of psychology at The University of Texas at Austin. He is a diplomate in clinical neuropsychology, American Board of Professional Psychology.

C. Munro Cullum received his PhD in clinical psychology from The University of Texas in 1986. He completed an internship in clinical psychology, with a focus in neuropsychology, at the University of California, San Diego, and the San Diego VA Medical Center. He then completed a two-year NIH postdoctoral fellowship in neuropsychology at the University of California, San Diego, and is now an assistant professor of psychiatry and associate director of the Neuropsychology Laboratory at the University of Colorado Health Sciences Center in Denver.

Ann V. Deaton received her PhD from The University of Texas at Austin in clinical psychology. She is the coordinator of psychological services at Cumberland, A Hospital for Children and Adolescents, a treatment facility designed for patients who have both medical diagnoses (e.g., brain injury, diabetes) and emotional or behavioral difficulties (e.g., physical aggression, noncompliance). Her research interests include evaluating the efficacy of treatment interventions designed to remediate the cognitive and social-emotional difficulties that often accompany brain injury and other chronic health problems.

Linda Ewing-Cobbs received a PhD in 1985 from the University of Houston–University Park. She is an assistant professor in the Department of Psychiatry and Behavioral Sciences and the Division of Neurosurgery at the University of Texas Medical School at Houston. Dr. Ewing-Cobbs has extensive clinical and research expertise in the area of head injury in children.

Jack M. Fletcher received his PhD in 1978 from the University of Florida. He is presently an associate professor of psychology at the University of Houston–University Park. Dr. Fletcher is a diplomate, American Board of Professional Psychology. He has authored numerous articles on the effects of brain injury on child development.

Elizabeth L. Glisky is a visiting assistant professor in the Department of Psychology at the University of Arizona. She received her PhD in experimental psychology from the University of Toronto where she was subsequently associated with the Unit for Memory Disorders. She is currently conducting research at the Amnesia and Cognition Unit, University of Arizona, concerning the nature of organic memory disorders and possibilities for rehabilitation.

Felicia C. Goldstein is an assistant professor in the Neurology Department at The University of Texas Medical Branch in Galveston, Texas. She received her PhD in developmental psychology from Emory University.

George W. Hynd, EdD, is research professor of educational psychology and psychology at the University of Georgia and assistant clinical professor of neurology at the Medical College of Georgia.

Pamela S. Klonoff, PhD, received her doctorate in clinical neuropsychology from the University of Victoria in 1984. Postdoctoral training was obtained at the Presbyterian Hospital in Oklahoma City under the supervision of George P. Prigatano, from 1984 to 1985. Her current position is manager of the Adult Day Hospital for Neurological Rehabilitation, an outpatient rehabilitation program for brain injured patients, at Barrow Neurological Institute, Phoenix, Arizona.

Julia Kuck is presently completing her doctoral degree in clinical psychology. She received an MA in clinical psychology in 1985 and completed an internship in clinical psychology at the University of California, San Diego, and the San Diego VA Medical Center in 1987. Currently she is the coordinator of the UCSD Outpatient Clinical Research Center.

Harvey S. Levin is a professor of neurosurgery at The University of Texas Medical Branch. He has a PhD in clinical psychology from the University of Iowa. He is engaged in research concerning neurobehavioral recovery following closed head injury.

Muriel D. Lezak is an associate professor of neurology and psychiatry at the Oregon Health Sciences University and diplomate in clinical psychology and in clinical neuropsychology. She is also the past president of the International Neuropsychological Society.

Tona L. McGuire is a clinical assistant professor of psychiatry and behavioral sciences at the University of Washington. She received her PhD in clinical psychology from Fuller Theological Seminary. Formerly the associate head, Division of Pediatric Consultation and Liaison, Children's Hospital and Medical Center, Seattle, she is now in private practice.

Thomas P. Marquardt, PhD, is a professor of speech communication and director of the Program in Communication Disorders at The University of Texas at Austin.

Darlene Aulds Martin is an assistant professor in community health care and health care ethics and law at The University of Texas at Austin School of Nursing. She received her PhD from The University of Texas School of Public Health at Houston and was a Joseph P. Kennedy, Jr., Fellow in Biomedical Ethics at Rice University. She has served on the professional advisory boards of numerous organizations for disabled persons and is the parent of a child with traumatic brain injury.

Reed Martin is an attorney specializing in rights of citizens with disabilities. Martin has represented several thousand individuals over the past 15 years in administrative trials and court cases, including the U.S. Supreme Court. He has also served as a consultant to schools and other agencies in 35 states. Martin has served on the board of 22 different organizations for rights of citizens with disabilities at the local, state, and national level. He is the author of four books on rights of disabled persons, including *Educating Handicapped Children: The Legal Mandate*, and numerous journal articles. Martin has worked extensively with brain injured and learning disabled students for 12 years. He is a recipient of the Pioneer Award from the National Association for Children and Adults with Learning Disabilities, for which he serves on the Professional Advisory Board, and the Texas Key Award from the Texas Association for Children with Learning Disabilities.

Richard I. Naugle received his PhD from The University of Texas at Austin and completed an internship specializing in clinical neuropsychology at the West Haven Veterans Administration Medical Center in West Haven, Connecticut. He is presently on staff in the Neuropsychology Section within the Department of Psychiatry at the Cleveland Clinic Foundation in Cleveland, Ohio.

Kevin P. O'Brien is a clinical neuropsychologist at the Barrow Neurological Institute and staff member of the Adult Day Hospital for Neurological Rehabilitation, an outpatient program for brain injured adults.

John E. Obrzut, PhD, is professor of educational psychology and director of school psychology at the University of Arizona.

George P. Prigatano received his PhD in clinical psychology from Bowling Green State University in 1972 and was a visiting scholar in the Department of Psychology, Stanford University, in 1978. Presently he is chairman of neuropsychology, Barrow Neurological Institute.

Ronald M. Ruff received his PhD in psychology from the University of Zurich in 1978. He was a postdoctoral fellow at Stanford University for two years and then joined the University of California, San Diego. Currently he is an associate clinical professor of psychiatry and neurosurgery at the University of California, San Diego, and is the director of the UCSD Head Injury Center/ Learning Services Center.

Daniel L. Schacter is an associate professor of psychology at the University of Arizona. He received his PhD in experimental psychology from the University of Toronto where he was subsequently associated with the Unit for Memory Disorders. He is currently conducting research at the Amnesia and Cognition Unit, University of Arizona, concerning the nature of organic memory disorders and possibilities for rehabilitation.

Julie Stoll, MS, is a doctoral student in speech/language pathology at The University of Texas at Austin.

Harvey Sussman, PhD, is a professor of linguistics and speech communication at The University of Texas at Austin.

Carrie E. Sylvester is director, pediatrics consultation/liaison and assistant professor of psychiatry at the Institute for Juvenile Research and the University of Illinois at Chicago. She received her MD and MPH from the University of Washington and is board certified in pediatrics and psychiatry.

Cathy F. Telzrow, PhD, is psychologist and coordinator of the Educational Assessment Project at the Cuyahoga Special Education Service Center in Cleveland, Ohio.

Rodger Ll. Wood obtained an honors degree in psychology at the University of Wales, Great Britain. He subsequently studied for a professional qualification in clinical psychology at the University of Wales, National School of Medicine, and later studied neurosciences at Downing College and Addenbrookes Hospital Cambridge, and the National Hospital for Nervous Diseases, Queen's Square, London. He obtained his PhD from Leicester University. Dr. Wood was consultant neuropsychologist and co-director of the Kemsley Brain Injury Rehabilitation Unit, St. Andrew's Hospital, Northampton, England, and is now Clinical Director of Brain Injury Rehabilitation Services at Casa Colina Hospital, Pomona, California. He has published a number of articles and chapters in the field of head injury and neuropsychological research. He is the author of a recent book entitled *Brain Injury Rehabilitation: A Neurobehavioral Approach.*

Author Index

Subject Index